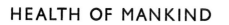

HEALTH OF MANKIND

HEALTH OF MANKIND

Ciba Foundation 100th Symposium

Edited by
GORDON WOLSTENHOLME
and
MAEVE O'CONNOR

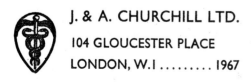

J. & A. CHURCHILL LTD.
104 GLOUCESTER PLACE
LONDON, W.I 1967

With 38 illustrations

Standard Book Number 7000 1318 0

Contents

v

CONTENTS

Manpower and education

Chairman: Sir Eric Ashby

Membership

Symposium on Health of Mankind held 8th-10th March, 1967

The Rt. Hon. Lord Adrian	Trinity College, University of Cambridge
Sir Eric Ashby	Clare College, University of Cambridge
A. L. Banks	Department of Human Ecology, University of Cambridge
H. Beer	The League of Red Cross Societies, Geneva
W. I. B. Beveridge	Department of Animal Pathology, University of Cambridge
D. Burkitt	External Scientific Staff, Medical Research Council, London
M. G. Candau	World Health Organization, Geneva
The Rt. Hon. Lord Cohen of Birkenhead	Royal Infirmary, Liverpool
I. Dogramaci	Hacettepe Science Center, Ankara
C. A. Doxiadis	Doxiadis Associates, Athens
K. Evang	The Health Services of Norway, The Royal Norwegian Ministry of Social Affairs, Oslo
G. Fanconi	Zürich
The Rt. Hon. Lord Florey	The Queen's College, University of Oxford
Victoria Garcia	School of Public Health, University of Chile, Santiago, Chile
J. H. de Haas	Department of Health Development, Netherlands Institute for Preventive Medicine, Leiden
P. E. A. Johnson-Marshall	Department of Architecture, University of Edinburgh
L. A. Kaprio	World Health Organization, Copenhagen
H. Katsunuma	Department of Public Health, Faculty of Medicine, University of Tokyo
T. A. Lambo	Department of Psychiatry and Neurology, University of Ibadan
W. H. le Riche	Department of Epidemiology and Biometrics, School of Hygiene, University of Toronto
Patricia J. Lindop	St. Bartholomew's Hospital Medical College, London
A. M.-M. Payne	World Health Organization, Geneva
H. Pequignot	Faculty of Medicine, University of Paris

The Ciba Foundation

The Ciba Foundation was opened in 1949 to promote international co-operation in medical and chemical research among scientists from all parts of the world. Its house at 41 Portland Place, London, has become a meeting place well known to workers in many fields of science. Every year the Foundation organizes from six to ten three-day symposia and three or four one-day study groups, all of which are published in book form. Many other informal meetings also take place in the house, organized either by the Foundation or by other scientific groups needing a place to meet. In addition, bedrooms are available for visiting scientists, whether or not they are attending a meeting in the building.

The Ciba Foundation owes its existence to the generosity of CIBA Ltd, Basle, who, realizing the disruption of scientific communication caused by the war and by problems of distance, decided to set up a philanthropic institution whose aim would be to overcome such barriers. London was chosen as its site for reasons dictated by the special advantages of English charitable trust law (ensuring the independence of its actions), as well as those of language and geography.

The Foundation's many activities are controlled by a small group of distinguished trustees. Within the general framework of biological science, interpreted in its broadest sense, these activities are well summed up by the Ciba Foundation's motto, *Consocient Gentes*—let the nations come together.

Introduction

MORE than one hundred meetings of one kind or another are held at the Ciba Foundation each year, but of our own major conferences, each lasting three or four days, the hundredth was held in March 1967, and this book contains the papers and discussions of that occasion.

I use the word "major" from a domestic point of view only: these symposia, which began in January 1950, have been notable for having a severely restricted membership of 30 or less, the intention being to provide at least as much opportunity and time for discussion as for the hearing of prepared papers. The members are always selected entirely on our own responsibility, and interdisciplinary contact is regarded as being as important as international co-operation.

Most of our symposia have been on research topics of acute interest. Given an excuse such as the 50th symposium, the opening of a new conference room, or a quinquennial birthday, we have allowed ourselves a little eccentricity and have organized meetings on such wide-ranging subjects as "Medical Biology and Etruscan Origins", "Man and his Future", "Man and Africa", and "Conflict in Society". For this 100th symposium we thought we could perhaps be even more foolhardy: I had tried to look at all Africa as one unit—why not attempt now to consider the health of the whole world?

We could assess the total burden of infectious and other physical diseases, the special problems of the care of mother and child, the incidence of mental and behavioural disorders, the injuries of environmental origin, and the relevance of animal diseases to human health. Then there were the factors which aggravate the task of health services: incomparably the greatest is the problem of population growth, but there are also questions of food variety and supply, the pollution of water and air, the inhumanity of cities, and the artificial boundaries produced by politics and traditions. We could consider also the present and anticipated world resources of medical manpower of all kinds, the facilities for education and training, and whether the great work of the World Health Organization might be extended into a World Health Service.

This most ambitious plan could hardly have become a reality if I had not received immediate encouragement from Dr. Candau, Professor Banks and Mr. Beer. Their unhesitating support and promise of personal participation gave me courage to go ahead in this attempt to draw the eyes of man upwards for a while from the prevalent squalor of preventable disease and starvation, and from all man's incomprehensible and continuing cruelty to man. If we cannot work together for the health of mankind, we are rightly doomed. If we can learn to collaborate in all the many aspects of medical care we may also begin to think healthily about race, politics, sovereignty, international use of resources of all kinds, and economic interdependence.

It was perhaps unfair to ask the speakers at this meeting to talk in global terms. But when the time came, they did so with courage and concern. The views expressed are those of individuals, not organizations.

This conference was the completion of a century. It is also a beginning.

G. E. W. WOLSTENHOLME

As this book was about to be printed, the sad news was received of the death of one of its contributors, Dr. Pincus. This symposium proved, therefore, to be the last of many occasions on which Dr. Pincus had joined generously and brilliantly in the Ciba Foundation's activities. We mourn him profoundly as a friend. Those who did not know him personally will nevertheless discern from his contributions to this book his sincere compassion and the tireless intellectual and experimental effort with which he tackled the supreme problem of population growth. His concern was as much for every individual as for the whole of mankind, and such very practical idealism is a striking example of what this publication is intended to encourage.

With all respect and affection this book is now dedicated

TO THE MEMORY OF

GREGORY PINCUS

I

WORLD INCIDENCE AND PREVALENCE
OF THE MAJOR COMMUNICABLE DISEASES

W. Harding le Riche
Department of Epidemiology and Biometrics,
School of Hygiene, University of Toronto, Toronto, Canada

"Youth is alive and once we too were young,
Dreamed we could make the world all over new,
Tossed eager projects lightly from the tongue,
And hoped the hurrying years would prove them true."
GAMALIEL BRADFORD: Wellesley at Fifty, 1881–1932.

D URING the last forty years the western world has certainly been
made anew as regards its communicable diseases—except, of
course, for the common cold and influenza, which are still very
much with us, and with the rest of the world as well.

History shows that, particularly in Western Europe, plague almost disappeared in the 17th century, only to have its place taken by typhus and smallpox. In the 19th century typhus was nearly conquered[1] but it fought a rearguard action during the wars of the 20th century. Smallpox and cholera caused widespread confusion and unnumbered deaths in the 19th century. Smallpox has maintained its stronghold in the East and in West Africa, and cholera has retreated to the delta of the Ganges at the present time. Typhoid came into prominence in the 19th century and made the proper disposal of sewage and the provision of pure water supplies an urgent problem for city dwellers. This particular battle is still being waged in many parts of the world.

The major killing diseases in the world today are pneumonia, tuberculosis and the diarrhoeal diseases, but cholera and smallpox remain. Plague is no longer epidemic in its sylvatic or rural form. The most spectacular outbreak of modern times was the great pandemic of influenza that swept across the world in 1918–19 and attacked an estimated 700 million people, killing over 20 million.[1] No doubt this sort of epidemic could happen again because we do not really know how to control such an onslaught.

In large areas of the world insect-borne disease is still a menace. Malaria and yellow fever and trypanosomiasis are by no means conquered and may return in full strength if preventive guards are let down. The discovery of new insecticides has, of course, been of great help in controlling insects, but these chemicals are poisonous to other creatures.

At present we have the technical knowledge required to control many infectious diseases, but we experience increasing difficulty in applying it because of administrative disorganization in many parts of the world. This is bound up with vast population increases, declining food production per head in many developing countries, and the inability of many countries to cope with a rapidly changing technology.

We cannot, of course, take a fatalistic view about these matters, but we should at least be completely realistic. Many people in public health and clinical medicine tend to consider only their own specialities, forgetting that the welfare of mankind is a far more complicated question than the prevention of disease and the care of the sick.

CONCEPTS OF HEALTH AND DISEASE

In discussing matters of health and disease we should keep our feet on the ground, although there is no reason why we should not now and again have our heads in the clouds. The following quotation from Dubos[2] is rather appropriate:

"The hope that disease can be completely eradicated becomes a dangerous mirage only when its unattainable character is forgotten. It can then be compared to a will-o'-the-wisp luring its followers into the swamps of unreality. In particular it encourages the illusion that man can control his responses to stimuli and can make adjustments to new ways of life without having to pay for these adaptive changes. The less pleasant reality is that in an ever-changing world each period and each type of civilization will continue to have its burden of diseases created by unavoidable failures of adaptation to the new environment."

As it is impossible to measure the "health" of a population, the best we can do is to measure "lack of health". The indices based on mortality, such as crude and age-adjusted death rates, infant mortality rates, and expectation of life have traditionally been used as measures of health. Quite clearly, they are crude measures which do not take into consideration anything but the most extreme situation, shown as death. These rates are an uncertain guide to the amount of illness (morbidity) in the community, a matter of greater economic importance than a measure of mortality. In the developed

Table I

POPULATION, RATE OF INCREASE, BIRTH AND DEATH RATES, AREA AND DENSITY FOR THE WORLD, MAJOR DIVISIONS AND REGIONS FOR SELECTED YEARS[6]

(Unless otherwise specified, all figures are estimates of the order of magnitude and are subject to a substantial margin of error)

Major divisions	Estimates of mid-year population (millions)						Rate of population increase* (%)		Birth rate (o/oo) 1958–63	Death rate (o/oo) 1958–63	Area† km² (ooo's) 1963	Density‡ 1963
	1930	1940	1950	1958	1960	1963	1958–63	1960–63				
WORLD TOTAL	2,070	2,295	2,517	2,875	2,990	3,160	1·8	1·9	34	16	135,761	23
Africa	164	191	222	262	273	294	2·3	2·5	46	23	30,227	10
Northern America§	134	144	166	192	199	208	1·6	1·6	24‖	9‖	21,515	10
Latin America	108	130	163	203	212	231	2·7	2·8	40	14	20,535	11
East Asia¶	591	634	684	772	793	828	1·4	1·4	33	19	11,725	71
South Asia**	529	610	697	826	858	920	2·2	2·4	42	20	15,896	58
Europe††	355	380	392	418	425	437	0·9	0·9	19	10	4,929	89
Oceania§	10·0	11·1	12·7	15·1	15·7	16·8	2·1‡‡	2·2‡‡	27	11	8,532	2
USSR	179	195	180	207	214	225	1·6	1·6	24‖	7‖	22,402	10

* Average annual per cent rate of population increase.
† Comprising land area and inland waters, but excluding uninhabited polar regions and some uninhabited islands.
‡ Population per square kilometre of area.
§ Hawaii, a state of the United States of America, is included in Northern America rather than Oceania.
‖ Weighted average of recorded rates.
¶ Excluding the USSR, shown separately below.
** Excluding the USSR, shown separately, but including both the Asian and European portions of Turkey.
†† Excluding the USSR, shown separately below, and the European portion of Turkey, which is included in South Asia.
‡‡ Rate reflects effect of natural increase and migration.

3

parts of the world we do have some morbidity statistics. These include notifications of infectious disease, with the clear limitations of such data; hospital separations, which give only a partial picture of disease episodes; and some special studies, such as the records of general practitioners or the records of medical insurance plans, that give an estimate of work carried out by physicians. The best general picture of the health of a community is provided by health surveys, such as the National Health Survey of the United States[3], the United Kingdom Survey of Sickness[4] and others. These surveys have the limitation that the diagnoses are those reported by patients rather than by physicians. The whole complex matter of the conceptual problems in the developing of an index of health has been discussed by Sullivan[5], to whose work reference should be made for additional information. Its concepts are applicable only in the developed countries of the world where it is possible to carry out sampling and other surveys of the health of the population.

WORLD POPULATIONS AND GEOGRAPHICAL AREAS

It is sound epidemiological practice to define the population at risk and this information is given in Table I, for the years 1930 to 1963. Only major geographical subdivisions are mentioned, with data derived from the United Nations Demographic Yearbook, shown in Tables I[6] and II[6].

Table II

COMPOSITION OF WORLD REGIONS[6]

AFRICA	Eastern Africa	Northern Africa
Western Africa	Burundi	Algeria
Cape Verde Islands	Comoro Islands	Ifni
Dahomey	Ethiopia	Libya
Gambia	French Somaliland	Morocco
Ghana	Kenya	Spanish North Africa
Guinea	Madagascar	Spanish Sahara
Ivory Coast	Malawi	Sudan
Liberia	Mauritius	Tunisia
Mali	Mozambique	United Arab Republic
Mauritania	Réunion	
Niger	Rwanda	*Middle Africa*
Nigeria	Seychelles	Angola
Portuguese Guinea	Somalia	Cameroon
St. Helena (including	Southern Rhodesia	Central African Republic
dependencies)	Uganda	Chad
Senegal	United Republic of	Congo (Brazzaville)
Sierra Leone	Tanzania	Congo (Democratic
Togo	Zambia	Republic of)
Upper Volta		Equatorial Guinea

4

Table II—Continued

Middle Africa—Cont.
  Gabon
  São Tomé and Principé

Southern Africa
  Basutoland
  Bechuanaland
  French Southern and
    Antarctic Territories
  South Africa
  South West Africa
  Swaziland

NORTHERN AMERICA
  Bermuda
  Canada
  Greenland
  St. Pierre and
    Miquelon
  United States (including
    Hawaii)

LATIN AMERICA
Tropical South America
  Bolivia
  Brazil
  British Guiana
  Colombia
  Ecuador
  French Guiana
  Peru
  Surinam
  Venezuela

Middle America (Mainland)
  British Honduras
  Canal Zone
  Costa Rica
  El Salvador
  Guatemala
  Honduras
  Mexico
  Nicaragua
  Panama

Temperate South America
  Argentina
  Chile
  Falkland Islands
  Paraguay
  Uruguay

Caribbean
  Antigua
  Bahama Islands
  Barbados
  Cayman Islands
  Cuba
  Dominica
  Dominican Republic
  Grenada
  Guadeloupe
  Haiti
  Jamaica
  Martinique
  Montserrat
  Netherlands Antilles
  Puerto Rico
  St. Kitts-Nevis and
    Anguilla
  St. Lucia
  St. Vincent
  Trinidad and Tobago
  Turks and Caicos Islands
  Virgin Islands (UK)
  Virgin Islands (US)

EAST ASIA
Mainland region
  China (mainland)
  Hong Kong
  Macau
  Mongolia

Japan

Other East Asia
  Bonin Islands
  China (Taiwan)
  Korea
  Ryukyu Islands

SOUTH ASIA
Middle South Asia
  Afghanistan
  Bhutan
  Ceylon
  India
  Iran
  Maldive Islands
  Pakistan

Middle South Asia—Cont.
  Nepal
  Sikkim

South-East Asia
  Brunei
  Burma
  Cambodia
  Indonesia
    West Irian
  Laos
  Malaysia
  Philippines
  Portuguese Timor
  Thailand
  Viet-Nam

South-West Asia
  Aden
  Bahrain
  Cyprus
  Gaza Strip (Palestine)
  Iraq
  Israel
  Jordan
  Kuwait
  Lebanon
  Muscat and Oman
  Protectorate of South
    Arabia
  Qatar
  Saudi Arabia
  Syria
  Trucial Oman
  Turkey
  Yemen

EUROPE
Western Europe
  Austria
  Belgium
  France
  Germany, Federal
    Republic of
  Liechtenstein
  Luxembourg
  Monaco
  Netherlands
  Switzerland
  West Berlin

Southern Europe
  Albania
  Andorra

Table II—Continued

Southern Europe—Cont.
Gibraltar
Greece
Holy See
Italy
Malta
Portugal
San Marino
Spain
Yugoslavia

Eastern Europe
Bulgaria
Czechoslovakia
East Berlin
Eastern Germany
Hungary
Poland
Romania

Northern Europe
Channel Islands
Denmark
Faeroe Islands
Finland
Iceland

Northern Europe—Cont.
Ireland
Isle of Man
Norway
Svalbard and Jan Mayen
Islands
Sweden
United Kingdom

OCEANIA
Australia and New Zealand

Melanesia
British Solomon
Islands
New Caledonia
New Guinea
New Hebrides
Norfolk Island
Papua

Polynesia and Micronesia
American Samoa
Canton and Enderbury

Polynesia and Micronesia
—Cont.
Christmas Island
Cocos (Keeling) Islands
Cook Islands
Fiji Islands
French Polynesia
Gilbert and Ellice
Islands
Guam
Johnston Island
Midway Islands
Nauru
Niue
Pacific Islands
Pitcairn
Tokelau Islands
Tonga
Wake Island
Western Samoa

*UNION OF SOVIET
SOCIALIST REPUBLICS*

Rates of population increase per year (1960–63) range from 2·8 per cent in Latin America, 2·5 per cent in Africa, down to 0·9 per cent in Europe. In these eight areas, the highest death rate, 23 per 1,000, is found in Africa, with South Asia a close second at 20 per 1,000. Many of these figures had to be based on estimates or on inspired guesses.

A LISTING OF COMMUNICABLE DISEASES

A communicable disease is an "illness due to a specific infectious agent or its toxic products, which arises through transmission of that agent or its products from a reservoir to a susceptible host, either directly as from an infected person or animal, or indirectly through the agency of an intermediate plant or animal host, a vector or the inanimate environment."[7]

These diseases are listed in Table III[7], indicating how many of these conditions are currently identifiable. The order relates to the potential danger of the infections, and ranges from the six internationally quarantinable diseases to those that may not be commonly notifiable.

Table III

CLASSIFICATION OF COMMUNICABLE DISEASES[7]

1. *Case report universally required by international sanitary regulations*
    Cholera
    Plague
    Relapsing fever, epidemic louse-borne (*see also* 3B)
    Smallpox
    Typhus fever, epidemic louse-borne (classical typhus fever)
    Yellow fever—mosquito-borne

2. *Case report regularly required wherever the disease occurs*

    (A) By telephone, telegraph or other rapid means:

    Anthrax
    Eastern equine ⎫
    Western equine ⎪
    Japanese B   ⎬ mosquito-borne encephalitis
    Murray valley   ⎪
    St. Louis   ⎭
    Diphtheria
    Botulism (food poisoning)
    Glanders
    Gonococcal vulvovaginitis of children
    Gonococcal ophthalmia neonatorum
    Meningitis, meningococcal
    Paratyphoid fever
    Poliomyelitis
    Psittacosis
    Rabies
    Scarlet fever
    Puerperal fever
    Tetanus
    Typhoid fever

    (B) By most practicable means:

    Brucellosis
    Chancroid
    Conjunctivitis, inclusion
    Gonorrhoea (gonococcal urethritis)
    Infectious hepatitis
    Serum hepatitis
    Leprosy
    Leptospirosis
    Malaria (or 3C)
    Measles
    Shigellosis
    Syphilis, venereal
    Trachoma
    Trichinosis
    Tuberculosis
    Typhus fever, endemic flea-borne (murine typhus)
    Whooping cough

7

3. *Selectively reportable in recognized endemic areas*

   (A) By telephone, telegraph or other rapid means:

   Haemorrhagic fever with renal syndrome (unknown, mite?)
   Argentinian ⎱
   Bolivian   ⎰ haemorrhagic fevers
   Scrub typhus

   (B) By most practical means:

   Russian spring-summer encephalitis ⎫
   Diphasic meningoencephalitis   ⎬ tick-borne encephalitis
   Louping ill   ⎪
   Powassan encephalitis   ⎭
   Bunyamwera   ⎫
   Bwamba   ⎪
   Chikungunya   ⎪
   Mayaro   ⎪
   O'nyong-nyong   ⎬ mosquito-borne viral fever
   Rift Valley   ⎪
   Venezuelan equine ⎪
   West Nile   ⎪
   Group C viral fevers ⎭
   Colorado tick fever
   Crimean haemorrhagic fever, tick-borne
   Omsk haemorrhagic fever   ⎱
   Kyasanur Forest disease   ⎰ tick-borne
   Bartonellosis
   Chickenpox in adults where smallpox is infrequent (*see also* 5)
   Coccidioidomycosis
   Echinococcosis (hydatidosis)
   Granuloma inguinale
   Histoplasmosis
   Leishmaniasis, cutaneous
   Leishmaniasis, visceral (kala azar)
   Meningitis, aseptic
   Paragonimiasis
   Pinta
   Q fever
   Relapsing fever, endemic tick-borne (*see also* 1)
   Rheumatic fever
   Rocky Mountain spotted fever
   Boutonneuse fever
   Queensland tick typhus
   North Asian tick-borne rickettsiosis
   Rickettsial pox
   Syphilis, non-venereal (Bejel, Dichuchwa, Njovera, Sibbens, Radesyke)
   Trypanosomiasis, African
   Trypanosomiasis, American
   Tularaemia
   Yaws

(C) Collective report weekly by mail:

Amoebiasis
Clonorchiasis
Dracontiasis
Fasciolopsiasis
Filariasis
Hookworm disease
Loiasis
Lymphogranuloma venereum
Malaria (or 2B)
Onchocerciasis
Sandfly fever (phlebotomus-borne)
Schistosomiasis (bilharziasis)
Strongyloidiasis
Toxoplasmosis

4. *Obligatory report of epidemics. No case report required*
Dengue fever
Haemorrhagic fevers of the Philippines and South-east Asia
Conjunctivitis, acute bacterial
Diarrhoea of early childhood
Epidemic diarrhoea in nurseries for the newborn
Food poisoning (a) Salmonellosis
               (b) Staphylococcal
               (c) Clostridium perfringens
Herpangina
Influenza
Keratoconjunctivitis, infectious
Mononucleosis, infectious
Pleurodynia
Pneumonia, pneumococcal
Pneumonia, bacterial (other than pneumococcal)
Pneumonia, mycoplasmal (PPLO)
Rat-bite fever, streptobacillus moniliformis disease (Haverhill fever)
Acute febrile respiratory disease
Ringworm of scalp (tinea capitis)
Ringworm of body (tinea corporis)
Rubella
Scabies
Staphylococcal disease in the community
Streptococcal disease, haemolytic; streptococcal sore throat; erysipelas

5. *Official report not ordinarily justifiable*

Actinomycosis	Lymphocytic choriomeningitis
Ascariasis	Mumps
Aspergillosis	Mycetoma
North American blastomycosis	Nocardiosis
Candidiasis	Paracoccidioidal granuloma
Cat scratch fever	Pediculosis
Chickenpox (*see also* 3B)	Common cold
Chromoblastomycosis	Ringworm of foot (tinea pedis)
Cryptococcosis	Ringworm of nails (tinea unguium)
Diphyllobothriasis	Sporotrichosis
Enterobiasis	Taeniasis and cysticercosis
Larva migrans, visceral	Trichomoniasis
Listeriosis	Trichuriasis

9

INCIDENCE AND PREVALENCE

In this paper we clearly need a discussion of the measures of frequency of disease. One of these measures is that of incidence, the occurrence of events during a given period of time in a certain population. This incidence, attack or inception rate may be expressed as follows[8, 9]:

$$\frac{\text{Number of new cases beginning during a defined period of time}}{\text{Average number in a defined population exposed to risk during that time}} \times 1,000$$

For instance, in the Canadian Sickness Survey 1950–51[10] a similar definition for incidence was used:

"Incidence is measured by the number of new illnesses commencing during the survey year and the number of persons reporting these illnesses. A new illness is any reported disturbance of health independent of any preceding illness. (Acute and infectious diseases were always treated as new illnesses. They were composed of the following numbers in the International Classification: 040–108, 470, and 480–483). Other illnesses, i.e. those reported as recurring attacks of previous illnesses, thus are not counted in the incidence of illness."

Incidence may of course be counted either in terms of new illnesses (spells of illness, sickness episodes) or in terms of persons reporting new illnesses. Particularly with the common cold and upper respiratory illnesses one person may have a number of new episodes of the same condition during the year under study. For instance, in the Canadian Sickness Survey under the heading "Illness Commencing in Survey Year", which is an expression of incidence, the rate in "Common Colds" for "persons" came to 398·8, but for "illnesses" the figure was 659·9, per 1,000 population at risk, meaning that each person started about two episodes of colds during the study year.

The meaning of the word "prevalence" has not always been clearly stated in surveys or studies. The "point prevalence rate" is commonly expressed as[8, 11, 12]:

$$\frac{\text{Number of cases ill at one point in time}}{\text{Defined population exposed to risk at that time}} \times 1,000$$

The "period prevalence rate" is a rather more difficult concept, because it embraces both "point prevalence" at the start of the study period and a more recent incidence.

In the Canadian Sickness Survey prevalence was defined as follows:

"Prevalence thus concerns illnesses (both new and recurring) which commenced at some time prior to the beginning of the Survey and which had not yet terminated at the time the Survey began. It is, therefore, a point prevalence, the point being the beginning of the Survey."[10]

In this Survey both "Persons reporting illness" and "Illnesses reported", are in the table on prevalence. For instance, under "Prevalence" the rate per 1,000 population for persons reporting illnesses (all causes) was 85, while for "illnesses reported (all causes)" the figure was 98, indicating that there was a slight excess of "illnesses" over persons at the beginning of the review period. This is due to the fact that one person may have two illnesses, such as a man with a fractured arm also developing pneumonia.

Both birth and death rates are examples of incidence in that each measures the frequency of a phenomenon per unit of time in a given mean population. They are also a measurement of something that is a new event or experience to each and every one of us. These rates are known reasonably well for most parts of the world. Illness or morbidity is much more difficult to determine.

For certain communicable diseases notifications provide some measurement of new cases. But notifications are not complete, even in the most highly developed countries. Stocks[13] examined the completeness of notification of certain communicable diseases in England and Wales, reaching the following conclusions:

Acute poliomyelitis Cerebro-spinal fever Diphtheria Scarlet fever	Notification is fairly complete
Respiratory tuberculosis	Probably nine-tenths notified
Typhoid and paratyphoid fevers	Probably four-fifths notified
Measles	About two-thirds notified
Pneumonia	From a third to a quarter notified
Whooping cough	From a quarter to a fifth notified
Erysipelas Non-respiratory tuberculosis	Defective to an indeterminate degree
Dysentery	Notification only fractional

Quite clearly, notification is far from adequate as a means of collecting data concerning the incidence of infectious diseases. A much more satisfactory method was introduced in the United States in 1957 when the

National Health Survey began monthly collections of material on current illness from a representative sample of that population[3].

One of the objectives in a study of incidence and prevalence is to develop some idea of persons ill with certain diseases, relative to the number who die from that particular condition. Tables IVa and IVb show, for Ontario 1963[14, 15, 16], the number of hospital separations and persons ill on one or more occasions per death during the year, and their relationships to the corresponding numbers of deaths. This is the kind of information that one would like for the whole world, but which is at present only available in countries with many data on morbidity. From the Ontario figures we may conclude, for instance, that for each death in the total grouping of diseases

Table IVa

PERSONS SICK DURING YEAR COMPARED WITH HOSPITAL SEPARATIONS AND MORTALITY, IN ONTARIO, 1963[14, 15, 16]

(Rates per 1,000 population)

		Rates		
Diagnostic group		Mortality[14]	Hospital separations[15]	Persons sick during year[16]
VII	Diseases of the circulatory system	3·452	12·1	103·34
II	Neoplasms	1·404	8·4	30·75
VI	Diseases of the nervous system and sense organs	1·016	6·9	155·35
XVII	Accidents, poisonings, and violence	0·653	13·6	171·20
VIII	Diseases of the respiratory system	0·544	24·4	505·88
XIV	Congenital malformations	0·467	1·8	13·61
XV	Certain diseases of early infancy			
IX	Diseases of the digestive system	0·299	19·7	158·89
XI	Deliveries and complications of pregnancy, childbirth and the puerperium	0·297	31·7	40·39
III	Allergic, endocrine system, metabolic and nutritional diseases	0·158	3·6	99·53
X	Diseases of the genito-urinary system	0·149	13·0	155·60
I	Infective and parasitic diseases	0·055	1·5	65·76
XVI	Symptoms, senility, and ill-defined conditions	0·026	3·5	131·41
V	Mental, psychoneurotic, and personality disorders	0·026	3·3	61·06
IV	Diseases of the blood and blood-forming organs	0·025	0·8	33·40
XIII	Diseases of the bones and organs of movement	0·024	5·0	91·00
XII	Diseases of the skin and cellular tissue	0·010	2·7	145·40
XVIII	Supplementary classifications for special admissions, live births, stillbirths, prophylactic inoculations, impairments, blindness, and deafness	0·000	0·9	181·49

Table IVb

ONTARIO 1963: RATIO OF HOSPITAL SEPARATIONS AND PERSONS SICK DURING YEAR TO
DEATHS[14, 15, 16]

	Hospital separations per death	Persons sick during year per death
VII Diseases of the circulatory system	4	30
II Neoplasms	6	22
VI Diseases of the nervous system and sense organs	7	153
XVII Accidents, poisonings and violence	21	262
VIII Diseases of the respiratory system	45	930
XIV Congenital malformations } XV Certain diseases of early infancy }	4	29
IX Diseases of the digestive system	66	531
XI Deliveries and complications of pregnancy, childbirth and the puerperium	107	136
III Allergic, endocrine system, metabolic and nutritional diseases	23	630
X Diseases of the genito-urinary system	87	1044
I Infective and parasitic diseases	27	1196
XVI Symptoms, senility and ill-defined conditions	135	5054
V Mental, psychoneurotic, and personality disorders	127	2348
IV Diseases of the blood and blood-forming organs	32	1336
XIII Diseases of the bones and organs of movement	208	3792
XII Diseases of the skin and cellular tissue	270	14,540

of the respiratory system there are 45 hospital separations and 930 persons ill on one or more occasions during the year. For infectious and parasitic diseases the figures come to 27 separations as against 1,196 sick persons. In diseases of the skin and cellular tissue there are 270 separations for each death and 14,540 sick persons. These figures include both new and old episodes of disease and are strictly speaking a combination of incidence and prevalence. Calculations have been made for various parts of the world of notifications per death, which give some idea of new cases (incidence). Such figures have been accepted with many reservations because notifications of certain diseases are not good in the most advanced countries, and are either non-existent or merely misleading in the other parts of the world.

A WORLD ESTIMATE OF DEATHS DUE TO THE LEADING COMMUNICABLE
DISEASES

I have attempted here to estimate the number of deaths from the leading communicable diseases[17] in the world (Tables V and VI). This is *not* merely a sum of sporadic and irregular reports from the valiant countries making attempts to assess their vital statistics.

Table V

DEATHS FROM COMMUNICABLE DISEASES

(Estimated World Totals, 1963 (see text for computation))

Cause of death	Number of deaths in thousands	Percentage of deaths from these causes
1. Pneumonia	5,701	33·12
2. Gastritis, duodenitis, enteritis, and colitis, except diarrhoea of the newborn	3,094	17·97
3. Tuberculosis of respiratory system	2,839	16·49
4. All other diseases classified as infective and parasitic	1,347	7·83
5. Infections of the newborn	1,131	6·57
6. Bronchitis	1,085	6·30
7. Measles	508	2·95
8. Malaria	326	1·90
9. Influenza	313	1·82
10. Dysentery, all forms	202	1·17
11. Smallpox	172	1·00
12. Diphtheria	127	·74
13. Whooping cough	112	·65
14. Typhoid fever	98	·57
15. Syphilis and its sequelae	68	·39
16. Acute poliomyelitis	35	·20
17. Meningococcal infections	31	·18
18. Cholera	12	·07
19. Typhus	7	·04
20. Scarlet fever and streptococcal sore throat	6	·03
21. Plague	0·5	—

Table VI

"ALL OTHER DISEASES CLASSIFIED AS INFECTIVE AND PARASITIC"[17]

030–039	Gonococcal infection and other venereal diseases
040	Paratyphoid fever
042	Other salmonella infections
044	Brucellosis (undulant fever)
049	Food poisoning (infection and intoxication)
052–054	Erysipelas; septicaemia and pyaemia; bacterial toxaemia
059–074	Tularaemia; leprosy; tetanus; anthrax; gas gangrene; other bacterial diseases; Vincent's angina; relapsing fever; leptospirosis; yaws; spirochaetal diseases except syphilis
081–083	Late effects of acute poliomyelitis; acute infectious encephalitis; late effects of acute infectious encephalitis
086–096	Rubella; chicken pox; herpes zoster; mumps; dengue; yellow fever; infectious hepatitis; glandular fever (infectious mononucleosis); rabies; trachoma; other diseases attributable to viruses
120–138	Leishmaniasis; trypanosomiasis; other protozoal diseases; schistosomiasis; other trematode infestations; hydatid disease; other cestode infestations; filariasis; trichiniasis; ankylostomiasis; infestation with worms of other mixed and unspecified type; dermatophytosis; actinomycosis; coccidioidomycosis; other fungus infections; scabies; pediculosis; other arthropod infestation; other infective and parasitic diseases

The countries of the world were divided into eight geographical areas designated as ''major divisions'', and these were subdivided into ''regions'', according to the scheme of Table 2 in the United Nations *Demographic Yearbook*, 1964[6] and ''Composition of Regions Set Forth in Table 2'' (Table II)[6].

The figures for population were taken from the United Nations *Statistical Yearbook*, 1964[18], the mid-year estimates for 1963 for each country of the world being used. These figures formed the basis of all further computations. Totals of populations for major divisions may not coincide exactly with figures quoted from summaries in the United Nations *Demographic Yearbook*, most of which are rounded off to three significant figures. Population data were used as counted or as estimated without taking into account the exceptions and qualifications in the footnotes, since these influenced the overall estimates only slightly.

The United Nations *Demographic Yearbook*, 1964, provided figures for deaths by cause for over a third of the countries of the world, but these were concentrated particularly in Europe and Northern America. Where the records were incomplete values were estimated for a region or a major division based on a ratio of the data from countries or regions reporting to the all-causes mortality for the area. In some instances the same procedure had to be used in order to derive a national figure for a country in which the mortality records related only to certain local populations.

Total estimated deaths were computed from population figures and the death rates per 1,000 as given in Table 2 of the *Yearbook*[6]. Populations by countries were added to give totals for regions, which when multiplied by the estimated death rate gave the estimated number of deaths for that region used throughout this paper. Totals of the regions within a major division multiplied by the United Nations estimated death rate gave the estimated number of deaths for that division—which is therefore not necessarily equal to the sum of deaths in the constituent regions. The total numbers of deaths for Western Africa and for Africa as a whole, for example, were estimated as follows:

	Population in thousands		Death rate per 1,000		Number of deaths
Western Africa	94,383	×	28	=	2,642,724
Africa (total)	296,259	×	23	=	6,965,453

In order to estimate the number and rate of total deaths and deaths according to cause, it was frequently necessary to make a calculation for a region or division based on very few countries reporting within that area.

To begin with it was necessary to correct the data to produce a figure that indicated deaths from assignable cause. Accordingly, the entries under B45—"Senility without mention of psychosis, ill-defined and unknown causes"—were subtracted from the total recorded deaths and this adjusted figure was used as the "total" figure in the calculations for deaths by cause. A ratio was then computed for each region of the total estimated deaths to the total number of deaths from assignable cause within that region. For example, Western Africa had a total of 6,733 deaths from the two countries reporting, and a total of 780 deaths from ill-defined causes (B45), leaving 5,953 deaths from assignable cause. In that region there were an estimated 2,642,724 deaths, giving a ratio of 443·93 : 1. This figure was used through-out the calculations of death by cause for that particular region to estimate the number of deaths from a specific disease. As an example, from the 166 cases of death from tuberculosis reported in the two countries providing statistics in Western Africa an estimate was made of 166 × 443·93 = 73,692 deaths from tuberculosis in that region. The ratio used as an illustration is a particularly high one, because of the scarcity of countries reporting, whereas in regions like Japan, Australia and New Zealand, North America, Western and Northern Europe, it is practically 1 : 1.

The death rate for a particular disease was calculated from the estimated number of deaths, as computed above, as a proportion of the population for the region or the major division, and expressed as deaths per 100,000 population. In Western Africa the death rate from tuberculosis was deter-mined as

$$\frac{73,692}{94,383,000} \times 100,000 = 78 \text{ per } 100,000.$$

The results of these calculations are shown in Table V. These figures should be considered against the background of deaths from all causes. Our estimates of deaths in the world in 1963, from all causes, is 52,500,798 in a population of 3,165,078,000, producing a rate of 16·6 per 1,000. Deaths from infectious diseases total 17,214,046, a rate of 5·4 per 1,000. Deaths from infectious diseases therefore amount to 32·6 per cent of deaths from all causes.

Among the communicable diseases, pneumonia heads the list, followed by tuberculosis. Obviously there is considerable overlap between these two categories, depending on the degree of medical sophistication of the countries concerned. In some countries of the world there would be over-lap between pulmonary tuberculosis and many of the other upper respira-tory diseases. In the diarrhoeal diseases, probably with the exception of

16

cholera, there would also be considerable overlap in diagnoses. Deaths from influenza were relatively low in 1963, although this situation may change very rapidly in an epidemic period. The total mortality occasioned by measles is likely to be much greater than any estimate based on death certificates; nevertheless our total of 508,000 makes it far the most lethal of the childhood communicable diseases. Diphtheria and whooping cough each account for only about a quarter of the deaths attributable to measles. Even malaria with a third of a million deaths ranks below measles in terms of total mortality.

This comparison of measles and malaria illustrates the limitations of the simple death count as an indicator of the relative importance of diseases. These figures, for example, give no measurement of the amount of incapacitating illness in the community or of the associated requirements for medical services.

THE SIX INTERNATIONALLY QUARANTINABLE DISEASES

The six internationally quarantinable diseases are cholera, plague, smallpox, yellow fever, louse-borne typhus fever, and louse-borne relapsing fever.

Our estimate of deaths from *cholera* in 1963 was 12,000, a very low figure. This is a far cry from the great cholera pandemics starting in 1817 in India and spreading to Europe, North America and North Africa. Paul[1] states that the number of cholera deaths in India averaged nearly 80,000 per year over the decade 1946–1955, although by the end of this period, as a result of control and immunization, the annual figure had fallen to 14,000. A notable spread of cholera in recent years was a brief invasion of Egypt in 1947. It is generally assumed that East Pakistan and the adjacent area of India (Calcutta) are the endemic focus where infection is always found and from where it may spread.

Cholera spread to 23 countries in 1965 and provisional figures indicate that there were 51,334 cases of the disease and 13,990 deaths. Starting from Indonesia in 1961, cholera has steadily progressed westwards and the situation is considered by the World Health Organization to be serious, owing to last year's invasion of new territories, particularly Iran (2,943 cases) and the Asiatic part of the USSR (570 cases). WHO warns that there is a threat of further spread of cholera to the west and that effective control measures have proved very difficult. The effectiveness of vaccines in current use has been proved to be low and of short duration[19]. There is no reason to suppose that cholera is completely under control; there may again be a recrudescence, especially as a result of civil commotion, mass population movements and consequent decline of preventive medical services.

The estimated number of deaths from *plague* in 1963 is 500. This disease is no longer a public health hazard of major importance under normal peace conditions, but remains an important threat in any catastrophe and the attendant breakdown in health standards. In 1965, 11 countries reported 1,326 cases and 120 deaths from plague[20]. For that same year, *Time* magazine reported 4,500 cases of bubonic plague with upwards of 200 deaths in South Vietnam as a result of increasing resistance of the flea population to available insecticides and of inadequate inspection of ships in the harbours[21]. In South America and even in the United States the disease persists in its sylvatic form, although in recent years human cases have been limited to a small number of cases:

REPORTED CASES OF PLAGUE

World totals[20]		Provisional figures in the Americas, 1965[22]	
1961	781	Bolivia	149
1962	1,443	Brazil	119
1963	861	Ecuador	374
1964	1,604	Peru	200
1965	1,326	United States	6

Smallpox remains a serious threat, with estimated deaths of 172,000 in 1963. Assuming a case fatality rate of 40 per cent, which occurred amongst unvaccinated persons in Sweden and England during the outbreaks of 1962–63, there were probably about 430,000 cases of smallpox in 1963. This is more than five times the number of cases actually reported in a year at the start of the world-wide eradication programme[23].

It would appear that the disease has now been almost or completely eradicated in North, Central and part of South America, Europe, North Africa, and the countries of the Eastern Mediterranean and the Pacific. The endemic areas include six countries in Asia (Afghanistan, Burma, India, Indonesia, Nepal and Pakistan), three in South America (Brazil, Colombia, Peru) and most of the African countries south of the Sahara (in these the lowest incidence occurs in Bechuanaland, South Africa and Mozambique). In general, incidence in Africa is higher than in Asia.

Of all the communicable diseases, smallpox best lends itself to eradication. It is readily detectable, especially in epidemic form, and the victims do not transmit virus for any great length of time; in addition, they become immune to further attacks. Adequate surveillance and co-operation between countries in eradication programmes are, of course, essential.

In the list of deaths from communicable diseases no estimates are given for *yellow fever* as the numbers concerned are so small at present[24]. This does not mean that this disease is unimportant. It is, however, a tribute to the campaign initiated by the Rockefeller Foundation half a century ago in co-operation with the United States Government, the Brazilian Government and other interested agencies. The apparent eradication of yellow fever in the Caribbean, Central and South American republics represents a great triumph of preventive medicine[25]. In Africa, however, the situation is by no means satisfactory[24]. In 1958 the first epidemic in 20 years was reported in the Congo, where it is enzootic in the forest monkeys[26]. Sixty cases were reported, with 23 deaths. The former Belgian Congo continues to be an endemic centre, while there has also been an epidemic in Ethiopia, with more than 3,000 deaths up to 1961. Under localized epidemic situations yellow fever is a serious disease with a very high case fatality rate. It may spread, as the chief urban vector, the mosquito *Aedes aegypti*, exists in many localities. At present, however, this disease does not appear to be a serious threat, except possibly in Africa, where the southern limit of the endemic zone was recognized by WHO as latitude 10°S, but including all of Angola and what was formerly Tanganyika[27].

We have estimated that there were 7,000 deaths from *typhus* (B15, "Typhus and other rickettsial diseases"). Of cases reported (all types of typhus) in 1957, 70 per cent were from Africa, 16 per cent from South Central and South East Asia, and 12 per cent from the Caribbean. In Africa, both louse-borne and flea-borne typhus occur, particularly in Ethiopia, Libya, the Congo, Ruanda-Urundi and Egypt[28].

Louse-borne *relapsing fever* does not appear to be a major public health problem. Most cases appear in Africa, with Ethiopia as the country of highest incidence and prevalence[29]. The only endemic focus of louse-borne relapsing fever in the world appears to be Ethiopia.

Colds and influenza

When discussing the major communicable diseases of the world, one could very easily fall into the trap of forgetting to mention what are probably the conditions of highest incidence. In the United States (1961–62) only 272 episodes per 1,000 population per year were due to the infective and parasitic diseases, which include the common infectious diseases of childhood, while no less than 1,277 per 1,000 were due to respiratory diseases, which include the common cold, influenza, pneumonia and bronchitis and similar conditions[3]. It is safe to assume from this and other studies that there will be at least one episode of a cough or cold for each person in the world per year, which would amount to about 3,500 million episodes in a normal year. This does not include allowance for the possibility, always to be feared, that a large-scale epidemic of influenza may emerge from this background of less serious conditions of the upper respiratory tract.

Bronchitis and pneumonia

Included in the general grouping of upper respiratory diseases are pneumonia and bronchitis. In Table V pneumonia, even without bronchitis, appears as the biggest single cause of death in the world. These categories would include many diverse types of acute pulmonary disease resulting in death. As diagnostic accuracy is limited by lack of trained medical personnel in many parts of the world there will also be considerable overlap between this group and other groups listed in Table V, particularly pulmonary tuberculosis, influenza and whooping cough. The variety of aetiological agents producing "pneumonia" is shown in Table VII[30].

From the United States National Health Survey we find a combined figure for pneumonia and bronchitis of 35 acute conditions per 1,000 population per year[3]. The corresponding rate under these headings for the Canadian Sickness Survey was 43[10]. For the world population of 3,165 million in 1963, we therefore estimate illnesses within the categories of pneumonia and bronchitis to be about 126·4 million assuming a rate of 40 per 1,000. Quite clearly, this is only a lower limit, as most Canadians and Americans are not exposed to the temperature extremes and other traumata suffered by people in poorer parts of the world, where one would expect more illness and deaths from acute pulmonary disease. An alternative form of estimate that leads to an upper limit may be based on Canadian data in Table VIII[31], where it is shown that for each death from diseases of the respiratory system, mainly pneumonia and bronchitis, about 50 persons were admitted to hospital. Applying this ratio to the world total of deaths, we arrive at a world figure of 350 million.

The diarrhoeal diseases

Under the general heading of "Gastritis, duodenitis, enteritis and colitis, except diarrhoea of the newborn" (B36), many diseases of this nature are included and there is overlap between this category, dysentery,

Table VII

THE PNEUMONIAS: AETIOLOGICAL CLASSIFICATION[30]

I. BACTERIA
  Pneumococcus
  Streptococcus
  Staphylococcus
  Klebsiella pneumoniae
  Haemophilus organisms
    1—*H. pertussis*
    2—*H. influenzae*
  Pasteurella organisms
    1—*Pasteurella pestis*
    2—*Pasteurella tularensis*
  Coliform, proteus and pseudomonas (Gram-negative)
  Salmonella group 1—typhoid
               2—paratyphoid A, B, C
  Brucella
  Anthrax bacillus
  Glanders bacillus

II. VIRUSES, KNOWN AND PROBABLE
  Primary atypical pneumonia virus
  Psittacosis
  Influenza A and B
  Measles
  Variola
  Varicella
  Rubella
  Lymphocytic choriomeningitis
  Primary pneumonitis of infants
  Infectious mononucleosis
  Erythema multiforme exudativum

III. RICKETTSIAE THAT CAUSE
  Typhus
  Rocky Mountain spotted fever
  Q fever

IV. MYCOSES THAT PRODUCE A PNEUMONIA-LIKE PICTURE
  Actinomycosis
  Histoplasmosis
  Blastomycosis
  Moniliasis
  Coccidioidomycosis
  Aspergillosis
  Cryptococcosis
  Nocardiosis
  Geotrichosis
  Penicilliosis
  Sporotrichosis

and probably typhoid and the other salmonelloses, in most parts of the world where proper diagnostic and laboratory facilities are lacking.

It is useful, as an epidemiological approach, to classify all the diarrhoeal diseases in a group as suggested by Cvjetanović[32]:

Table VIII

CANADIAN SICKNESS SURVEY 1950–51:
INCIDENCE OF ILLNESS DURING SURVEY YEAR

(*Rates per 1,000 Population for Principal Diagnostic Groups* [from Chart 4, ref. 31])

Persons	Diagnostic groups	Illnesses
398·8	Common cold	659·9
348·4	Influenza with respiratory and nervous manifestations and influenza unqualified	423·7
67·7	Disorders of function of stomach and other diseases of stomach and duodenum	79·8
59·7	Acute pharyngitis	68·5
42·6	Headaches	66·1
42·4	Symptoms referable to limbs and back	52·2
42·1	Influenza with digestive manifestations	46·9
34·2	Measles	34·4
29·5	Bronchitis	32·4
28·2	Other ill-defined symptoms and conditions	31·1
27·7	Symptoms referable to abdomen and lower gastro-intestinal system	30·8
26·5	Lacerations and open wounds	29·7
26·5	Other and unspecified effects and external causes including foreign bodies and poisonings	28·3
26·4	Symptoms referable to respiratory system	29·7

Persons reporting new illnesses, both sexes, per 1,000 population = 776·2

New illnesses reported by both sexes, per 1,000 population = 2,231·7

"Diarrhoeal diseases would comprise (besides certain less common conditions in which diarrhoea may appear) the following broad groups:

(1) Parasitic diseases caused by (a) bacteria (*Escherichia*; *Salmonella*; *Shigella*; *Vibrio*), (b) protozoa (*Amoeba*, *Giardia*), (c) viruses (ECHO, *Coxsackie*) and (d) helminths.

(2) Intoxications and allergies caused by bacterial toxins, chemicals, etc.

(3) Malnutrition and improper feeding leading to deficiency diseases (kwashiorkor, sprue, pellagra, coeliac disease).

"Diseases enumerated in the International Classification[17] under cross heading INFECTIOUS DISEASES COMMONLY ARISING IN INTESTINAL TRACT do not contain all diarrhoeal disease and yet comprise others which do not belong to this group. Nevertheless, when original statistical data are available, a compilation of diarrhoeal diseases could be attempted by using the International list of three-digit categories with four-digit subcategories.

"Diarrhoeal diseases would thus comprise: (040) typhoid, (041) paratyphoid, (042) other salmonelloses, (043) cholera, (045) bacillary dysentery, (046) amoebiasis, (047) other protozoal dysentery, (048) unspecified forms of dysentery, (049) food poisoning (excluding 049·1 botulism), (764) diarrhoea of newborn, (785·6) diarrhoea (age 2 years and over), (571) gastro-enteritis and colitis, (788·0) dehydration (when due to diarrhoea) and perhaps including (286·0) steatorrhoea and (286·6) kwashiorkor.

"The term 'diarrhoeal syndrome' could be used to distinguish between 'diarrhoeal disease' and diarrhoea as a symptom. The term 'diarrhoea' is often used to indicate a symptom that may occur in many diseases. Diarrhoeal syndrome, in addition to the symptom of diarrhoea, includes such other general and local symptoms or pathological changes as: loss of body liquids, imbalance of electrolytes and dehydration, intestinal lesions, abdominal pains and other symptoms which regularly or sometimes accompany this condition. From the practical point of view, diarrhoeal syndrome is what matters more than simple diarrhoea.

"Most cases of diarrhoeal diseases pass unrecorded and are not registered in national health statistics. Differences in this respect are great among various countries and therefore true comparison is impossible."

However, mortality data are more comparable. The differences between the rich countries and the poor are striking. Without entering into details of accuracy and significance, it is clear that higher mortality rates exist among the less developed countries. Again, in a particular country, mortality is lower in well-to-do and educated communities than among the poorer ones. Diarrhoea of the newborn is a major contributor to mortality in many countries and racial groups. In this paper we are primarily concerned with diarrhoeal disease of infectious origin, but quite clearly this problem cannot be separated from the problems of malnutrition and deficiency diseases.

In Table V we estimate that world deaths in 1963 in the grouping "Gastritis, duodenitis, enteritis and colitis, except diarrhoea of the newborn", numbered 3,094,000, with dysentery accounting for 202,000, typhoid for 98,000 and cholera for 12,000. In Table IX[1, 22, 33, 34, 35] we provide

23

estimates of world incidence of diarrhoeal disease based on rather flimsy evidence, shown in the table. These figures exclude diarrhoea of the new-born, which runs to tens of millions per year.

Table IX

DIARRHOEAL DISEASES:

ESTIMATED WORLD INCIDENCE, 1963[1,22,33,34,35]

Group of diseases	Estimated cases per death	Estimated cases, annual world incidence
Typhoid	20[1,22]	2,000,000
Cholera	2[35]	24,000
Dysentery	250[33,34]	50,000,000
Gastritis, enteritis, duodenitis, colitis group except diarrhoea of the newborn	250*	750,000,000

* Pure guesswork.

In considering the diarrhoeal diseases attention must be given to the question of world supplies of water. Wealthy industrial parts of the world now use about 200 gallons per person per day. Even in New York there are already signs of water shortage. In parts of South America, Africa, India and Australia the factor limiting population growth may be water rather than food, which itself needs water for its production. Add pollution to limited water supplies and the stage is set for diarrhoeal diseases on a grand scale. The time may be close when disposal of sewage by means other than water may become imperative in many communities.

Table X

SHIGELLA PREVALENCE ACCORDING TO AVAILABILITY
OF WATER SUPPLY AND ECONOMIC STATUS[36]

Group	Economic status	Water supply	Bacterial cultures	Number positive	Prevalence rate
A	Moderate	In home	278	1	0·4
B	Low	In home	376	8	2·1
C	Low	15 per faucet	2,182	116	5·3
D	Low	15 per faucet	1,057	97	9·2

"The relationship of water supplies to the incidence of bacillary dysentery in camps and town fringe areas in California has lately been demonstrated."[36] As Table X shows, "prevalence rates of *shigella* carriers among children up to 10 years of age rose steadily from group A to D as running water became more inaccessible. This finding raises the question as to which is more important in environmental sanitation—adequate clean water supplies or proper disposal of sewage—as control measures in such specific infections as enteric fever, bacillary dysentery and cholera.''[37]

In the southern parts of the United States, as in other warm areas, flies play an important part in spreading the organisms of gastrointestinal infection. Insecticidal sprays reduce the incidence of bacillary dysentery, but not of salmonella infections in the child population. This reduction stops, however, when flies develop resistance to the particular insecticide used, and more cases of diarrhoeal disease then again occur[38].

Salmonella organisms, apart from the typhoid-paratyphoid group, are common pathogens of animals, wild and domestic. Control should therefore be aimed at cleanliness in abattoirs and reduction of contamination in other foodstuffs for human consumption. An important need here is for vastly improved refrigeration, clearly beyond the financial capacity of most of the world's population. Simple hygienic measures, such as hand-washing, are however, perfectly practical, provided the reasons are known and accepted. But even in modern hospitals educated physicians and nurses do not wash their hands as often as they should, especially if they have to walk some distance to the nearest washbasin[39]. And when four gallons of water, carried ten miles or more, are all that many people in the drier parts of Africa, India and South America can obtain per day, advice about frequent hand-washing becomes pointless.

Certain communicable diseases of childhood

High on our list of deaths from communicable diseases are three childhood infections. These are measles, with an estimate of 508,000, whooping cough 112,000, diphtheria 127,000. Smaller in numbers are 31,000 for meningococcal infection, 35,000 for poliomyelitis and 6,000 for scarlet fever. Most of these estimates may be too low.

While *measles* is a serious disease in North America and Europe, it can be devastating in Asia and Africa and South America, where it is superimposed on parasitism, anaemia and malnutrition, and where it may attack non-immune populations living under primitive conditions. The complications of measles include bacterial pneumonia, otitis media, enteritis and encephalitis. There is also evidence that measles may reduce resistance to tuberculosis[40].

In 1952 there were two epidemics of measles amongst Indians and Eskimos in the Canadian Arctic, both with attack rates of over 99 per cent at all ages and mortality rates of 7 per cent and 2 per cent, about 20 per cent of cases being complicated by pneumonia[41].

In certain crowded areas in India, South America and Africa, the case fatality from measles may be as high as 7 per cent, comparable with the rates in Britain during the last century. In a five-year study in Western Nigeria, 19 per cent of the children admitted to hospital had measles, with a quarter of them dying. The estimated case fatality for all ages was 5 per cent, half the cases being under 17 months of age[42].

There are many shortcomings in the reporting of measles deaths and even more so of measles morbidity. If we follow the classical method of Chapin[43], postulating that 90 per cent of the population experience the disease and knowing that each year about 100,000,000 susceptibles are added to the world population, the annual incidence should be in the region of 90,000,000 as a world estimate. This would represent about 180 cases per death actually ascribed to measles. Deaths from this disease have declined in the wealthier countries of the world, particularly since the introduction of the sulphonamides and the antibiotics for the treatment of complications, but it is still a serious problem in areas with large populations of malnourished children. Measles is a disease that can be prevented, and encouraging progress has been made by using both live attenuated and inactivated vaccines in various combinations[44].

According to our world estimates, *whooping cough* produced about a quarter of the number of the deaths shown for measles. It is a serious disease in infants and young children, especially in malnourished populations where it probably predisposes to pulmonary tuberculosis. If we assume that about 70 per cent of the population experience this disease and use Chapin's reasoning we arrive at an annual incidence of about 70,000,000 cases in the world. Immunization is said to be about 70 per cent effective in the prevention of whooping cough.

Our estimates suggest a figure of 127,000 for *diphtheria* deaths. Since cases of this disease are missed even where good laboratories are available, this figure is undoubtedly an underestimate. Although diphtheria has been brought under control in many countries, it is still a continuing problem in the tropics. Edsall[45] has expressed the view that this disease is a growing problem in these communities and that it will become more serious with urbanization. Diphtheria can be controlled by immunization, especially if all children are immunized in infancy and early childhood. In the United States at present there are about 10 cases per death from diphtheria[22]. This is a favourable situation. In countries where treatment is limited or absent, case fatality will be higher. Using this ratio, however, we arrive at an annual incidence of 1,270,000 cases of diphtheria per year.

Table V gives an estimated figure of 31,000 deaths in the world due to *meningococcal meningitis*. It is well known that this is a disease of crowding, as was illustrated amongst troops in Britain during the First World War. In Britain there was also an epidemic during the Second World War, with considerably more cases than in the previous conflict. The case fatality rate in the earlier period was about 85 per cent, falling to about 20 per cent during the last few years, having been reduced by the use of sulphonamides (sulphadiazine) and penicillin. In Britain, during recent years for each death from this disease about five cases have been notified[1], and in this situation notification can be considered accurate. Using this ratio, we then estimate an incidence of about 150,000 cases in the world. One would expect the case fatality rate to be considerably higher in the tropics where medical aid may not be readily available. However, in certain tropical areas where 8,276 deaths from meningococcal meningitis were notified in 1957, the number of cases reported was 43,748[22]. This also gives a ratio of one death in five cases, as in Britain.

In Africa south of the Sahara, meningitis represents quite a different picture. There we find that devastating epidemics spread in the dry savannah area including Ghana, Nigeria, the French-speaking countries and the Sudan. Waddy[46] reports that the attack rate during a cycle of epidemics between 1943 and 1950 was 81·9 per 1,000 per year. The disease apparently dies out completely during inter-epidemic periods, with new cycles recurring from an endemic focus in the Republic of the Sudan. Without going into a detailed discussion of aetiological agents it should be pointed out, however, that acute purulent meningitis may be caused by organisms other than the meningococcus. Senecal, Dupin and Charpentier[47], studying 202 consecutive cases in West Africa, found the most common offending organism to be *Haemophilus influenzae*, followed by the pneumococcus.

As Sabin[48] has recently pointed out, *poliomyelitis* as a paralytic disease has become an increasingly important problem in many subtropical and tropical areas of Africa, Asia and Latin America, especially since 1950. In his view, some of this increase has resulted from increasing population mobility and consequent spread of infection. In recent years extensive oral vaccine programmes have been carried out in many subtropical and tropical areas including those of the USSR, the Republic of South Africa, Mexico, some states of Brazil, Chile, North Vietnam, Ceylon, Japan, Israel and the United Arab Republic. Our estimate of deaths in 1963 from poliomyelitis is 35,000. As this is but the tip of the iceberg, the number of maimed surviving cases must be considerably larger. Gear[49] also points out that the incidence of poliomyelitis appears to be increasing, especially in the

27

underdeveloped parts of the world. It would probably also be increasing in the countries with high standards of living were it not for immunization programmes.

While *scarlet fever* appears low in our list of causes of death (Table V) there is increasing evidence that *rheumatic fever* is a major cause of organic heart disease in tropical and subtropical areas. This has been noted in India, and the Philippines. A survey of cardiovascular disease among Africans living in the vicinity of the Albert Schweitzer Hospital, Lambaréné, showed rheumatic heart disease to be frequent. At the Baragwanath Hospital, Johannesburg, Chesler and his colleagues[50] found a high hospital frequency with 10·6 cases per 1,000 admissions of Bantu children under the age of 10 years with acute rheumatic fever. In that hospital surgical treatment for mitral stenosis is carried out. In Johannesburg the mean annual death rate (1963) for mitral valve disease came to 0·055 per 1,000 for whites and 0·067 per 1,000 for Bantu. A large proportion of the Bantu deaths occurred below an age of 20 years.

While *tetanus* is not strictly one of the common childhood communicable fevers, it may be extremely important in some countries. It is stated by Pai[51], for example, to be one of the four main causes of death in rural India, where it replaces tuberculosis as the leading cause of death. Neonatal tetanus is far more frequent than any other type, doubtless due to cultural and environmental factors discussed by Learmonth[52], a situation that finds parallels in other parts of the world. In Latin America, for example, two-thirds or more of deaths from tetanus occur before one year of age, principally in newborn infants. In the United States, in 1962 only a quarter of the deaths were in this age group[22].

INFECTIOUS DISEASES OF MORE CHRONIC NATURE

In this group of diseases, tuberculosis clearly heads the world list. Next in importance is malaria, but African sleeping sickness should also be included in this category, with a brief mention of certain other diseases. The next section on "The Silent Diseases" will include the venereal diseases, leprosy, and conditions like yaws, worm infestations, and brucellosis, that tend to be forgotten.

Horwitz and Palmer[53] have presented an excellent study on the dynamics of pulmonary *tuberculosis* morbidity and mortality in Denmark, furnishing details of the disease not previously available on a nation-wide basis. For instance, the official statistics show a mortality rate of 3·8 per 100,000—174 deaths in 4·5 million people. Actually 314 deaths occurred from the so-called Pool of Active Cases, but 140 of these were certified as due to other diseases. This would suggest that official figures for tuberculosis death rates, even in a sophisticated country like Denmark, greatly underestimate the ravages of this disease. Our world estimate of 2,800,000 annual deaths from tuberculosis is almost certainly a marked underestimate of deaths caused by this disease, or in association with this disease (Table V).

The Danish data show 1,221 cases of active respiratory tuberculosis diagnosed and reported during 1960. This incidence rate of 27 per 100,000 includes "first-timers" (21 per 100,000), "relapses" (5 per 100,000), additional "relapses" (1 per 100,000) not recorded in the "File of Previous Cases". Prevalence for Denmark is measured by the number in the "Pool of Active Cases", which was 7,859 in 1960. This means about 45 persons ill with the disease per death certified to the disease. In most parts of the world deaths would be higher relative to existing cases, because of overcrowding, malnutrition and lack of medical care.

Prevalence studies on tuberculosis are not simple to interpret. Whereas practically all persons found to excrete tubercle bacilli reacted to a low dose of tuberculin in the WHO-assisted studies, a considerable fraction of bacteriologically negative persons with radiological evidence of lung infiltrate did not[54]. From the experience of these prevalence surveys it was found that such tuberculin negatives with lung shadows are not likely to be tuberculous, since children in contact with them have a very much lower prevalence of tuberculous infection than those in contact with tuberculin positives with lung infiltrates. Clearly, then, prevalence surveys should consist of tuberculin testing followed by chest photofluoroscopy and sputum examination. This should give true point prevalence, provided sampling methods have been adequate.

During recent years interpretation of the tuberculin test has become complicated, especially in tropical areas, by the existence of mycobacteria of low pathogenicity. In temperate and subtropical regions the test is effective when a suitable reactive size is used as the limit between positive and negative reactors. In tropical regions the efficacy of the test is sharply reduced, as it is only from a very small or a very large reaction that a diagnosis can be made with some confidence. This whole complex matter has recently been discussed by Nyboe[55].

Tuberculin testing was amongst the methods used by Frimodt-Møller in his study of a South Indian rural community[56]. In this community prevalence of active pulmonary tuberculosis diagnosed by photofluoroscopy was 5·4 for males and 2·8 for females, per 1,000 population. This prevalence is remarkably low and it does not seem that the area is representative of the

2*

situation in India, since it has an unusually good nutritional status. The Indian morbidity figures were remarkable for the absence of any "youth peak" such as has been observed in Western countries, including England and Wales, as seen in Table XI[53, 57, 58].

Table XI

INCIDENCE (ATTACK RATE) IN TUBERCULOSIS:

NEW CASES PER YEAR PER 1,000 POPULATION[53,57,58]

Country	Morbidity rate per 1,000 population by photofluoroscopy
England and Wales[58]	Females Age 15 to 24: 2·8 25 to 34: 0·7 Males—Without pneumoconiosis Age 15 to 24: 4·7 25 to 34: 1·0
Yugoslavia[57]	3·4 Females all ages 3·4 Males all ages
Denmark[53]	0·27 Both sexes all ages

Table XI shows certain incidence figures for active tuberculosis in Yugoslavia[57], England and Wales[58] and Denmark[53]. The figures in this table cannot be said to provide any firm basis for an estimate of world tuberculosis incidence. However, if we take it as axiomatic that the rates in underdeveloped parts of the world, especially in overcrowded cities with increasing industrialization, must be higher than in Europe, then it may be reasonable to assume a 1 per 1,000 incidence for Europe, North America and the USSR and a 5 per 1,000 incidence for the rest of the world. This would yield a world total of just over 12 million cases in 1963.

A prevalence estimate that has at least the merit of consistency with our incidence estimate may be obtained by using the Danish ratio of prevalence to incidence (6 : 1) for Europe, North America and the USSR, and an arbitrarily chosen value of 3 : 1 for the rest of the world. This leads to a figure of 40 million currently active cases. It will be noted from Table XII[53, 56-63] that the prevalence found by Simeonov in Yugoslavia was considerably higher than the figure here suggested for Europe, probably because it includes quiescent cases.

As Maegraith[64] has recently pointed out, falciparum *malaria* is potentially the most dangerous of all exotic diseases, particularly in non-immune persons. In immune individuals, such as African seamen based in tropical Africa, the disease is mild. In tropical regions where malaria is common a

Table XII

PREVALENCE STUDIES IN PULMONARY TUBERCULOSIS[53,56-63]

Country	Population group	Morbidity rate per 1,000 population by photofluoroscopy
Canada Ontario[59]	Canadian-born Whites Canadian Indians Foreign-born Whites	0·20 1·95 0·48 (active tuberculosis)
England & Wales[58]	White	1950-51—10·3 females 1953— 6·9 females (active & infectious)
Denmark[53]	White	1960—1·72 (active tuberculosis)
Yugoslavia[57]	White	1959—23·5 males 1959—17·7 females 1960—29·0 males 1960—26·7 females (active & quiescent cases)
Africa Ghana[60]	African	10—General 3—Farming village 30—Coastal village (active pulmonary tuberculosis)
Bechuanaland[61]	African	13—active pulmonary tuberculosis
Transkei (South Africa)[62]	African	23—active pulmonary tuberculosis
South Africa[63]	White	0·9 11·2—26·1 (active pulmonary tuberculosis)
South India Madanapalle[56]	Indian	5·4 males 2·8 females (active pulmonary tuberculosis)

considerable proportion of children die early but the survivors acquire a fair degree of immunity, after some years of miserable ill-health[65]. In general, while malaria may not have a spectacularly high death rate, it has a marked debilitating effect on many millions of people in the tropical and subtropical parts of the world. In 1955 Pampana and Russell[66] estimated that of the approximately 2,500 million persons on earth at that time more than 250 million had clinical attacks of malaria, and possibly 2·5 million died of the disease each year. Our estimated figure for deaths in 1963 is considerably lower, at 326,000.

From data gathered in Middle America[22] we may assume that there are about 75 reported cases of malaria per death. This suggests a world occurrence of about 25,000,000 clinical cases per year. From this report it is not clear whether these are new cases or not.

As Hinman[24] observes, it was in Mexico City in 1955 that the World Health Organization took the step of embarking on a world-wide eradication programme of malaria. In Mexico malaria had prevented the settlement of potentially rich agricultural lands and there were periodic epidemics of the disease, particularly after hurricanes. This is the sort of tale that could be told of countless other countries where the climate is suitable for the propagation of malaria.

Of an estimated population in 1965 of 1,576 million people living in the originally malarious parts of the world, 1,214 million people live in areas where the disease has been eradicated or eradication programmes are in operation. The population of areas in the maintenance and consolidation phases who are thus freed from the risk of endemic malaria now amount to 905 million, or over 57 per cent of the population in originally malarious areas.

There are still 184 million people living in countries undertaking pre-eradication programmes, while 86 million, mainly in Africa, have not yet decided on campaigns against malaria.

Setbacks have occurred in certain programmes, notably in Ceylon, Jordan, Iraq, Syria, British Honduras, Costa Rica, Guatemala, and others. The difficulties which have arisen are both technical and administrative, the latter arising from lack of money, a dearth of good administrative and technical people, and, even more seriously, political instability[64].

The terrible potential danger of invasion by an insect vector is well illustrated by the crossing of *Anopheles gambiae*, probably late in 1929 or early in 1930, from Dakar to Natal, Brazil, on a French destroyer. A distance of over 2,000 miles was covered in four days. An explosive malaria epidemic occurred in Natal during three months, with an attack rate of 100 per cent. The species then spread within the area, and it was not until 1940 that it was beaten back and destroyed. This success was due to the splendid work of the International Health Division of the Rockefeller Foundation and the Brazilian government. The whole campaign is described in the publications of Dr. Fred L. Soper, Dr. D. Bruce Wilson and their colleagues[68].

African *trypanosomiasis* is still a serious disease in West and Central Africa, extending from approximately latitude 15°N to 20°S. The Gambian form of the disease is transmitted by the riverine tsetse flies; Rhodesian sleeping sickness is transmitted by the "savannah woodland" tsetse flies[28]. The latter disease is found in East Africa, Zanzibar, Rhodesia and Ruanda-Urundi, with a small focus in Bechuanaland.

In 1957, 11,442 cases of trypanosomiasis were reported, with 1,058 deaths[28]. The disease has shown some signs of receding in the face of campaigns of treatment and insect control, but the potential for new outbreaks is high. There can be no relaxation of effort on the part of governments.

THE SILENT DISEASES

This section deals briefly with those diseases concerning which people prefer to be silent, such as the venereal diseases and leprosy, and the other serious conditions like trachoma and worm infestations, which cause a great deal of debility but which do not kill very many people.

Determination of world incidence and prevalence of *venereal disease* is an almost impossible task. Even in highly sophisticated countries with adequate medical services, notification of these diseases is inadequate. In a survey in the United States[69] it was estimated that nine out of ten cases of infectious syphilis and gonorrhoea are treated by private physicians and are not reported to health departments. If we accept this, the incidence figures for these diseases for the United States and Canada, and probably for Western Europe and other countries with similar levels of medical care, should be multiplied by 10 to obtain a closer idea of incidence. For the rest of the world, particularly the tropical countries (population 1,200 million) with considerably more limited treatment and probably more chances of spread due to social and family dislocation, such as migrant labour, incidence figures are almost certainly considerably higher than in North America.

The venereal diseases are gonorrhoea, syphilis, chancroid, lymphogranuloma venereum and granuloma inguinale. Only the first two of these conditions will be discussed here.

It would appear that the incidence of venereal disease has been increasing in many parts of the world during the last few years[70]. Many factors are no doubt involved in this, such as population movement, complacency on the part of health authorities, and possibly an increase in alleged irresponsibility of youth. In many instances, particularly in females, both gonorrhoea and syphilis may be hidden, leading to increasing spread if there is promiscuity.

As regards *gonorrhoea*, diagnosis has improved by use of the delayed fluorescent antibody test, and the present problem is that of the increasing resistance of the organism to penicillin. Amies[71] has recently shown that 27 per cent of strains now isolated in Ontario need a very high concentration of penicillin for control, requiring intramuscular soluble penicillin in a high dosage of 2–8 million units. Furthermore, many of the penicillin-resistant strains are resistant to tetracycline as well. It would therefore appear that talk about eradication of gonorrhoea is somewhat optimistic.

Table V estimates the world total of deaths from *syphilis* as 68,000 in 1963. This is certainly a marked under-estimate of deaths due to this disease, manifested as aneurysm of the aorta, other cardiovascular syphilis, general paralysis of the insane, tabes dorsalis and other syphilis of the central nervous system. It has been estimated[72] that the outlook for untreated syphilis is that 1 patient in 13 will develop syphilitic heart disease, 1 in 25 will become crippled or incapacitated, 1 in 44 will develop syphilitic insanity and 1 in 200 will become blind. This situation, in a world population often lacking adequate medical care, is serious, in spite of valiant efforts being made in prevention and treatment.

As regards prevalence, some indication is given by serological tests. Without entering into a discussion concerning the detailed interpretation of such tests, it suffices to say that in the United States the National Health Survey[73] has produced data for 1960–62, on the Kolmer-Reiter protein test, which shows a prevalence in the age group 18–79 years of positive reactions in white males and females of 4·4 and 3·6 per cent respectively, as against 22·9 and 16·3 for negro males and females respectively. There are certainly many parts of the world with a higher prevalence of the disease than in the United States. Such serological data would also be influenced by interval since infection, and by treatment. But it does give some reasonably accurate information on prevalence of primary and secondary syphilis. As far as incidence figures for early syphilis are concerned, recent surveys show a marked increase. Estimated maximum and minimum incidence rates per annum between 1950 and 1960 were as shown in Table XIII[70].

With venereal syphilis we should also consider the non-venereal type of endemic syphilis, called "dichuchwa" in Bechuanaland, with various synonyms such as bejel, njovera, sibbens or radesyke. This condition is found in the Balkans and eastern Mediterranean, with numerous foci in Africa. The Bechuanaland study carried out by Murray, Merriweather and Freedman[74] found that dichuchwa is a family and childhood disease, with a seropositive rate of 37 per cent (Kolmer cardiolipin complement-fixation test). In this study, cardiovascular and neurological late lesions are described, but they are rare.

Table XIII

RANGE OF ANNUAL INCIDENCE RATES PER 100,000 ADULT POPULATION OVER 15 YEARS OF AGE, MAXIMA AND MINIMA OF EARLY SYPHILIS FOR EACH WORLD REGION, 1950–60[70]

Region	Highest and lowest rates in 1950	Highest and lowest rates in 1960	Minimum rate during decade	Maximum rate during decade
Africa	Senegal 1,156.5 Tanganyika 0.5	Togo 729.8 Mauritius 8.0	Tanganyika 0.02 (1959)	Basutoland 1,232.0 (1951)
Americas	Colombia 340.0 Guatemala 8.9	El Salvador 180.0 British Guiana 2.0	Canada 1.6 (1956)	Colombia 340.0 (1950)
Eastern Mediterranean	Sudan 3,687.5 Israel 7.2	Ethiopia 82.2 Jordan 2.0	Jordan 0.01 (1959)	Sudan 3,687.5 (1950)
Europe	Yugoslavia 53.6 France 8.4	Turkey 41.1 Finland 0.7	Czechoslovakia 0.2 (1958)	Yugoslavia 53.6 (1950)
South-east Asia and Western Pacific	Malaya 246.5 Philippines 2.6	New Caledonia 44.3 Fiji 2.0	Philippines 0.2 (1960)	French Polynesia 250.8 (1952)

One method of studying the epidemiology of syphilis is by means of serological surveys and in recent years WHO has conducted a number of studies along these lines. One of the difficulties encountered in this work is that of distinguishing between reactions due to syphilis and those from yaws and even from false seroreactions unconnected with the treponematoses.

About 20 years ago some 200 million people were living in rural areas affected by endemic treponematoses and about 50 million were suffering from these infections. Yaws was endemic throughout large areas of the tropics, where active clinical prevalences ranged from 5·6 per cent (Cameroon) to 30 per cent (Liberia) in Africa, from 2·5 per cent (Brazil) to 50 per cent (Haiti) in the Americas, from 3·1 per cent (Thailand) to 17·2 per cent (Indonesia) in South-East Asia, and from 3·6 per cent (Laos) to 40 per cent (New Hebrides) in the Western Pacific Region[75].

As a result of co-operative efforts between the countries concerned, and agencies such as WHO and UNICEF, great changes have been brought about in reducing the prevalence not only of yaws but of pinta in South America and endemic syphilis in other parts of the world. In the endemic treponematoses surveys of this type 42,245,000 persons had been treated up to 1963. The number of infected people in these areas is now estimated at only 10–15 million. The low-cost penicillin-treatment campaigns have markedly reduced the transmission of infection and prevalence of these diseases[75]. What remains now is for the individual governments to carry on with the work, which must essentially be run by the administrations of the countries concerned, with guidance and help from the World Health Organization. Table XIV[70] provides additional summarized information on the treponematoses.

It is difficult to find accurate information on the prevalence of *leprosy*, but a good recent study of this question has appeared[76]. In all, there are 2,831,775 registered patients and an estimated 10,786,000 active cases, which may be an underestimate. About 2,097 million people live in areas with prevalence rates of 0·5 per 1,000 or higher. In these areas nearly one million new cases of the disease may be expected during the next five years. Estimates of cases by continent are, in order of magnitude: Asia, with 6,475,000 (excluding Mongolia); Africa, 3,868,000; America, 358,000; Europe, 52,000; and Oceania, 33,000. The estimated world total of disabled patients is 3,872,000. Leprosy is a disease of long duration and treatment is extremely expensive, particularly if reconstructive surgery is attempted. Moreover, the age-old prejudice against the disease aggravates the suffering, not only of the patient but also of his family. While we cannot

Table XIV

A MEASURE OF THE DISTRIBUTION, EXTENT AND IMPORTANCE OF ENDEMIC TREPONEMATOSES[70]

	Venereal syphilis: adults	*"Endemic" syphilis ("bejel"): children*	*Yaws: children*	*Pinta: children*
Distribution	Sporadic; world-wide; all climates; all socio-economic groups; urban; seaports; migration; traffic arteries	Focal; familial; endemic; underdeveloped, isolated communities; all regions except the Americas; prevalent in Mediterranean belt, Africa, Australia	Endemic; rural; tropical humid belt; all regions except Europe; disease "at the end of the road"; not above 6,000 feet	Focal; endemic; rural; only in the Americas; in semi-arid, hot and humid tropical areas; all altitudes
Extent of problem following Second World War	Post-war peak 1946–1948 in most countries; wide variations between regions and countries; annual incidence 15–500 new cases per 100,000 over 15 years of age; estimated total number of cases in world in 1948: 20 million	Varying prevalence in existing foci; sometimes 5 to 10% infectious lesions; 20–50% seroreactivity	Estimated 50 million active and 150 million latent cases; 5–10% infectious lesions; seroreactivity up to 60–70% in rural populations; frequent infectious relapses from latency	Varying prevalence in existing foci; seroreactivity high
Social and economic importance	Reduced manpower; absenteeism; incapacitation; cost of medical care; physical and mental invalidism	Reduced manpower in adolescents and young age-groups; incapacitation; late invalidism; cost of medical care	Invaliding sequelae in 10% of infected; ankylosis, destructive lesions; reduced manpower pool in developing countries; social and economic burden on community; cost of medical care	Cosmetic aspect, also mental health repercussions from pigmentation and dyspigmentation; cost of medical care

37

Table XV

THE CALCULATED NUMBER OF HUMAN HELMINTHIC INFECTIONS, IN MILLIONS (FROM "THIS WORMY WORLD")[78], P. 15, FIGURES ADJUSTED TO 1963 POPULATION OF 3,165 MILLION)

	Northern America	Middle and South America	Africa	Europe (without USSR)	USSR	Asia (without USSR)	Oceania	Total
Trichinella spiralis	30·6	2·3	·4	4·4	1·7			39·4
Taenia saginata	0·1	1·2	24·0	0·9	25·3	8·9	0·2	60·6
Taenia solium			1·0		1·1	1·8		3·9
Hydatid								
Hymenolepsis nana	0·1	1·2	1·2	1·8	4·2	20·9		29·4
Diphyllobothrium latum				3·2	8·4	1·8		13·4
Clonorchis sinensis						28·3		28·3
Opisthorchis felineus				0·1	1·3			1·4
Fasciolopsis buski						14·9		14·9
Paragonimus westermani						4·8		4·8
Schistosoma japonicum						68·6		68·6
Schistosoma haematobium			78·1			0·3		78·4
Schistosoma mansoni		10·8	46·0					56·8
Dracunculus medinensis			30·0		4·4	44·7		79·1
Onchocerca volvulus		1·4	38·0					39·4
Mansonella ozzardi		12·2						12·2
Acanthocheilonema perstans		13·9	38·0					51·9
Loa loa			26·0					26·0
Wuchereria bancrofti and malayi	26·1	15·7	44·0	69·9	42·9	234·1	1·7	295·5
Enterobius vermicularis	2·6	27·9	17·8	1·6	3·7	105·9	0·7	291·2
Hookworm	4·4	73·0	98·1	36·1	26·3	535·3	1·3	715·6
Ascaris lumbricoides	0·6	73·0	118·1	38·3	35·9	727·7	0·8	986·4
Trichuris trichiura	0·6	66·2	56·0	0·7	1·2	338·5	0·8	536·3
Strongyloides stercoralis		15·0	6·6		1·2	31·3	0·2	55·6
Trichostrongylus spp.					1·3	6·7		8·0
Total infections	65·1	313·8	623·3	157·0	157·7	2174·5	5·7	3497·1
Population (millions)	208·4	227·8	296·2	436·6	224·8	1754·4	16·8	3165·0
Per cent infections of population	31	138	210	36	70	124	34	110

discuss the epidemiology of leprosy in this presentation, one important point that should be stressed is that the secondary attack rate can be considerable in household contacts of this disease[77].

The *worm diseases* are a tremendous burden in vast areas of the world. Table XV is an updating of the well-known paper "This Wormy World" by Stoll[78]. While there has certainly been a reduction in the United States of America in the prevalence of trichinosis and hookworm, the position in most other parts of the world has probably remained the same, with some deterioration regarding schistosomiasis in Africa.

One of the most debilitating and widespread chronic diseases in the tropics today is *schistosomiasis* (bilharziasis)[79]. It shares its position with malaria and ankylostomiasis. Schistosomiasis does not kill, but it weakens countless millions of people in Africa, the Eastern Mediterranean, China, Japan, the Philippines, Celebes and parts of South America. The loss due to this disease is tremendous and cannot readily be expressed in monetary values. In the same areas where it is endemic, there is often a heavy infestation with ankylostomiasis and other parasitic worms, as well as malaria.

This disease is increasingly man-made. Schistosomiasis was unknown until the introduction of perennial irrigation in many areas such as the Qena and Aswan provinces of Egypt. In Southern Rhodesia the Umshandige Irrigation Scheme costing £3,000,000 had to be abandoned in 1949, ten years after its commencement, mainly because the prevalence of schistosomiasis had reached such vast proportions. It is tragic that in many countries the agricultural experts apparently take little notice of the danger of schistosomiasis and ignore the advice of health authorities, who are competent to make recommendations on the control of the snail vector. The irrigation engineer must co-operate with the snail expert and the epidemiologist in designing snail control measures applicable to irrigation systems.

The other greatly debilitating parasitic worm disease is *ankylostomiasis* (hookworm), estimated to infest more than 50 per cent of the population in the moist tropical countries and nearly one-fourth of the world's population[7]. This amounts to about 700,000,000 persons. The disease may be caused either by *Ankylostoma duodenale* or *Necator americanus*. Clinically one would distinguish between primary infection, re-infection or super-infection. The worst effect of the condition is iron-deficiency anaemia and consequent debility.

Trachoma is one of the very serious silent diseases[80, 81, 82]. It causes partial and complete blindness, but it does not kill. The populations worst affected are those of North Africa, the Middle East, the northern part of the Indian

39

sub-continent and large areas of the Far East, such as Vietnam and China. There is a high or moderate prevalence over large parts of Africa, Southern India, the Far East and parts of Australasia. The disease is also found, to a lesser extent, in Southern Europe, the Soviet Union, Japan, South America and the North American Indian reservations. It is probable that the only countries virtually free of trachoma are Canada, Iceland, Norway, Sweden, Denmark, the United Kingdom, the Benelux countries, Switzerland, Germany and Austria[83].

The micro-organisms of trachoma and inclusion blennorrhoea are usually referred to as viruses. Gear and his colleagues have recently suggested the acronym TRIC (TR = trachoma, IC= inclusion conjunctivitis) for these agents. The extent of disability resulting from trachoma and associated infections is frequently understated. It is a not uncommon finding where virtually whole populations are afflicted with trachoma and seasonal conjunctivitis that more than 1 per cent of adults are totally blind, more than 4 per cent are unable to perform work for which sight is essential, and a large number have visual defects. The economic loss due to this situation is staggering[80]. It is well known that what is needed for trachoma prevention and cure is a good clean water supply and in most cases certain sulphonamide eyedrops. For primary treatment of existing lesions tetracycline is probably the most effective agent.

Manson-Bahr[65] describes *undulant fever* (brucellosis)—the melitensis type, derived from infected goat's milk—as being a disease of low mortality, indefinite duration and irregular course. Common complications are a rheumatic-like affection of joints, profuse sweating, anaemia and liability to orchitis and neuralgia. It is rarely fatal, but causes much inefficiency and invalidism. This disease is closely associated with goats and sheep and it is difficult to state its exact geographical range or the number of patients affected. The abortus type of the disease is derived from cattle and particularly from milk. The disease is of shorter duration than the melitensis variety. In countries where high standards of hygiene exist and where milk is pasteurized this disease is uncommon[84].

Amongst the "silent diseases", *infectious hepatitis* is coming into greater prominence, partly no doubt because of improved diagnosis and more complete notification. Estimates of world incidence are not worth attempting, because so many cases will be missed, especially in tropical areas where so many people may have other conditions associated with jaundice. The largest water-borne outbreak on record occurred in Delhi, India with an estimated 29,300 icteric cases in a six-week period between November 1955 and January 1956[85]. Among 33 countries for which some recent incidence figures have been published[22, 86, 87], it is notable that five that have considerably higher rates than any others form a continuous territory from the Baltic to the Adriatic Sea.

There are many more diseases that plague man but they are not sufficiently important, with the world as our stage, to be included in the present discussion. They may, however, be very serious in particular localities at particular points in time.

The greatest, most horrifying, and most intractable "silent disease" of them all is *hunger*, which is gnawing at the vitals of perhaps two-thirds of the world's population. This is a condition that we should never be allowed to forget.

A CONCLUDING VIEW

I have discussed diseases one at a time, but that is not of course how they are experienced. "When sorrows come, they come not single spies, But in battalions." In subtropical and tropical regions multiple pathology is the rule rather than the exception. This was the situation found years ago by Kark and le Riche[88] in the Bantu Nutrition Survey, and there is no reason to believe that it has changed in any substantial manner.

In Table XVI an attempt is made to summarize the incidence and prevalence of certain diseases. The data on worm infestations are not repeated, except for ankylostomiasis, and schistosomiasis. The figures are the best I could find and for their inaccuracies I crave the indulgence of my audience.

The World Health Organization has made a good start on the great project of controlling and reducing communicable disease in the entire world. We will serve these aims best if we cultivate the ecological view that encompasses the whole welfare of man in terms of his health, his work, his living conditions, his food—and his remarkable propensity for multiplication. The task of checking population growth is only one of many that now confront governments in the new countries, and which call for a degree of understanding as well as for technical skills that these countries may lack. Some populations may even lack the necessary motivation to attack their disease problems, because of a fatalistic view of conditions that they regard as "normal" and cannot hope to change.

Others in the more comfortable circumstances of the developed countries find that the task of studying, let alone solving, these problems is more than they feel inclined to undertake. Some such failure of stamina is evident in what is probably the most complete report on tropical health ever attempted, namely the United States National Academy of Sciences—National Research Council study to which frequent reference has already

Table XVI

ESTIMATES OF WORLD INCIDENCE, DEATHS AND PREVALENCE OF
COMMONLY OCCURRING COMMUNICABLE DISEASES

(from data in text)

Disease	World incidence (recent year)	World deaths (1963)	World prevalence
1. Common cold	3,500,000,000	Low	Not applicable
2. Gastritis, duodenitis	750,000,000	3,094,000	Not applicable
3. Pneumonia	125–350,000,000	5,701,000	Not applicable
4. Bronchitis		1,085,000	Not applicable
5. Measles	90,000,000	508,000	Not applicable
6. Whooping cough	70,000,000	112,000	Not applicable
7. Dysentery	50,000,000	202,000	Not applicable
8. Malaria	25,000,000	326,000	Not known
9. Tuberculosis (respiratory)	13,000,000	2,800,000	40,000,000 active cases
10. Typhoid	2,000,000	98,000	Not applicable
11. Diphtheria	1,270,000	127,000	Not applicable
12. Smallpox	430,000	172,000	Not applicable
13. Leprosy	200,000		10,786,000 cases
14. Meningococcal meningitis	150,000	31,000	Not applicable
15. Cholera	24,000	12,000	Not applicable
16. Yaws			10–15,000,000 cases
17. Helminthic infestations:			
Ankylostomiasis (hookworm)			715,600,000 cases
Schistosomiasis			203,800,000 cases
Taenia saginata (beef tapeworm)			60,600,000 cases
Taenia solium (pork tapeworm)			3,900,000 cases

been made[28]. This document contains many numerical errors and inconsistencies of a type that the distinguished authors would have been unlikely to overlook when dealing with any question for which they felt a scholarly concern. Greater intellectual efforts are now required of those with a responsibility for proposing plans of action, while governments of the new countries must also appreciate that much hard work and perseverance are needed in order to bring about those favourable changes that they so much desire for their peoples.

If these changes are achieved then we may feel that Man truly merits the encomium of Robert Ardrey[89], "... *we were born of risen apes, not fallen angels, and the apes were armed killers besides. And so what shall we wonder at? Our murders and massacres and missiles, and our irreconcilable regiments? Or our treaties whatever they may be worth; our symphonies, however seldom they may be played; our peaceful acres, however frequently they may be converted into battlefields; our dreams, however rarely they may be accomplished. The miracle of man is not how far he has sunk but how magnificently he has risen. We are known among the stars by our poems, not our corpses.*"

DISCUSSION

Candau : You are to be congratulated on having the courage to present those world figures, Professor le Riche. It is extremely difficult to generalize from such figures. Large areas of the world have no doctors, so what is put on the death certificate is an unknown cause of death ("fevers of unknown origin" account for most deaths in developing countries), or else the cause is something written by lay people and has no meaning at all. The only published statistics for Brazil, which you mentioned, refer to 21 cities and to generalize from these to the rest of the country is impossible.

The new wave of cholera to which you referred has now reached the frontier of Turkey. Probably sporadic cases will occur in Europe some time during the next few years. This is more or less the same trend as was followed by the last wave in 1899–1923.

The widespread epidemic of yellow fever in Senegal, starting in 1965 and transmitted by *Aedes aegypti*, is something completely different from what we had in earlier years. *Aedes aegypti* is at the moment one of the most interesting vectors of disease, and it has been responsible for very severe epidemics of haemorrhagic fever and dengue fever in Asia, and dengue fever in the Caribbean.

Pequignot : Clinicians and statisticians or epidemiologists do not speak quite the same language. I cannot understand why statisticians speak of pneumonia as the cause of death, for deaths from pneumonia always occur in people who have other diseases as well. The developing and the developed countries both have the problem of infectious disease but it is not the same problem. Tuberculosis in Africa, for instance, is often very acute tuberculosis, while in England or France death from tuberculosis occurs after a man has had the disease for twenty or thirty years. In the developing countries, people have many illnesses and the final infection is added to many others. In statistics it is very important to separate the different types of underlying morbidity.

Kaprio : That is certainly something that has to be remembered when preventive action is being considered, especially in the developing countries.

In the rapidly increasing city populations of the world, the problem is not necessarily one of industrialization but of lack of industrialization. Especially when there is lack of work the places where people live become breeding places for new diseases. We have to be prepared, with modern traffic and communications, for the greater mobility of certain infectious diseases over the whole globe. That means we must be much more alert to our responsibilities concerning infectious diseases, even though some of them are now much better controlled than formerly.

Evang: Closer co-operation between public health authorities and agricultural authorities, for example in the attempt to check schistosomiasis, opens up a very broad field. Diseases like plague, smallpox, cholera, diphtheria, etc., are now a long way down the ranking list of killing diseases, because we have been able to fight them. Other communicable diseases, for example tuberculosis, leprosy and enteric infections, are not in the same process of being fought. So far we have been reaping the harvest which is easiest to reap. Professor le Riche touched on a very fundamental problem—that is, we have had excellent results in fighting those communicable diseases where the understanding and co-operation of the public was not needed, and no economic or political changes were needed, or any changes in habits or environment—one just vaccinated, or used DDT, etc. But now we are approaching this area of greater complexity and involvement.

Can you improve on the definition of health in the World Health Organization constitution ("Health is a state of complete physical, mental and social wellbeing and not merely the absence of disease or infirmity.")?

le Riche: The WHO definition is the sort of definition which says that one is against sin or in favour of virtue, but it can't be used as a measure. I can't give a better definition but I think that some people have repeated this one like a sort of dogma, until now they think it is a big truth, yet many dogmas are not necessarily true. They try to get away from really trying to measure the situation. To the clinician the only way to measure health is by the absence of disease. When you get into this positive health business you lose me.

Garcia: As a health educator I believe the definition of health is very important. We have to set some kind of standard to reach, because in our underdeveloped countries many people are perfectly happy when they are not in hospital, even though they have diarrhoea, headaches and so on. The cultural background and the pattern of life in any particular group are of tremendous importance in deciding what is the state of good health or bad health. We have the problem of fatalism—"it is God's will"—but a kind of conformity is something that really helps people.

le Riche: You mean you must have a gospel even if it is not true?

Wolman: The definition of health serves certain useful purposes, but it is actually a universal description of man and his fate. We have just convinced ourselves as public health workers that all the welfare of man means is "health", when in fact it actually means everything that man does.

Candau: But health cannot be separated from other conditions in society.

Johnson-Marshall: As a physical planner who is interested in environmental health I wonder just how much physical planning can help. The problem is partly one of causes and priorities and I would like to list one or two points.

(1) What degree of priority should the community place on slum clearance and direct action of this kind?

(2) Could one focus on schools for positive health education?

(3) Should particular kinds of employment be provided for particular places?

(4) In terms of better space conditions and the planning dilemma between urban decentralization and the convenience of concentration, do we know enough about the relationship of space conditions to health factors?

(5) How much urban ill-health is due to the greater wear and tear of metropolitan over-concentration, causing serious debilities and lack of physical resistance?

(6) Is there a danger that some communicable diseases might be accelerated in any way by affluence?

le Riche: I don't think affluence increases the incidence of communicable diseases, except perhaps if people go to hospital too often, as it may be dangerous to go to hospital if infection is acquired there. If we take a world picture, the most important thing with regard to health is the production of wealth, which we medical people have tended to forget. We have gone for the easiest things first, as Dr. Evang said, and we also think that we can produce change without starting at the beginning. England started the industrial revolution and people here didn't get too concerned about health until they had produced quite a considerable measure of wealth. The rest of the world should learn from this. The whole process cannot be telescoped too rapidly, and neither can the Americans go on paying for the rest of the world for ever. All the countries in the world should as soon as possible be standing on their own feet, though possibly with some help. But a dependent attitude is developing which I think is wrong. Countries should develop their own wealth by whatever means are most appropriate.

Wolman: The ultimate prevention of all the communicable diseases you mentioned is subject to the whole gamut of sociological, economic and physical adjustments. Nothing in the history of public health evolution discloses more clearly how the communicable disease incidence declined.

45

Many of the diseases of the developing world are the familiar ones which in early English history were finally readjusted by social reform, with all that that meant—a rise in the standard of living and a change in the physical complex of living. In Dr. Dubos's phrase, a constellation of causes was inherent in the prevention. The decline in tuberculosis, for example, even in the developed countries, was really in no small measure the result of socioeconomic improvement as much as anything else. Although we have been helped a tremendous amount by vaccines and all the therapeutic aids, they alone are not going to eliminate diseases such as schistosomiasis. These require a total change in what I call the geometry and hygiene of living, and in the whole socioeconomic status.

REFERENCES

1. Paul, H. (1964). *The Control of Diseases (Social and Communicable)*. 2nd edn. Edinburgh & London: Livingstone.
2. Dubos, R. (1965). *Man Adapting*. New Haven: Yale University Press.
3. National Center for Health Statistics (1963). Acute conditions, incidence and associated disability: United States: July 1961–June 1962. *Vital and Health Statistics*, Series 10, No. 1. Washington, D.C.: U.S. Dept. of Health, Education, and Welfare.
4. Logan, W. P. D., and Cushion, A. A. (1958). Morbidity statistics from general practice vol. 1. *Studies on Medical and Population Subjects*, No. 14. London: H.M.S.O.
5. National Center for Health Statistics (1966). Conceptual problems in developing an index of health. *Vital and Health Statistics*, Series 2, No. 17. Washington, D.C.: U.S. Dept. of Health, Education, and Welfare.
6. United Nations (Statistical Office) (1965). *Demographic Yearbook*, 1964. New York: United Nations.
7. Gordon, J. E. (ed.) (1965). *Control of Communicable Diseases in Man*, 10th edn. New York: American Public Health Association.
8. Dorn, H. F. (1957). A classification system for morbidity concepts. *Public Health Reports*, **72**, 1043–1048.
9. Reid, D. D. (1960). Epidemiological Methods in the Study of Mental Disorders. Geneva: WHO, Public Health Papers No. 2.
10. Department of National Health and Welfare and Dominion Bureau of Statistics (1960). Illness and health care in Canada. In *Canadian Sickness Survey*, 1950–1951. Ottawa: Queen's Printer.
11. MacMahon, B., Pugh, T. F., and Ipsen, J. (1960). *Epidemiologic Methods*. Boston: Little, Brown.
12. Densen, P. M. (1965). Statistical reasoning. In *Maxcy-Rosenau, Preventive Medicine and Public Health*, ed. Sartwell, P. E., pp. 20–44, 9th edn. New York: Appleton-Century-Crofts.
13. Stocks, P. (1949). Sickness in the population of England and Wales in 1944–47. *Studies on Medical and Population Subjects*, No. 2. London: H.M.S.O.
14. Dominion Bureau of Statistics (1963). *Vital Statistics* 1963, Table D8. Ottawa: Queen's Printer.
15. Le Riche, W. H., Bond, C. A., Stiver, W. G., and Csima, A. (1965). *A Linkage of Data on Physicians' Services and Hospital Separations for 1960 in Ontario*. Special Report No. 2. Appendix 2. Toronto: Physicians' Services Incorporated.

16. Le Riche, W. H., Bond., C. A., and Stiver, W. B. (1965). *A Study of a Comprehensive Non-profit Prepaid Medical Care Plan in Ontario*, 1963. Special Report No. 3. Appendix 3. Toronto: Physicians' Services Incorporated.

17. World Health Organization (1957). *Manual of the International Statistical Classification of Diseases, Injuries and Causes of Death*. Based on the recommendations of the Seventh Revision Conference, 1955, and Adopted by the Ninth World Health Assembly under WHO Nomenclature Regulations. 2 vols. Geneva: WHO.

18. United Nations (Statistical Office) (1965). *Statistical Yearbook*, 1964. New York: United Nations.

19. Editorial (1966). Around the world with WHO—cholera. *Medical Services Journal, Canada*, **22**, 290.

20. Department of National Health and Welfare (1966). Plague. *Epidemiological Bulletin*, **10**, 65. Ottawa: Department of National Health and Welfare.

21. *Time* magazine (1966). Medicine. A plague on both houses. *Time*, **88** (10).

22. World Health Organization (1966). *Health Conditions in the Americas*, 1961–1964. Scientific Publication No. 138. Washington: Pan American Health Organization (Pan Am. San. Bur.)—WHO.

23. World Health Organization (1966). Nineteenth World Health Assembly—2. *Chronicle of the World Health Organisation* **20**, 275–282. Geneva: WHO.

24. Hinman, F. H. (1966). *World Eradication of Infectious Diseases*. Springfield, Ill.: Charles C. Thomas.

25. Soper, F. A. (1963). The elimination of urban yellow fever in the Americas through the eradication of *Aedes aegypti*. *American Journal of Public Health*, **53**, 7–16.

26. United States Department of Health, Education, and Welfare. Public Health Service (1961). *Republic of the Congo (Formerly the Belgian Congo). A Study of Health Problems and Resources*. Washington, D.C.: United States Department of Health, Education, and Welfare. P. H. S. Publication No. 806.

27. World Health Organization (1961). *International Sanitary Regulations*, 2nd annotated edn. Geneva: WHO.

28. National Academy of Sciences—National Research Council (1962). *Tropical Health— A Report on a Study of Needs and Resources*. Washington, D.C.: NAS–NRC, Publication No. 996.

29. Sparrow, H. (1962). The relapsing fevers. In *Tropical Health—A Report on a Study of Needs and Resources*, pp. 499–500. Washington, D.C.: NAS–NRC, Publication No. 996.

30. Gregoire, F. (1960). Treatment of pneumonia. *Canadian Medical Association Journal*, **82**, 139–143.

31. Dominion Bureau of Statistics and the Department of National Health and Welfare. (1957). Illness frequency by diagnostic classification. National estimates. *Canadian Sickness Survey* 1950–51, No. 10. Ottawa: Queen's Printer.

32. Cvjetanović, B. (1963). An epidemiological approach to the study of diarrhoeal diseases. In *Epidemiology: Reports on Research and Teaching*, 1962, ed. Pemberton, J., pp. 49–59. London: Oxford University Press.

33. Dominion Bureau of Statistics (1964). *Annual Report of Notifiable Diseases*, 1964. p. 19. Ottawa: Queen's Printer.

34. Dominion Bureau of Statistics (1964). *Vital Statistics*, 1964, p. 112. Ottawa: Queen's Printer.

35. The Health Survey and Planning Committee (1962). *Report*, Aug. 1959–Oct. 1961. Vol. 1. Delhi: Ministry of Health.

36. Hollister, A. C., Beck, M. D., Gittelsohn, A. M., and Hemphill, E. C. (1955). Influence of water availability on shigella prevalence in children of farm labor families. *American Journal of Public Health*, **45**, 354–362.

37. Cruickshank, R. (1963). Diarrhoeal diseases in the United Kingdom. In *Epidemiology Reports on Research and Teaching*, 1962, ed. Pemberton, J. pp. 60–73. London: Oxford University Press.

38. Watt, J., Hollister, A. C., Beck, M. D., and Hemphill, E. C. (1953). Diarrhoeal diseases in Fresno County, California. *American Journal of Public Health*, 43, 728–741.

39. Le Riche, W. H., Balcom, C. E., and van Belle, G. (1966). *The Control of Infections in Hospitals with Special Reference to a Survey in Ontario*. Toronto: University of Toronto Press.

40. Babbott, F. L., Jr., and Gordon, J. E. (1954). Modern measles. *American Journal of Medical Science*, 228, 334–361.

41. Peart, A. F. W., and Nagler, F. P. (1954). Measles in the Canadian Arctic—1952. *Canadian Journal of Public Health*, 45, 146–156.

42. Morley, D., Woodland, M., and Martin, W. J. (1963). Measles in Nigerian children. A study of the disease in West Africa and its manifestations in England and other countries during different epochs. *Journal of Hygiene*, 61, 115–134.

43. Chapin, C. V. (1925). Measles in Providence, R.I., 1858–1923. *American Journal of Hygiene*, 5, 635–655.

44. World Health Organization (1963). Measles vaccines: Report of a WHO Scientific Group. *World Health Organization Technical Report Series*, No. 263.

45. Edsall, G. (1964). New aspects of immunization against smallpox and other diseases. In *Industry and Tropical Health V*, pp. 133–141. Boston: Harvard School of Public Health.

46. Waddy, B. B. (1962). Research problems in connection with meningococcal infections. In *Tropical Health*, pp. 466–467. Washington, D.C.: NAS–NRC, Publication No. 996.

47. Senecal, J., Dupin, H., and Charpentier, P. (1957). A propos de 202 cas de méningites aiguës du nourrisson. Considérations épidémiologiques, cliniques et thérapeutiques. *Bull. méd. de l'A. O. F. Dakar*. 2, 241–247. (Also *Bulletin of Hygiene* (1958). 33, 439.)

48. Sabin, A. B. (1964). Immunization against poliomyelitis with particular reference to the tropics. In *Industry and Tropical Health V*, pp. 74–80. Boston: Harvard School of Public Health.

49. Gear, J. H. S. (1955). Poliomyelitis in the under-developed areas of the world. In *Poliomyelitis*, pp. 31–58. Geneva: WHO Monograph Series, No. 26.

50. Chesler, E., Levin, S., Du Plessis, L., Freiman, I., Rogers, M., and Joffe, N. (1966). The pattern of rheumatic heart disease in the urbanized Bantu of Johannesburg. *South African Medical Journal*, 40, 899–904.

51. Pai, D. N. (1964). Tetanus mortality in India. *Journal of the Indian Medical Association*, 42, 239–241.

52. Learmonth, A. T. A. (1965). *Health in the Indian Sub-Continent 1955–64. A Geographic Review of Some Medical Literature*. Canberra, Australia: Dept. of Geography, A.N.U. School of General Studies, Occasional Papers No. 2.

53. Horwitz, O., and Palmer, C. E. (1964). Epidemiological basis of tuberculosis eradication. 2: Dynamics of tuberculosis morbidity and mortality. *Bulletin of the World Health Organization*, 30, 609–621.

54. World Health Organization (1965). WHO Activities in Tuberculosis, 1949–1964. Pts. 1–2. *Chronicle of the World Health Organization*, 19, 309–325; 365–374.

55. Nyboe, J. (1960). The efficacy of the tuberculin test: an analysis based on results from 33 countries. *Bulletin of the World Health Organization*, 22, 5–37.

56. Frimodt-Møller, J. (1962). The tuberculosis situation in India today. *Tubercle* 43, 88–94.

57. Simeonov, L. A. (1962). The results of two mass radiography surveys in a small urban population in Yugoslavia. *Tubercle*, 43, 386–391.

58. Cochrane, A. L., Cox, J. G., and Jarman, T. F. (1955). A "follow-up" chest X-ray survey in the Rhondda Fach. *British Medical Journal*, **1**, 371–378.
59. Grzybowski, S., and Allen, E. A. (1964). The challenge of tuberculosis in decline. *American Review of Respiratory Disease*, **90**, 707–720.
60. Koch, A. B. P. W. (1960). Tuberculosis in Ghana. *Tubercle*, **41**, 282–289.
61. Schechter, M. (1954). Mass X-ray survey. Bechuanaland Protectorate. *South African Medical Journal*, **28**, 351–356.
62. Wiles, F. J., and Rabie, C. J. (1955). Tuberculin and X-ray surveys in the Transkei. *South African Medical Journal*, **29**, 866–888.
63. Dubovsky, H. (1955). A mass miniature X-ray and tuberculin survey in Orange Free State and Northern Cape. *South African Medical Journal*, **29**, 992–997.
64. Maegraith, B. (1965). *Exotic Diseases in Practice*. London: William Heinemann Medical Books, Ltd.
65. Manson-Bahr, P. H. (1966). *Manson's Tropical Diseases: a manual of the diseases of warm climates*, 16th edn. London: Baillière, Tindall & Cassell.
66. Pampana, E. J. and Russell, P. F. (1955). Malaria—a world problem. *Chronicle of the World Health Organization*, **9**, 31–100.
67. World Health Organization (1966). Malaria eradication in 1965. *Chronicle of the World Health Organization*, **20**, 286–300.
68. Soper, F. H., and Wilson, D. B. (1943). *Anopheles gambiae in Brazil, 1930–1940*. New York: Rockefeller Foundation.
69. Curtis, A. C. (1963). National survey of venereal disease treatment. *Journal of the American Medical Association*, **186**, 46–49.
70. Guthe, T. (1964). Measure of treponematosis problem in the world. In *Proceedings of World Forum on Syphilis and Other Treponematoses*, Sept. 4–8, 1962. Atlanta, Ga.: Communicable Disease Center.
71. Amies, C. R. (1967). Development of resistance of gonococci to penicillin: an eight-year study. *Canadian Medical Association Journal*, **96**, 33–35.
72. Communicable Disease Center, Venereal Disease Branch (1963). *Proofs about Syphilis in the United States*. Atlanta, Ga.: U.S. Dept. of Health, Education, and Welfare.
73. National Center for Health Statistics (1965). Findings in the serologic test for syphilis in adults: United States: 1960–1962. Vital and Health Statistics, Series 11, No. 9. Washington, D.C.: U.S. Dept. of Health, Education, and Welfare.
74. Murray, J. F., Merriweather, A. M., and Freedman, M. L. (1956). Endemic syphilis in the Bakwena Reserve of the Bechuanaland Protectorate. A report on mass examination and treatment. *Bulletin of the World Health Organization*, **15**, 975–1039.
75. World Health Organization (1964, 1965). *International Work in Endemic Treponematoses and Venereal Infections*, 1948–1963. 1. Endemic treponematoses of childhood; 2. Venereal syphilis; 3. Gonococcal infections. *Chronicle of the World Health Organization*, **18**, 403–417; 451–462; **19**, 7–18.
76. Bechelli, L. M., and Martínez Dominguez, V. (1966). The leprosy problem in the world. *Bulletin of the World Health Organization*, **34**, 811–826.
77. Newell, K. W. (1966). An epidemiologist's view of leprosy. *Bulletin of the World Health Organization*, **34**, 827–857.
78. Stoll, N. (1947). This wormy world. *Journal of Parasitology*, **33**, 1–18.
79. World Health Organization (1959). International work in bilharziasis, 1948–1958. *Chronicle of the World Health Organization*, **1**, 1–56.
80. Expert Committee on Trachoma (1962). Third report. *World Health Organization Technical Report Series*, No. 234. Geneva: WHO.
81. Scientific Group on Trachoma (1966). Fourth research report. *World Health Organization Technical Report Series*, No. 330. Geneva: WHO.

82. Thygeson, P. (1958). *Trachoma Manual and Atlas.* Washington, D.C.: U.S. Dept. of Health, Education, and Welfare, Public Health Service, Division of Indian Health.
83. Sowa, S., Sowa, J., Collier, L. H. and Blyth, W. (1965). Trachoma and allied infections in a Gambian village. *Special Report Series Medical Research Council*, No. 308, London: H.M.S.O.
84. Joint FAO/WHO Expert Committee on Brucellosis. (1964). Fourth report. *World Health Organization Technical Report Series*, No. 289. Geneva: WHO.
85. Viswanathan, R. (1957). Epidemiology. *Indian Journal of Medical Research*, **45**, (supplementary no.: Infectious Hepatitis in Delhi, 1955–56; a critical study), 1–29.
86. WHO Expert Committee on Hepatitis (1964). Second report. *World Health Organization Technical Report Series*, No. 285. Geneva: WHO.
87. Stoller, A., and Collman, R. D. (1965). Incidence of infective hepatitis followed by Down's syndrome nine months later. *Lancet*, **2**, 1221–1223.
88. Kark, S. L., and le Riche, W. H. (1944). Study on nutrition and health of Bantu school children. *Manpower*, **3**, 1–141.
89. Ardrey, R. (1963). *African Genesis. A personal investigation into the animal origins and nature of man.* New York: Dell Publishing Co.

2

CARE OF MOTHER AND CHILD

Ihsan Dogramaci
Hacettepe Medical Centre,
Ankara, Turkey

I n the days before scientific medicine, and to some extent even today, health and welfare were felt to be "in the hands of the gods". One became ill and died if the gods were angry, and the only recourse was to placate them with prayers, incantations and gifts. Preventive and protective activities varied from time to time and from people to people, but always, of course, remained within the limits of man's knowledge and ability.

We know that, throughout history, man has not hesitated to endanger his own life to save his child's. Fossil bones have been uncovered showing an adult holding a child above his head, seemingly in an attempt to preserve its life, if only for a second longer, from rising flood waters. In certain areas of Africa today, extremely undernourished mothers will continue to breast-feed their babies for several years, at the cost of their own health and lives, to give the baby the food they think is necessary.

TWO-THIRDS OF THE PEOPLE

In a developed country like the United Kingdom, where the average life-span is about 70 years, children under 14 constitute 20 per cent of the population. But in less developed countries where the average life expectancy is 35 years, children under 14 constitute some 50 per cent of the population. If the other 50 per cent is composed of adult men and women in roughly equal proportions, it is evident that mothers and children may constitute more than two-thirds of the total population in these countries. Because such a large percentage of humanity is involved, every country must plan to fulfil the basic needs of its mothers and children. The quality and intensity of effort directed to the solution of this problem cannot fail to affect the future of the whole world.

Children are, after all, the future of the nation. This is not a nationalistic or a sentimental statement. Today's children are the statesmen, planners, administrators, industrial and commercial leaders, professional workers, and investigators who will plan and direct the social, cultural and economic affairs of the future world.

Thus, concern for protection of mother and child is, and must be, universal. The fact that everyone wants to do "something" for mothers and children does not mean that achievements everywhere are satisfactory or comparable. Two-thirds of the world's people, including more than three-quarters of all of the children in the world, live in countries that have not yet reached a socioeconomic level of development sufficient to ensure to mothers and children even minimum care. In the less developed countries, and especially in their rural areas, where centuries of tradition, poverty and disease have gone hand in hand, medical services remain rudimentary. A constant supply of safe drinking water is often lacking. Diets generally provide less than the minimum allowance of foods necessary for maintaining health. For under-privileged people living in the large cities and in the peri-urban shanty towns, health conditions may be even worse, because intense overcrowding facilitates the spread of infectious diseases. Where such conditions prevail, children are the principal sufferers because they are the most vulnerable.

The concept of maternal and child health has become broader in our day. Both preventive and curative obstetrics and paediatrics are now considered to be well within the purview of maternal and child health. The concept also includes nutrition, mental health, health education, training of personnel, education of the public and research. Maternal and child health programmes must be adapted to the needs and resources of the community they serve. They must be conceived in terms of the specific needs and limitations of the local cultures. They must undertake to supervise the well-being of mothers and of children through adolescence. They must foster parental responsibility and ensure education and opportunity to the maximum potential of the particular community.

MATERNAL HEALTH

Maternal mortality in some of the less developed countries that do furnish statistics is ten times as high as it is in the economically advanced countries. For other areas of our world where vital statistics are not available, maternal mortality is suspected to be even higher.

Maternity care services in countries which have greatly reduced their maternal mortality are increasingly emphasizing perinatal mortality, problems related to pregnancy, and the importance of preconceptional defects and the emotional disturbances of pregnancy. On the other hand, the less developed countries, where maternal mortality is still high, might well define different aims corresponding to their more limited resources. They might start by providing, for as many women as possible, some form of prenatal supervision including treatment of infections and diseases, correction of anaemia and inadequate nutrition, and education in mother-craft. Faced with the obvious necessity to establish priorities, they will have to institute a system of screening procedures which will determine those pregnancies most likely to result in complications requiring service and attention beyond routine care. They will have to focus on the training of existing indigenous birth attendants until enough professional midwives are available. They will have to provide facilities and personnel capable of handling complicated and emergency deliveries.

CHILD HEALTH AND INFANT MORTALITY

In developing countries, undernutrition and malnutrition affect half of the population and more than half of the children. The highest mortality rates prevail among the youngest groups of children: about one-third of them die before they reach the age of five. The infant mortality rate is regarded as a sensitive index of the status of child health in a community. Available data indicate that infant mortality is as high as 400 per 1,000 in some African and Asian communities. In the advanced countries, infant mortality rates range from about fifteen deaths per 1,000 live births during the first year at best, to 50 at worst.

In the past 50 years, there has been a decrease in infant mortality in all countries in varying degrees. This we see clearly in Table I. The relatively low infant mortality rates of highly developed countries should not blind us to the fact that in these countries there are still children who do not benefit from the affluence of their society. As recently as 1953, the infant mortality rate in the United Kingdom was 27 per 1,000 live births, but the risk of death to a labourer's child under one year of age was about twice as great as the risk to a professional person's child. Unfortunately, reliable and comparable statistical data are not always available in developing countries. It may, therefore, be reasonably assumed that the actual rate is higher than the official figures.

Deaths before one year of age are usually subdivided into the neonatal period (under 28 days) and post-neonatal period (28 days to one year).

Table I

DECREASE IN INFANT MORTALITY RATES PER 1,000 LIVE BIRTHS FOR
SELECTED COUNTRIES AND PERIODS OF TIME[1,2]

	1921–1925	1951–1955	1962	% Decrease
Norway	52	23	18	65·4
USA	74	28	25	66·2
UK (England & Wales)	76	27	22	71·1
Denmark	82	27	20	75·6
Finland	96	32	21	78·1
Canada	99	35	28	71·7
Belgium	106	44	28	73·6
Italy	127	58	42	66·9
El Salvador	135	81	71	47·4
Austria	138	51	33	76·1
Japan	159	48	26	83·6
Ceylon	190	75	53	72·1
Chile	239	132	121	49·4

Neonatal deaths are those believed to be mainly due to prenatal and natal factors, while post-neonatal deaths are believed to be largely due to various environmental factors. In those countries where the infant mortality rate has dropped to 20 or less per 1,000 live births, the period in which these relatively few deaths occur is gradually being narrowed down to early neonatal. The major obstacle encountered by these countries is the slow and difficult search for the causes of death during this period. These countries are fortunate in having both the facilities and the will to carry out the necessary research.

In the less fortunate areas of the world, however, where infant mortality rates are still high, the pattern of infant mortality is quite different. That neonatal mortality rates are much higher than in the developed countries is hardly surprising. Intrauterine development often occurs in a permanently undernourished mother, whose exposure to numerous infections and infestations has weakened her general health, and whose culture may impose further limitations of diet and activity.

On the other hand, there is a dramatic difference among post-neonatal mortality rates in the developed and developing countries and the difference is found to be closely related to socioeconomic levels, to the extent of control of environment, and to existing health services. The causes of post-neonatal mortality which were once potent in the developed countries still prevail in the developing ones. In addition to those causes of death, the special hazards of a tropical or subtropical climate further affect the mortality rate. Incomplete as they are, the available data indicate that infections and parasitic diseases are important causes of death in the post-neonatal period.

PRE-SCHOOL AND SCHOOL CHILDREN

In countries where high health standards have been achieved, mortality among toddlers and the pre-school group has declined radically and now runs to about 1 per 1,000 per year or less. On the other hand, in the less developed countries, mortality in this age group may be as much as 40 times greater as a result of exposure to common childhood diseases, parasitic infestations and infections. Children in developing areas may succumb to any one of these illnesses easily because they are under-nourished or malnourished at a stage when their nutritional needs are at a high level in order to sustain rapid growth. Furthermore, they are exposed to these hazards while still largely dependent upon their parents for protection and care. The parents themselves, however, may be ill-prepared to provide this care because of poverty, overwork, lack of knowledge of the child's needs, and child-rearing practices peculiar to the culture.

Malnutrition, particularly protein-calorie malnutrition, affects an estimated 70 per cent of the pre-school-age children in developing regions of the world today, impairing their growth and development, sometimes irreversibly. The problems of providing proper nutrition for these children alone is enormous, and they become greater in proportion to the increased growth rate of the population, internal migration, and industrial development.

Another major handicap of the school-age children is the lack of educational facilities. Of those children who do manage to survive the early years, only half receive an elementary education, and a much smaller proportion go on to have more advanced schooling, with the training and guidance they need in order to participate effectively in the rapidly changing world they will eventually inherit. For many different reasons—lack of facilities, lack of teachers, lack of motivation, lack of economic means— the great reservoir of potential trainees is reduced to a tiny pool. Because there is often no school to attend, or because of the pressure of economic conditions, children may join the labour force at the age of 12 years or less. Life expectancy, as well as what one expects from life, depends not only on what happens to the individual as an adult, but also on the nurture he had as a child.

OBSTACLES TO PROGRESS

Since considerable progress has been made in lowering the high morbidity and mortality among mothers and children in the developed countries, some progress should be possible in the developing countries.

Yet this is not as easily done as said. There are many limiting factors in developing countries and to eliminate them all sound planning, time, hard work and patience are essential.

Economic conditions are a major obstacle. Despite the fact that as much as two-thirds of the labour force in developing countries may be engaged in agriculture, the population is inadequately fed because agricultural productivity is extremely low. For example, in Asia it is estimated that more than 100 man-days of labour are required to bring an acre of ground to harvest as opposed to two man-days of labour in the United States. The combined income of the developing countries, excluding mainland China, is of the order of US $175,000 million. It is increasing by $5,000 to $10,000 million a year. The average weekly income per head in these countries is about $2. The combined national income of the developed countries, on the other hand, is of the order of $1,000,000 million and is growing each year by $40,000 to $50,000 million. The developed countries annually spend the equivalent of more than two-thirds of the total income of the developing countries on armaments alone.

The population of the developing countries is generally increasing by two to three per cent per year. If the rate of natural increase of a country is, let us say, 2·5 per cent per year, then 10 per cent of the nation's income must be reinvested each year just to maintain the *status quo*. Any limitation of the number of children born depends on the decisions of hundreds of millions of families.

In the developing countries there is usually an acute shortage of trained people, including doctors, other health personnel, supervisors, teachers and technicians.

One very rough indication of the extent of health services in a given area is the number of inhabitants per physician (Table II). The situation in rural areas is much worse than even these figures suggest. It is not only the supply of physicians that must be considered, but the supply of other health workers, as well as the organization and quality of services available. It is clear that in most of these countries, decades will be required to extend even

Table II

INHABITANTS PER PHYSICIAN IN SELECTED COUNTRIES[3]

USSR	310	India	2,400
United States	780	Burma	15,000
Canada	900	Ghana	21,000
Japan	930	Nigeria	32,000
Brazil	2,100	Niger	103,000

rudimentary services throughout the rural areas and the fringe areas surrounding the rapidly growing cities.

I must also refer here to the indispensable role of community leaders such as midwives, doctors, teachers and administrators in improving local health conditions.

Elaborate means are not necessarily essential to significant results. The achievements of one dedicated man can be monumental. For example, Dr. David Morley's work in Nigeria can be cited. In a village with the simplest possible facilities and equipment he has, in five years, reduced the infant mortality rate from nearly 300 to 77 per 1,000, and in the age group 1–4 years from nearly 70 to 31.

ORGANIZATION OF HEALTH SERVICES FOR CHILDREN AND MOTHERS

The World Health Organization recommends that health services for children should be developed as an integral part of a nation's or community's general health services. The needs of mother and child must be provided for and supervised by some kind of central organization responsible for maternal and child health. In practice, owing to insufficient financial resources and shortages of doctors and nurses, it is occasionally more feasible to develop certain branches of health services before others. These services might include national action programmes against specific diseases that can be carried out by auxiliary personnel using relatively simple techniques. Midwife services are usually developed before the broader health services because of the possibility of using midwives to deliver babies in the home and of training indigenous birth attendants to deal with normal births. Furthermore, it is sometimes feasible to develop maternal and child health services in selected areas. These services have indeed proved to be one of the best ways of arousing the interest of a rural population in better health care and of convincing them they should provide facilities and voluntary support. Any or all of these services may be used to prepare the way for permanent health services to meet the needs of the entire population.

Most countries have plans to combine preventive and curative services and to extend these into rural areas. This means strengthening the infrastructure and establishing a network of health centres and subcentres.

Of all the needs of the developing areas, that for personnel is the most pressing. Outside assistance is particularly useful in meeting this need. The training of nurses and midwives, at both the fully qualified and auxiliary levels, also needs to be reoriented in many countries. All too often their

57

present training remains under the influence of Western nursing patterns, sometimes those already discarded by the West. Modern curricula in the developing countries today need more emphasis on public health, maternal and child health and on paediatrics, including growth and development and nutrition.

CONCLUSION

I have tried to contrast the conditions of maternal and child health in the developing countries with those in developed countries. It may have seemed that I was describing two different worlds, so diverse are the conditions. The uneven distribution of "the good things in life" is not new but it has become more striking in our time. The increasing speed and ease of travel and communications have made the world irrevocably a "neighbourhood", and with this comes the responsibility of neighbourliness. Part of that responsibility, for those of us who have the knowledge and the means, is to make available to everyone the best that our "neighbourhood" has to offer.

SUMMARY

Significant differences in the quality and extent of maternal and child care exist between the developing and the developed countries. Because the level of general health and medical services is closely related to other socioeconomic conditions, any attempt to raise it must be integrally related to the country's overall development plans. Furthermore, specific programmes of improvement must be formulated in the light of the country's traditions and culture.

The major obstacle to advances in maternal and child care in the developing countries is lack of trained personnel. Other problems are related to environmental factors, such as endemic disease and parasitic infestation, poor nutrition, low level of economic development, lack of elementary educational facilities and an exploding population.

DISCUSSION

Fanconi : At the Children's Hospital in Dakar the mothers are instructed for a few days on how to treat and feed their children. When these mothers go home to the country they spread their knowledge around to the rest of

58

the population. This is one of the reasons why child mortality is going down rapidly even in underdeveloped countries.

le Riche: Some years ago in Zululand we were able to reduce infant mortality and total mortality markedly when health centres were set up. The mistake we made was that we didn't aim at a total development of the area. In other words we produced a food deficit in that community within about five years. So when we think of reducing mortality we must at the same time think of the extra food and the extra economic development needed by that community. In the past many people only looked at the one end, but one has to take a total view of human welfare.

Lindop: The increasing number of children surviving to old age may eventually be an added burden to the community, and this must be considered now. The problem has two sides to it: in the developed countries we know that we are not likely to increase the lifespan much at the moment, but we also know that we have made very little progress in improving health in old age. In other words, if we extend the lifespan we may only be extending the non-productive period. But if we extend the lifespan in developing countries, which is much more possible, then unless we look now at the type of diseases and problems which might develop during this period of extended lifespan, we may make the same mistake of creating a very large proportion of the population who are not productive. When we increase the labour force by improving child health we must also think of how to increase productivity in old age.

Candau: The whole problem is one of manpower and the use of manpower. If the necessary health manpower exists in a developed country and if it can be properly utilized, old age presents only the normal problem of what to do, of how to fill up the time of the aged. If we are talking about increasing manpower which we cannot utilize, I think the problem is indeed going to be extremely serious at the other end of the line.

Pincus: That problem is of course raised every time anything to do with the control of population is discussed. The problem of population is straightforward: either you increase the mortality rate or you decrease the birth rate. Who will advocate increasing the mortality rate? When we talk about child health in a population practising fertility control, we really mean the health of a limited number of children.

Dogramaci: If we are afraid of overpopulation why *should* we make so much effort to save the babies and children? This question used to be asked sometimes in my country by the officials of the Ministry of Finance when we wanted some money! Leaving aside the humanitarian aspects, one reason is that if the children are left without care it is not necessarily true that the fittest survive and the others disappear. What happens is that many children remain crippled mentally and physically, and thus burden the country because they are not productive. Secondly, the burden on mothers during pregnancy and on health services which have to take care of diseased children is very great.

Lambo: Childhood morbidity in fact is the basis for the quality of the manpower to which Dr. Candau referred. Seventy per cent of the children who reach us for any form of psychiatric help have sustained irreversible brain damage through acute infections or even malnutrition.

Kaprio: Dr. Dogramaci's examples about what can be done were related to a situation where an enthusiastic and knowledgeable person is working permanently in a community. I would like to link that with the population problem. One of the great problems at this moment is making people feel secure with their families and in their surroundings. One priority is to convince ministers of finance that families need good health services for their children so that they can be convinced it is worth having a small family. This includes making people believe that such a change is actually taking place.

Many of us believe that investment in the child health services should be undertaken both for humanitarian reasons and also because there should be equality for future generations. If children below a certain nutritional status have their potential mental capacities permanently damaged, then things we neglect now may cause a repetition of the same problems in later generations.

Banks: In 1867 maternal mortality in England was about 6 per thousand, working out at 3,600 maternal deaths a year. Infant mortality was about 155 per thousand live births. The birth rate was 35 per thousand in the south, going up to 41 in the mining villages of the north. The death rate was about 22 per thousand. The emigration rate was interesting: some 500 people a day were leaving these islands and they were assisted to emigrate by their relatives overseas to the extent of half a million pounds a year! The picture was therefore as black as one could paint for any country. It didn't improve very fast, either, because in 1904 in the London borough in which I was born, the Mayor's fund to provide breakfast for starving children was in a flourishing condition, and the infant mortality rate was still 155 per thousand live births. Nearly all the advances have come within the last 60 years.

Querido: But you are talking about a country which had already experienced the industrial revolution, which is a completely different situation from that in the developing countries now. The actual benefits, as shown by statistics, didn't begin to become obvious until after 1900 in England, but the country then had its industrial revolution behind it. Furthermore it was a country with Christian ethics, that is, with a basis for trying to achieve something for all people on an equal basis. Those two factors— industrial revolution and equality for all—are lacking now in some countries. In that context their situation is far more serious than the situation in England in 1900.

Banks: I agree. I just wanted to make the point that improvements do take time and that we should keep the situation in perspective.

de Haas: In the so-called developed countries the lowering of infant mortality certainly progressed rather slowly, but if somebody in 1900 had been given large sums to reduce infant mortality, which at that time was as high as 20 per cent, down to 2 or even 5 per cent, it would have been practically impossible to reach this goal for the whole population. The difference with the developing countries now is that we know exactly how to reduce infant mortality, even under difficult and economically weak conditions. If we want to do it, we can do it and we can even do it in a short time. In Indonesia before the war, we were able to reduce infant mortality in the poor children of our welfare centres from 20 to 5 per cent in a few years.

It is even less difficult to reduce maternal mortality. At the beginning of this century maternal mortality was still high in industrialized countries, but it has now been reduced to two or three per 10,000 births, while in countries where there is virtually no obstetrical care it may even now be as high as 2 per cent. One of the most shocking medical experiences I can remember is a woman dying in childbirth without any obstetrical aid in primitive conditions. It must be our duty to reduce drastically both maternal mortality and infant mortality in developing countries. Experience has taught us how to do this, but we are still not putting this experience into practice in the underprivileged part of the world.

REFERENCES

1. World Health Organization. (1960). *Epidemiological and Vital Statistics Report*, **13**, 54. Geneva: WHO.
2. World Health Organization. (1964). *Epidemiological and Vital Statistics Report*, **17**, 545–549. Geneva: WHO.
3. World Health Organization. (1962). *Annual Epidemiological and Vital Statistics*, 1959, **15**, 651–660. Geneva: WHO.

GENERAL READING

Williams, C. D. (1964). Maternal and child health services in developing countries. *Lancet*, **1**, 345–348.

REFERENCES

Committee Report. (1964). How is a nation's health level measured? *Journal of the American Medical Association*, **189**, 321–323.
Winnicka, W. (1965). *The Major Health Problems of Children in Developing Countries*. Third Jessie M. Bierman Annual Lecture in Maternal and Child Health. Delivered 19th March, 1965, at School of Public Health, University of California, Berkeley.
Keeny, S. M. (1957). *Half of the World's Children: a Diary of UNICEF at Work in Asia*. New York: Association Press.
World Health Organization. (1959). *First Report on the World Health Situation, 1954–1956*. Geneva: WHO, No. 94.
World Health Organization. (1963). *Second Report on the World Health Situation, 1957–1960*. Geneva: WHO, No. 122.
United Nations International Children's Emergency Fund. (1964). *Children of the Developing Countries: a Report*. London: Nelson.
Hyde, H. van Z. (ed.) (1966). Manpower for the world's health. *Journal of Medical Education*, **41**, no. 9 (part 2).
United Nations Children's Fund. (1966). *Children and Youth in National Planning and Development in Asia*. Report of a conference held in Bangkok, Thailand, March, 1966. New York: United Nations Children's Fund.

3

ANIMAL HEALTH AND ITS IMPLICATIONS
FOR MAN

W. I. B. BEVERIDGE

Department of Animal Pathology, University of Cambridge

A NIMAL health affects man in three ways: (1) disease in livestock depresses production and thus aggravates the shortage of human food, especially animal protein; (2) some diseases of animals are transmissible to man; and (3) study of disease in animals produces knowledge with applications in medicine.

The first point I shall discuss only very briefly because it is an aspect of the general problem of world food supply, which will be covered here by Sir Norman Wright.

The simplest way of assessing the magnitude of the animal disease problem and of seeing it in perspective is to reduce it to economic terms. The Food and Agriculture Organization has collected data from a number of countries on the annual value of animal products and the estimated losses caused by disease. In the USA, Britain and France the losses were estimated at US $3,500 million or 15 per cent of production. In less developed countries the percentage losses were higher, frequently over 30, thus the effect was greatest in regions where food is short[1]. Some of the loss was due to animals dying but the greater part was due to the depressing effect of disease. An animal burdened with parasites or suffering from an infection or malnutrition may survive but produce only a fraction of what it could if healthy.

There are a number of diseases which decimate herds and flocks and play havoc with production unless they are kept in check by appropriate means. For example, foot-and-mouth disease in Europe in 1952 is estimated to have caused a loss of £200 million. Provided that funds and skilled manpower are available, it is generally easier to combat diseases in domestic animals than in man, because the movement and lives of animals are more subject to control than those of men. Quarantine measures can be effectively employed to confine many livestock diseases, vaccination programmes can be enforced and, when the occasion demands, infected animals can be killed and destroyed. By such methods, coupled with specific diagnostic techniques, some of the worst bacterial and viral diseases have been completely eradicated from the more advanced countries and others are kept in check. Eradication, total and permanent, is entirely feasible with certain diseases on a regional basis, and there is no scientific reason why it should not be extended over the globe. Glanders, rinderpest, contagious bovine pleuropneumonia and sheep pox were once firmly entrenched in the British Isles but were eradicated many years ago. Apparently we have already the first example of a disease having been banished from the world: vesicular exanthema of swine appeared as a new disease in California in 1932 and spread throughout the USA, but it was stamped out in 1955.

Although in the western world the more serious epizootic diseases have been successfully combated there are many insidious diseases which continue to depress production without killing the animals. As an example of their significance, mastitis in cows in the USA is estimated to have caused an annual loss of £70 million worth of milk and meat in the decade 1942–1951. Crowd diseases flourish under modern methods of intensive husbandry, just as in man after industrialization. There are several endemic respiratory and intestinal infections which are of little or no importance under traditional farming conditions but which become epidemic diseases with serious economic consequences when large numbers of young animals are gathered together from different farms and crowded into enclosed spaces. Chronic respiratory infections due to mycoplasma have been estimated to cause in Britain an annual loss of £10 million in chickens and a similar figure in pigs. Before intensive methods of husbandry were introduced these diseases were unknown.

Although there is an enormous gap between what is possible even with our present knowledge and what is in fact practised throughout the world today, the gap is gradually narrowing. FAO is making an important contribution by helping developing nations to improve their means of coping with livestock diseases, both by applying known techniques and by promoting research on their special problems. However, to my mind, it is the problems which we are encountering in developed countries which have the most interesting implications for a future in which animal production will be of an ever more concentrated nature. The problems involved in combating these diseases have much in common with some modern problems in medicine and there may even be analogous psychological problems created by living in a crowded world, as is shown by an experiment which I shall refer to later. The time for an all-out investigation of these problems is now, because, apart from the comparative value of such work, the toll of disease will otherwise rise alongside the technological advances in farming.

The second point at which animal health impinges on human health is through the transmission of disease from animals to man. There are over 100 zoonoses, as these diseases are called. Many affect man only occasionally but about a dozen are prevalent and serious enough to constitute significant public health problems in many countries. I shall discuss briefly the changes that have occurred in recent years in some of the worst of these diseases.

The most widespread zoonosis is *salmonella food poisoning*. This disease has been on the increase in nearly all western countries and four reasons have been advanced for this deterioration in the situation. Firstly, international trade in human foods and animal feedstuffs has increased. Secondly, there is a higher incidence of salmonella in farm animals, partly due to the importation of feedstuffs mentioned and partly due to modern intensive farming, and hence more carriers in the animals being slaughtered with more contamination of meat. Thirdly, the widespread use of household detergents has interfered with effective processing of sewerage, and effluents now commonly contain salmonella. Fourthly, the industrial centralization of food processing and manufacture accompanied by wide distribution of half-preserved or frozen "prepared" foods has extended the possible range of outbreaks of food-borne disease. Instead of incidents being confined to households, institutions or parties, we now sometimes see cases from one source scattered over a wide area, with numbers occasionally assuming serious epidemic proportions.

The industrial trends which have been largely responsible for the greater frequency of salmonellosis in animals and in man fortunately have certain advantages from the point of view of application of control measures such as bacteriological surveillance. Also vaccines have recently been developed which are giving encouraging results in calves and pigs. Vigorous action on the part of multidisciplinary teams could check salmonellosis and there are encouraging signs that the position may be improving in the United Kingdom, where the number of incidents reported is declining.

Another aspect of salmonellosis that has attracted attention lately is that these organisms may acquire multiple resistance to antibiotics and sulphonamides from contact with other species of bacteria which are resistant.

Two antibiotics—penicillin and tetracycline—are commonly added to the feed of pigs and poultry, and this practice leads to the wholesale development of strains of *Escherichia coli* which are resistant to a wide range of antibacterial drugs. These strains of *E. coli*, themselves harmless, may pass on their resistance to salmonella strains by transferring episomes during conjugation. The discovery of this surprising phenomenon of infectious, multiple resistance poses new problems in animal health and human health, the implications of which have not yet been fully explored.

Bovine tuberculosis at one time was responsible for about 20 per cent of human cases of tuberculosis. National campaigns for the eradication of the bovine disease by tuberculin test and slaughter have been put into effect during the last 50 years in USA, Canada, Britain, the Netherlands, the Scandinavian countries, Switzerland, Portugal, Austria, Germany and Japan. In these countries the percentage of animals reacting to the tuberculin test has been reduced to a fraction of 1 per cent. The complete eradication of this insidious disease from a region has proved very difficult. Several other countries have embarked on a similar programme but there are still many developing countries where the disease is prevalent, to the detriment of both animal and human health. For these latter countries control of tuberculosis has been rather less urgent than some other animal diseases and it is much more expensive in terms of skilled manpower and animals than, say, mass immunization against cattle plague.

Brucellosis is a world-wide disease. In 1947 it was estimated that possibly as many as 100,000 persons were infected in the Americas. In recent years brucellosis due to *Brucella abortus* has been virtually eradicated from some countries by test and slaughter of infected cattle. In Britain, however, the infection is still widespread and recent reports have shown that the chronic form of this unpleasant disease is not uncommon here in veterinary surgeons and farmers. *Brucella melitensis* continues to be a major problem in man and animals in several countries in the Mediterranean and Middle East and in Mongolia. There are now good prospects of controlling this disease by vaccinating sheep and goats, but the practical problems are still formidable as there are some 350 million goats in the world, about a third of which are believed to be infected and most of which are in underdeveloped countries and kept under primitive conditions. Extensive trials have been conducted in Russia on the immunization of people in high-risk occupations against *Brucella* but this does not appear to be a satisfactory solution to the problem because the live vaccine used is not entirely innocuous.

Leptospirosis has a global distribution and affects a very large range of domestic and wild animals, which form a vast reservoir making eradication out of the question. Progress has been made in epidemiological studies but the prevention of this disease is still difficult. Vaccines give some protection but the main precautions continue to be keeping down the rodent population and providing protective clothing for people whose occupation exposes them to infected environments.

Rabies has been on the increase over the last few years in several separate epidemiological foci. The greater incidence is mainly due to an increase in the population of wild carnivorous animals which constitute the reservoir. In some areas the explanation is a curious one: fashions have changed and fox furs are no longer in favour, hence the foxes have multiplied. The number of people treated annually against rabies after being bitten is estimated at about half a million, although the fatal cases reported are numbered in the hundreds.

The common tapeworm *Taenia saginata* with the cystic stage in cattle is said to have greatly increased in both developed and developing countries. Reasons for the increase are thought to be the growing popularity of camping with consequent contamination of pastures with human faeces, an increase in the consumption of meat, often not well cooked, and the adverse effects of detergents on sewerage processing.

Encephalitides and fevers due to various arboviruses are increasingly recognized as of public health importance as more investigations are undertaken, especially in tropical and subtropical regions. The reservoir hosts are usually wild animals and birds and prevention depends mainly on vaccines, which fortunately are effective against most of these diseases.

Outbreaks of pneumonia due to *ornithosis* have occurred in a number of poultry-packing plants since the mass production of turkeys began. The same persons may be affected two or three years in succession as there is practically no immunity to this organism. Infection can be largely prevented by efficient air hygiene in the packing plant.

There is no need for me to catalogue all zoonoses. No doubt the pattern will continue to change, and not always for the better. It is even possible that new diseases may arise: a micro-organism which perhaps causes little or no disease in its natural reservoir host and escapes notice may spread to man and cause serious disease. Examples of such having already happened are yellow fever and several other arboviruses, plague and tularaemia. One suspects that the sudden emergence of vesicular exanthema of swine in 1932 in California, mentioned above, is also to be explained on this basis. Similarly, the highly lethal disease of pigs known as swine fever arose apparently *de novo* in America in 1833 and spread throughout the world. The source of the virus causing this disease has never been found. Possibly myxomatosis in rabbits provides the most striking example of how devastating a disease can be when a virus finds a new susceptible host.

Yet another possibility is that human and animal strains of microbes may hybridize and produce a strain with a new combination of characters capable of causing an epidemic. Take for example the implications of such happening with the influenza virus. There have been 28 global epidemics of influenza in the last 300 years—about one every decade on the average. Each epidemic is believed to be due to the appearance of a strain immunologically different from any that has been prevalent for at least a generation. The source of these subtypes is a matter for speculation and three possibilities are: (a) a grand mutation from a previous subtype, (b) emergence from an animal reservoir as yet unknown, or (c) hybridization between an old human and an old animal strain.

The very first influenza A virus discovered was that isolated from pigs, and during the last few years subtypes have been found in other species besides man. Of the 11 subtypes at present known, three come from man, one from pig, two from horse and five from birds (chickens, turkeys, ducks, quails and seagulls). It has been shown in the laboratory that animal strains and human strains can exchange genetical material. Some of the avian strains are extremely virulent for birds, causing practically 100 per cent mortality, and it is alarming to think that they could possibly acquire the ability to infect man by hybridizing with human strains.

Most classes of virus have representatives in both animals and man and I feel that the possibility of new hybrids arising gives a new dimension to zoonoses which we should look at seriously. More laboratory investigations are needed to show the various possibilities so that we can be forewarned.

COMPARATIVE MEDICINE

In the first two parts of my paper I have discussed the ill-effects of animal disease, but there is another side to the coin to which I shall now turn: a great deal of medical knowledge has been gained by studying diseases in animals. I think it is not generally appreciated that our present-day knowledge of infectious diseases of man is based on concepts which were largely derived from investigations of diseases of domestic animals. May I remind you of some of the historical facts?

The truth of the all-important germ theory of disease itself was first convincingly demonstrated by Pasteur and Koch, working with anthrax in sheep. The concept of artificial immunization with attenuated vaccines originated in Jenner's work with cowpox and Pasteur's experiments with fowl plague. In 1886 the possibility of immunization by injection of killed cultures was discovered in the course of investigations with swine plague by Salmon and Smith. Within the last decade researchers at the Glasgow veterinary school have found out how to produce immunity against certain worm parasites and the method is now being tried with hookworm in man.

The fact that disease agents may be transmitted by arthropods was first shown in experiments with Texas fever of cattle, and the discoveries with malaria and yellow fever followed. The first viral encephalitis to be shown to be transmitted by mosquitoes was a disease of horses.

Mycoplasma have been familiar to veterinarians as a cause of disease since the end of the last century but only of recent years have they been recognized in human disease. In 1898 Loeffler and Frosch's discovery that a microbe smaller than bacteria, i.e. a virus, caused foot-and-mouth disease was the forerunner of the discovery of viruses as a cause of diseases in man. Today we seem to be witnessing another breakthrough of great biological and medical significance, namely, that the disease of sheep called scrapie is apparently caused by a replicating agent still smaller than viruses and fundamentally different in that it has no nucleic acid[2].

This remarkable series of key discoveries made during investigations on animal disease is not to be explained as due to there being more research on animals than man because the contrary is true. I submit that they show that the principles of disease can be revealed more readily in animals, and for much the same reason as diseases of animals can be more readily controlled.

These discoveries are examples of some of the incidental "fall-out" from investigations on communicable diseases of animals, undertaken in most instances because of their economic importance. The degenerative diseases are of little economic importance in animals so there has been no corresponding fall-out in these diseases. Research in this field needs to be sponsored in the deliberate expectation of findings relevant to human problems.

A traditional method in medical research is to attempt to reproduce a disease in an experimental animal, usually one of the laboratory rodents. This method has been very fruitful in communicable and nutritional diseases but has met with only limited success in the chronic degenerative diseases, because they are more difficult to reproduce. The modern approach is to search for species in which counterparts of human disease occur naturally and use these as models for research. Many animal species are involved in these investigations but non-human primates are receiving particular attention and in my opinion will play an increasingly important part in future medical research.

The advantages of an animal model are obvious but bear re-statement: all manner of experimental procedures and intervention studies not permissible in man become feasible. Human pathology is often handicapped by being confined largely to the terminal stages of a disease whereas study of the early stages is usually more informative. Furthermore, changes spread over half a century in the life of a man may be observed in a few years in a dog, pig or chicken. A deeper insight into the nature of the disease processes involved can be gained by investigating them in a wider context, as they occur in animals with different physiological processes and different ways of life. An analogous disease in another species is often not an exact replica of the human disease, even when the cause is identical, and the differences may be as significant and revealing as the similarities.

Since the conquest of most lethal epidemic diseases of man in the developed countries, cancer and cardiovascular diseases have become the main targets in medical research and it is in these two fields that most effort is being directed in comparative medicine.

The first need in comparative studies on atherosclerosis has been to survey as many species as possible for spontaneous lesions resembling the condition in man. During the last five years or so a good deal of potentially useful information has been accumulated. Lesions of atherosclerosis closely similar to the human disease occur in certain non-human primates, and lesions comparable to the uncomplicated lesions in man are to be found in the aortae of pigs. Chickens, turkeys and pigeons also develop atherosclerosis resembling human lesions in many respects.

In 1965 a book entitled "*Comparative Atherosclerosis*"[3] was published. This authoritative work by a number of contributors brings together for the first time what is known of this condition in animals and compares the lesions found in the various species with those in man. To my mind this marks the graduation of comparative studies in atherosclerosis. Models are now available for an experimental attack on this disease which was not possible just a few years ago and furthermore the natural development of the disease can be observed in a variety of physiological contexts.

But the recent discovery in comparative cardiovascular studies which I find most exciting is Dr. Hans Luginbühl's demonstration that very old pigs (10–14 years) quite commonly have extensive atherosclerosis of the cerebral arteries, often with associated cerebral infarcts[4]. Thus for the first time there is now available a model for studying cerebrovascular disease.

Another thought-provoking line of investigation has been Dr. Herbert Ratcliffe's work with chickens submitted to various forms of social stress[5]. He kept chickens in groups of different sizes and varying proportions of the sexes. When males and females were caged individually there was a minimum of vascular disease, but in groups consisting of twice as many males as females there were many deaths and a considerable amount of myocardial infarction associated with disease of the intramural coronary arteries, the males being worst affected. Experiments of a similar nature are being done with pigs and experiments with monkeys are in the planning stage.

Cancer calls for a rather different approach. Neoplasia is a common biological phenomenon found throughout the animal kingdom and many counterparts of human tumours are already known. All types of tumours occur in domestic animals, but the really significant thing is that the prevalence and site of origin of each type varies enormously from one species to another and in some instances from one breed to another and from one geographical region to another. If we can identify the particular physiological and environmental factors with which these patterns of incidence are specifically associated, it will add significantly to our understanding of the causes of neoplasia and the pathogenesis of tumours. Some tumours are more malignant in one species than in another and a study of these may throw light on factors involved in malignancy. Finally, spontaneous tumours in animals provide opportunities for testing new therapeutic methods.

The tremendous activity in research on human leukaemia today stems to a large extent from discoveries in animals. A lot of attention was attracted by the finding that the disease is caused by a virus not only in chickens but also in rodents. It now seems highly probable that leukaemia in cats also has a viral aetiology and there is suggestive evidence in the same direction regarding the disease in dogs and in cattle. Isolated incidents have been reported which seemed to indicate transmission of the disease from dogs to children, but the true significance of these observations is still in doubt. In one country it is claimed that areas with a high incidence of bovine leukaemia also have a high incidence of human leukaemia, but such an association could not be established in other countries.

The World Health Organization has been active in encouraging and co-ordinating comparative studies in cardiovascular diseases and oncology and centres in many countries are collaborating.

Those diseases grouped together under the general terms rheumatism and connective tissue disorders form another large field where comparative studies are making a useful contribution. The finding of systemic lupus erythematosus occurring spontaneously in New Zealand B mice has provided a valuable tool for research on autoimmune diseases generally. The more recent finding of this condition in dogs offers further possibilities which are now being taken up. Several other diseases of animals, for example, Aleutian disease of mink, have features in common with connective tissue diseases of man and offer possibilities of an experimental approach to these puzzling conditions[6].

Before leaving the subject of degenerative diseases I wish to mention also the opportunities for comparative studies in neuropathology. Of special topical interest is a possible relationship between scrapie of sheep and disseminated sclerosis of man. Sheep inoculated with material from a case of disseminated sclerosis have developed a scrapie-like condition[7].

I would like to conclude with one more illustration, this time from comparative microbiology, to show how research following reasoning by analogy can also be fruitful here.

Members of the Bedsonia or psittacosis group of agents are found in many species of animals where they cause several pathological conditions, with a distinct tendency in several species to localize in the respiratory tract, eyes, placenta and joints. Human diseases due to these agents affecting the respiratory tract or the eyes are well known but none affecting the placenta or joints. Recently investigations prompted by the analogy have found Bedsonia in the joints of four patients with Reiter's syndrome[8] and in four placentas from spontaneous abortions in women[9]. It is not suggested that in either Reiter's syndrome or the human abortions the infection came from animals: all that has been transferred is knowledge of the parallel disease in animals.

We have seen that medicine has gained much from research on communicable diseases of animals over the last 100 years. It is not too much to hope that comparative studies of the degenerative diseases, which are just beginning, will make a similar contribution over the next 100 years.

SUMMARY

Animal health affects man in three ways: disease in livestock depresses food production, some diseases of animals are transmitted to man, and study of diseases in animals produces knowledge with applications in medicine.

The health of food-producing animals has a profound effect on the supply of some of the most important components of the human diet. The Food and Agriculture Organization has estimated that the annual loss due to animal disease is of the order of 15 per cent of production in developed countries and often twice that figure in the less developed countries.

There are over 100 zoonoses, or diseases transmissible from animals to man; many affect man only occasionally but there are about a dozen that are significant public health problems. Some zoonoses are on the increase in developed as well as developing countries and the problems are continually changing.

Many important contributions to medicine have been, and continue to be, made from research on animal disease. Four notable examples of such discoveries are: the first animal virus, the first killed vaccine, the first recognition of transmission of disease by an arthropod, and helminth vaccines. At present comparative studies are being developed in the degenerative diseases, especially cardiovascular diseases and cancer.

DISCUSSION

Evang : The resistance of salmonellae which you mentioned is worrying. Animal feedstuffs now very often include antibiotics. Do you think it is time we had international regulations in this field? Some foods used in international trade are contamined with salmonellae, and in England during the war we had of course the advantage of having several new salmonella strains imported in dried eggs, for example!

In certain parts of the world where wild animals are killed for food the question of transportation is a problem. In Norway, we have been approached with the idea that the meat of game killed in the mountains and forests should be infused with antibiotics to preserve it, but we have stopped that, again because various strains of bacteria may develop resistance.

Beveridge : You emphasize once again the continually changing nature of these problems: like the girl in *Alice in Wonderland* we have to run fast in order to stay in the same place. The question of whether there should be international regulations concerning the use of antibiotics in animal feedstuffs is very controversial and a problem for the experts. Antibiotics in feeds are now becoming less popular in this country, but they are still widely used in some other countries. Restrictions would arouse a great deal of resistance from both the manufacturers and the users, who say antibiotics help to produce more food. They certainly give a fillip to food production under certain conditions but opponents of their use say that this added production can be achieved by better husbandry methods alone. There is an endless argument both ways. Many batches of fishmeal contain salmonellae. Certain countries have regulations to prevent the importation

73

of infected feedstuffs, which means at present that the infected shipments are diverted to those countries that are not so efficient in controlling imported feeds.

Lindop: Is there research on fish pathology commensurate with the use of fish as a future source of food?

Beveridge: There is no commercial fish production in this country in the sense that there is, for example, in Poland, where they have a very considerable industry. Such countries of course study fish diseases much more intensively than is done here.

Wolstenholme: Pesticides are being used in increasing amounts even in remote areas of the world. Are these practices in agriculture likely to prove more and more inimical to the health of man?

Beveridge: This subject is attracting attention in the veterinary world from the point of view of food hygiene. Some countries which export meat, for example New Zealand, have difficulty in meeting the American standard that imported meat should have no trace of DDT in it. I would not like to express an opinion about the seriousness of the world problem of contamination of human goods with pesticides, but so far they have not had deleterious effects on the health of farm animals.

Evang: The experiments on stress in chickens are most interesting. I submit that the tremendous benefits which we have had from work on animals in understanding somatic human disease might perhaps have contributed to some extent also to the underestimation of the mental factors in human disease. Formerly, however, no account was taken of it in animals. Now, through the Pavlovian school and other developments, we are entering a period in which these methods are being refined in experiments on animals.

We have experienced the thalidomide tragedy, where the drug-producing firms stated correctly that they followed 100 per cent the pattern of experiments with animals that was acceptable at that time. Something must have been missed here.

Adrian: The use of monkeys and other animals in the investigation of degenerative nervous diseases opens up the possibility that treatments may be found for things like disseminated sclerosis which are the bane of almost any age group.

Beveridge: Animal experiments and observations on animals generally have become much more sophisticated than they once were. A new attitude has developed and the appraisal of a food factor, drug or vaccine is no longer only in terms of freedom from clinical disease. The measure now includes the efficiency of production, that is, of growth rate and food conversion.

This is a very refined technique of getting the most out of the animal through the food and the environment generally. Not only the nutrition but also the effect of temperature of the environment, ventilation, the amount of floor space available, and so on, are assessed in this way.

Wolman: It was suggested earlier that either malnutrition or under-nutrition could result in permanent mental and physical impairment. Could you comment on that, Professor Beveridge?

Beveridge: The effects of early nutrition on ultimate physical development have been studied in animals for a long time. For example, if pigs when very young are severely underfed or suffer from a disease, they never catch up with their fellows and remain smaller as adults.

Lindop: On the other hand, if rats are underfed their lifespan can be increased by about 20–30 per cent. This might be a difference between deficient underfeeding and balanced underfeeding.

Kaprio: A group of psychologists, psychiatrists and biologists supported by WHO has been following up animal psychology and development to compare it with human development[10]. There is quite a lot to be learnt, through very sophisticated and systematic observation, about the normal development pattern.

Fanconi: Toxoplasmosis is probably one of the most important causes of mental impairment if the human foetus is infected. Have you any experience of the spread of toxoplasmosis in animals?

Beveridge: The epidemiology of toxoplasmosis is still very unclear. It is not certain how it spreads from one animal to another and how it infects the foetus, but it is a very widespread disease in almost all species. In this country it has been found to be quite common in sheep, sometimes causing abortion. Whether the infected animal constitutes a serious danger to man I do not think anybody knows at present.

Candau: Trypanosomiasis is one of the important problems for certain regions of Africa, especially at present. Have you any comments on that, Professor Beveridge?

Beveridge: FAO has estimated[1] that it would add a capital value of $5,000 million to African grazing land if the tsetse fly, which transmits trypanosomiasis, were eradicated. It is of course being cleared from many areas.

Candau: Eradication of certain diseases is perfectly possible in large contiguous areas of the world, but experience has shown that it is practically impossible to eradicate a disease from the whole world. We cannot assume that we can solve medical problems with blueprints. Once we thought that DDT would eradicate malaria, but we underestimated the intelligence of the mosquito and of the plasmodium. The problems of resistance arise there. However, in reality we have cleared large areas of the world and can clear more.

Another point is: should we carry out eradication in areas which do not even have a minimum health service? If eradication is carried out in such a place the whole effort of the country is concentrated on one disease, when not even the minimum services are available to provide medical care for the population or to ensure that the area concerned remains free of the disease which has been eradicated. It is more an administrative problem than a problem of feasibility. Eradication is feasible in large areas of the world. Moreover, certain campaigns of eradication have apparently stimulated governments to do something and to reduce some diseases to a certain level where they are no longer a public health problem. The fire brigade tactics are then used to deal with any case that might occur!

Too little attention is being paid to this very close connexion between human and animal disease which Professor Beveridge pointed out. Even in the last few years many diseases that were considered to be diseases of man have been found to be diseases of animals, where man plays just a part in the cycle of the disease. We thought at first that yellow fever was a disease of man and that it could be eradicated, but then we discovered that this was an animal disease existing in the forest. Human malaria has been seen in animals and although so far this has no epidemiological importance we don't know what will happen in the future. Recently Dr. C. J. Hackett referred[11] to the findings by Fribourg-Blanc and colleagues of pathogenic treponemes, apparently of the *pallidum-pertenue* type, in a baboon. Maybe tomorrow we shall discover that some of the diseases that we thought peculiar to man— for instance, smallpox—are not so. In the end I think the biologists are going to help us to have a better understanding of all these mutations and adaptations arising from the ecological conditions or the microclimate created for the different causal agents and vectors.

Beveridge: Many years ago Sir Macfarlane Burnet pointed out that although the human species evolved rather a long time ago, man existed only in small groups until a few thousand years ago: such a host population and time period were hardly suitable for the evolution of new parasites causing epidemic disease. Burnet therefore postulated that human pathogens were probably derived from already existing strains in older species of animals. If this is so, the animal prototypes very likely are still present and capable of again throwing off strains pathogenic for man.

Evang: There is no answer in principle to the question of "eradication". If the ecological situation is very complex, no eradication is possible at present, although theoretically in the future it may be possible. If the ecological situation is very simple then obviously eradication, both nationally and internationally, is possible. If only one reservoir of the causative agent is known, as for example in gonorrhoea, and also if the mode of transmission is well known and controllable, eradication of that disease is only a question of health services, administration and discipline. Since so many species of animals are involved it seems at present impossible to eradicate malaria.

Beveridge: Many diseases of course cannot be eradicated, but in my paper I emphasized that *certain* animal diseases can be. The veterinarian has an advantage over his medical colleague in that he can eliminate foci of infection by slaughter. Furthermore, quarantine can be very effective in animals although it is very difficult to apply to people.

Banks: How much work is going on, and are there any concrete results yet, on neoplasms in domestic and caged animals? I am thinking again of the environmental influences.

Beveridge: The World Health Organization has set up a number of centres to try to get uniform classifications, and a number of surveys are being done in different countries to estimate the prevalence of certain types of tumour. Attempts are being made to introduce widely a more sophisticated method of keeping records in veterinary clinics. We are in the early stage of collecting data. We are aware of a few types of tumour which have a distinct regional distribution, such as oesophageal cancer in cattle in one part of Africa and in parts of Brazil. A report appeared in the public press a few months ago that there had been a great increase in lung cancer in dogs. This arose from a misunderstanding. There has been no increase. The proportion of squamous-cell carcinoma to adenocarcinoma in dogs seems to be about 1:1, which it was in man 40 years ago, whereas now in man it is about 10:1. There is no good evidence that there has been a change in dogs as a result of exposure to polluted air.

REFERENCES

1. Food and Agriculture Organization (1963). *Animal Health Yearbook*, (1962), pp. 284–313. Rome: FAO.
2. Pattison, I. H. (1966). Scrapie. *Science Journal*, 3, 75–79.
3. Roberts, J. C., and Strauss, R. (eds.) (1965). *Comparative Atherosclerosis*. New York: Harper & Row.
4. Fankhauser, R., Luginbühl, H., and McGrath, J. T. (1965). Cerebrovascular diseases in various animal species. *Annals of the New York Academy of Sciences*, 127, 817–860.

REFERENCES

5. Ratcliffe, H. L., and Snyder, R. L. (1964). Myocardial infarction: a response to social interaction among chickens. *Science*, **144**, 425–426.
6. Leader, R. W. (1964). Lower animals, spontaneous diseases, and man. *Archives of Pathology*, **78**, 390–404.
7. Palsson, P. A., Pattison, I. H., and Field, E. J. (1965). Transmission experiments with multiple sclerosis. In *Slow, Latent and Temperate Virus Infections*, pp. 49–54, ed. Gajdusek, D. C., Gibbs, C. J., Jr., & Alpers, M. Washington, D.C.: U.S. Dept. of Health, Education & Welfare, NINDB Monograph No. 2.
8. Schachter, J., Barnes, M. G., Jones, J. P., Jr., Engleman, E. P., and Meyer, K. F. (1966). Isolation of Bedsoniae from the joints of patients with Reiter's syndrome. *Proceedings of the Society for Experimental Biology and Medicine*, **122**, 283–285.
9. Schachter, J., Mayer, K. F., and others (1966). Personal communication.
10. Conferences on *Concepts of Developmental Regulation in the Foetus and Child*, held in 1964, 1965 and 1966: organized by Dr. J. M. Tanner, London.
11. Hackett, C. J. (1967). Yaws eradication. *Transactions of the Royal Society of Tropical Medicine and Hygiene*, **61**, 148–152.

4

GEOGRAPHICAL PATHOLOGY OF
THE MAJOR KILLING DISORDERS:
CANCER AND CARDIOVASCULAR DISEASES

J. H. de Haas
Department of Health Development,
Netherlands Institute for Preventive Medicine, Leiden

THE title of this paper implies that cancer and cardiovascular diseases are the main causes of death in the world. But global epidemiology teaches us that less than 10 million out of the some 60 million people who die every year succumb from cardiovascular diseases and cancer, or about the same number as die from malaria and tuberculosis. Nearly half the total deaths in the world relate to newborns, infants and toddlers in Asia, Africa and Latin America. These underprivileged children, whose resistance is undermined by malnutrition, fall prey to infectious diseases or die from so-called tropical diseases.

The proposition that cancer and cardiovascular diseases are major killing disorders only applies to industrialized countries, where less than one-third of mankind lives and people have a life expectancy of 65–75 years.

This restriction does not mean that mortality from cardiovascular diseases and cancer does not exist in developing countries—the euphemistic modern word for technically underdeveloped starving countries—without a real infrastructure of public health. The contrary is true: cancer and cardiovascular diseases do occur in these poor countries, not as major killing diseases but as more or less rare disorders compared with the dominant position of infectious and parasitic diseases, in interrelation with malnutrition. People die before cancer and cardiovascular diseases are dominant causes of death, as their life expectancy at birth is about 50 years.

Epidemiologically, the study of cancer and cardiovascular diseases in developing countries is highly interesting, although their prevalence is low. Primary liver carcinoma in Asia and Africa associated with chronic protein deficiency, lymphoreticular tumours in Africa, differences of cancer by site between ethnic groups in the same country, and classical cases of heart infarction among well-to-do males of older age in developing countries, are well-known facts in geographical pathology.

Geographical pathology is not a felicitous term, as—historically—difference in place actually means difference in time[1]. But in this short paper this traditional but sometimes confusing term will be adopted. And as death certificates do not exist or are less reliable in medically underdeveloped regions, our analysis must confine itself to the mortality pattern in industrialized countries after 1950.

Are cancer and cardiovascular diseases really great killers in countries going through the second industrial revolution? To answer this question we must examine which part of total mortality originates from these two groups of causes of death, differentiated by sex and age. For this purpose and for the comparison of rates in different countries, national mortality statistics, compiled from medical death certificates, can be used with benefit[2, 3, 4].

Some basic facts on the two killers, cancer and cardiovascular diseases, will be produced, comparing the changing mortality patterns in different parts of the world. The rates are taken from the Annuals of World Health Statistics[5].

BIG KILLERS

Figs. 1–4 show the proportion of mortality from malignant neoplasms and cardiovascular diseases to total mortality in England and Wales, USA, the Netherlands and Japan, by sex.

In all industrialized countries and in both sexes the proportion of cardiovascular diseases increases with age. At the age of 40–44, for men 30–40 per cent (Japan 22 per cent) of total mortality is caused by cardiovascular diseases and for women 15–25 per cent; at the age of 70–74 this proportion is 50–60 per cent for both men and women.

At the age of 50–54 neoplasms are responsible for 20–30 per cent of total mortality in men and for 30–50 per cent in women. In both sexes these percentages decrease with ageing.

In industrialized countries cardiovascular diseases and neoplasms account for two-thirds of total mortality in both sexes, and in Japan for 50 per cent. It seems justified to say that cardiovascular diseases and cancer are the major killing diseases in technologically developed regions.

Nearly the same role as is performed by cardiovascular diseases and cancer as causes of death at middle and old age is taken over by accidents.

FIGS. 1-4. Mortality from neoplasms, cardiovascular diseases and accidents (percentage of total mortality per age group, by sex, 1962-63).

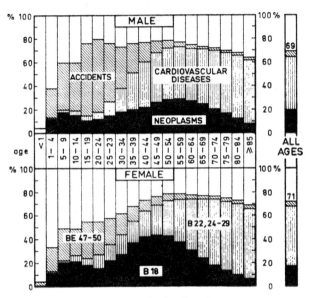

FIG. 1. England and Wales.

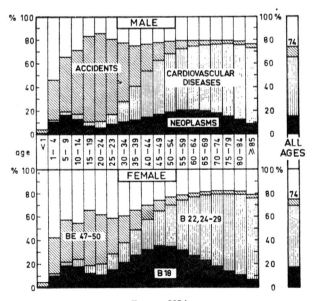

FIG. 2. USA.

81

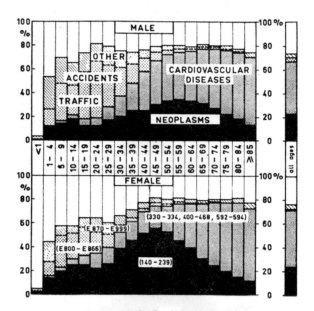

FIG. 3. Netherlands (1962–64).

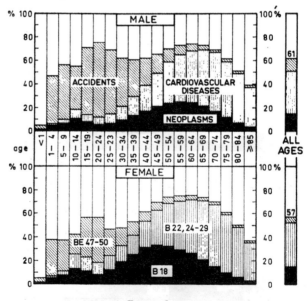

FIG. 4. Japan.

mainly traffic accidents, in young adults and children, especially in males (Figs. 1–4). Cardiovascular diseases, neoplasms and accidents therefore dominate the mortality pattern from childhood to old age. These three big killers have in common the fact that medical prevention is still in its infancy.

The mortality pattern differs from country to country. In this paper only international differences will be discussed. Disparity in rates within the same country—by province or occupation and between rural and urban areas—must be left aside, notwithstanding their great epidemiological importance[6, 7].

RATES AND TREND

To get a clear picture of recent developments in different regions the analysis of mortality from cancer and cardiovascular diseases as major killing diseases must be extended to the trend of the death rates for all neoplasms and cardiovascular diseases, and for one or two subgroups, over a certain period of time. In this paper the term death rate means age-specific death rate, by sex.

In all age groups the death rates for cardiovascular diseases are higher in men than in women. The same holds true for neoplasms, except in the age group 30–50 when mortality from all neoplasms is higher in women than in men.

In both sexes and in all countries the death rates for cardiovascular diseases and neoplasms increase with age. In nearly all industrialized countries the rates in men continue to rise and in women to fall.

The countries that have the highest death rates for cardiovascular diseases (Finland, USA and Australia) usually have high death rates for neoplasms (Figs. 5 and 6). England and Wales take a middle position in mortality from cardiovascular diseases, but have one of the highest death rates for neoplasms. Sweden shows a special pattern for cardiovascular diseases, having the lowest rates under the age of 60, but rising to the same level as Czechoslovakia and above the Dutch rates over the age of 60.

Czechoslovakia, the Netherlands and Sweden show relatively low cardiovascular disease rates in men, but Holland has a sharp increase under the age of 70. The death rates for all neoplasms in Czechoslovakia are as high as in Finland. Japanese death rates for cardiovascular diseases and neoplasms show a middle position.

The trend of total mortality, mortality from cardiovascular diseases and from neoplasms over the last decade or so greatly differs with sex. In

FIGS. 5–6. Mortality from cardiovascular diseases and neoplasms in selected countries, by sex (1953–55 and 1961–63, per 100,000).

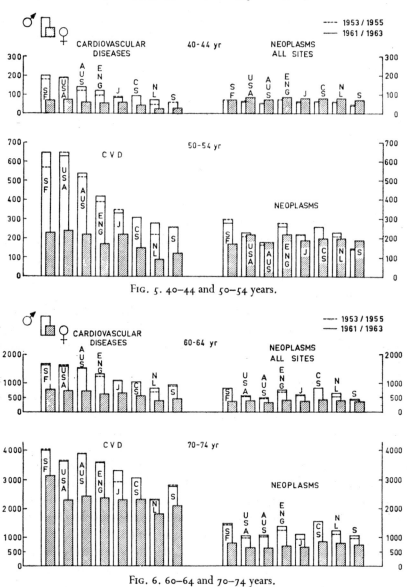

FIG. 5. 40–44 and 50–54 years.

FIG. 6. 60–64 and 70–74 years.

industrialized countries total mortality in men increases or remains constant from the age of about 50 onwards, while for women of all age groups mortality keeps falling. My monograph on changing mortality patterns points out that the increase of total mortality in older men is caused by the increase in mortality from cardiovascular diseases and neoplasms and a small portion from aspecific respiratory diseases and accidents. This increase is no longer compensated by the decrease from other causes of death, such as tuberculosis, diseases of the digestive system and other diseases[8].

The increase of mortality in men and the decrease in women result in the death rates for the two sexes diverging further over the age of 40–50.

Japan's total mortality in men continues to decrease because the increase for cardiovascular diseases and neoplasms is still overcompensated by a decrease from other causes, as was the case in western countries one or two decades ago.

CARDIOVASCULAR DISEASES BY SUBGROUPS

Figs. 7–11 show the death rates in two three-year periods, for all cardio-vascular diseases and main subgroups, ischaemic heart disease and hyper-tensive diseases (= cerebrovascular and hypertensive disease) and for neo-plasms of the lung, bronchus and trachea, in three age groups by sex.

Generally speaking, the death rates for ischaemic heart disease show the same ranking order as for all cardiovascular diseases, except in Japan (and Czechoslovakia). The rates in Finland are among the highest in Europe[7]. In

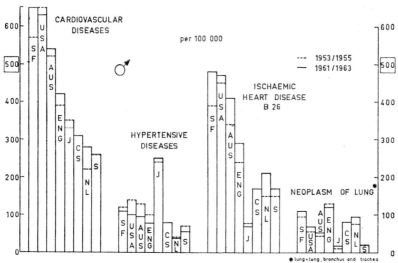

FIG. 7. Mortality from cardiovascular diseases by subgroups and from neoplasm of lung in selected countries (males, 50–54 years; 1953–55 and 1961–63).

FIGS. 8–9. Mortality from cardiovascular diseases by subgroup and from neoplasm of lung in selected countries (1953–55 and 1961–63).

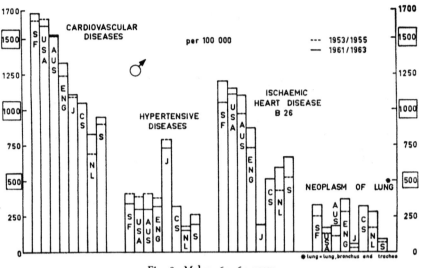

Fig. 8. Males, 60–64 years

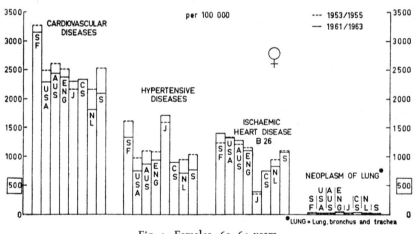

Fig. 9. Females, 60–64 years

men ischaemic heart disease accounts for two-thirds of deaths from all cardiovascular diseases, in women for about half.

In nearly all countries in men two to four times more deaths are registered from ischaemic heart disease than from hypertensive diseases (the

FIGS. 10–11. Mortality from cardiovascular diseases by subgroup and from neoplasm of lung in selected countries (1953–55 and 1961–63).

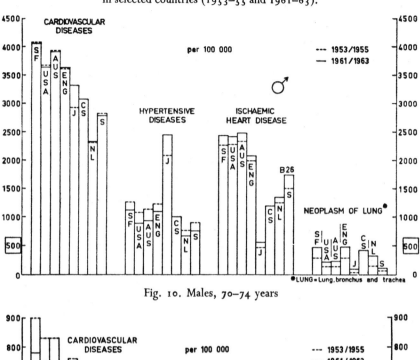

Fig. 10. Males, 70–74 years

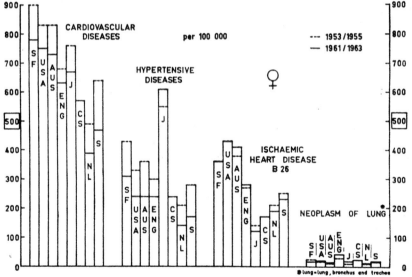

Fig. 11. Females, 70–74 years

ratio decreases with increasing age), and in women one to two times. In Japan the reverse holds true: for both sexes death rates for cerebrovascular and hypertensive disease are three to four times as high as for ischaemic

87

heart disease. In all age groups Japanese death rates for ischaemic heart disease are extremely low, but for hypertensive diseases they are extremely high and increasing. In the other countries the death rates for cerebro-vascular and hypertensive disease are decreasing in both sexes.

From the analysis of autopsy series in Hiroshima and Nagasaki it follows that the ratio between cerebrovascular disease and coronary heart disease " ... is not very different from the ratios based on the death certificate statements of underlying causes. . . . It seems reasonable to conclude, therefore, that in Japan deaths from cerebrovascular disease probably outnumber deaths from coronary heart disease by a factor of the order of 2 or 3 to 1, and that the explanation for the difference between Japanese and U.S. mortality patterns is not to be found in erroneous certifications in Japan, although, to be sure, local customs in both countries may tend to exaggerate the difference."[3]

Due to lack of reliable mortality statistics, Japanese rates cannot be compared with those of neighbouring countries, but autopsies and clinical figures in India indicate " . . . a higher incidence of cerebrovascular disease than ischemic heart disease in both sexes, the disparity being more marked in women."[8, 9] Recent autopsy studies in Africa confirm that the occurrence rate of myocardial infarcts in Uganda and Nigeria is virtually nil[10].

In the early fifties in European countries the death rates for cerebrovas-cular and hypertensive disease in women were higher than for ischaemic heart disease, as is still the case in American Negro women, whose mortality pattern from cardiovascular diseases shows an exceptional picture: very high rates both for hypertensive diseases and ischaemic heart disease, the rates for hypertensive diseases being even higher than in Japanese women.

The sex ratio in mortality from ischaemic heart disease differs by period, by age and by country (Fig. 12). In all countries the sex ratio in mortality from ischaemic heart disease falls with age: from 7 or 5 under the age of 50 to 2 at 70. The sex ratio in mortality from hypertensive diseases is much lower than in mortality from ischaemic heart disease and is nearly the same (1–1 · 5) in all countries, independent of age.

In Japan, which has low death rates for ischaemic heart disease and high rates for hypertensive diseases in both sexes, the sex ratio in mortality from ischaemic heart disease is much lower (1 · 5) and in mortality from hyper-tensive diseases hardly higher than in the other countries. Thus both sub-groups have more or less the same low sex ratio.

In the geographical pathology of cardiovascular diseases, especially of ischaemic heart disease, the high death rates of Finland, the relatively low rates of neighbouring Sweden, the comparison between Sweden and the

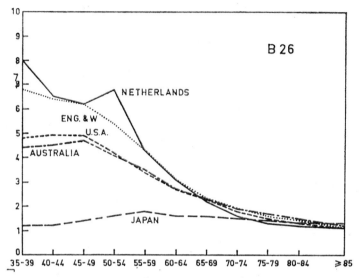

FIG. 12. Sex ratio by age in mortality from ischaemic heart disease in selected countries (1961–63).

Netherlands, and last but not least the situation in Japan, deserve special attention, not to speak of the differences by sex and age in all industrialized regions and the high rates in Anglo-Saxon countries.

The increasing mortality from ischaemic heart disease in males (Fig. 13 illustrates the trend in the Netherlands), spreading to younger and younger age groups, is becoming one of the most oppressive public health problems in industrialized countries.

NEOPLASMS BY SITE

In most countries mortality from neoplasms (all sites) shows the following pattern (Figs. 5 and 6):

(1) Death rates are increasing in men and decreasing in women;

(2) Over the age of 50 rates in men are higher than in women (the reverse holds true at the age of 30–50);

(3) Rates in men are lower than for mortality from cardiovascular diseases;

(4) Rates in women under 60 are as high as or higher than corresponding cardiovascular disease rates;

(5) Rates in women over 60 are lower than corresponding cardiovascular disease rates;

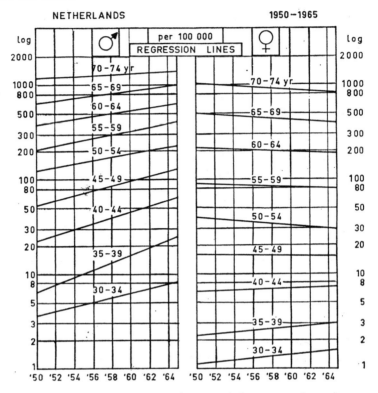

Fig. 13. Mortality from arteriosclerotic and degenerative heart disease
(420–422 = B26).

(6) The rates in different countries differ very little in women and somewhat more in men, but less than cardiovascular disease rates.

When mortality from neoplasms is differentiated according to the site
of the tumour some general rules become evident[11].

Mortality from cancer of the stomach, rectum, liver and uterus is
decreasing in most countries. While in nearly all countries a (sharp)
decrease in mortality from neoplasms of stomach and liver occurs, both in
men and women, the (high) rates in Japan remain stable in both sexes. The
death rates for stomach cancer in Finnish men and women are very high
(second to Japan), but decreasing.

In Japan the (low) death rates for cancer of the rectum are increasing
somewhat in males and females. Japan follows the general tendency of
(steep) decreasing death rates for neoplasms of the uterus, but the rates are
still high.

The death rates for neoplasms of the pharynx, larynx, oesophagus, intestine, skin and thyroid gland increase in some countries, decrease in other countries, or remain at the same level, independent of sex. Space does not permit the analysis of these irregular trends, however important they may be in the study of geographical pathology. Their importance arises from the fact that the death rate for neoplasm of the breast in women (which is increasing in some countries and remaining constant in others) is extremely low in Japan, relatively low in Finland and relatively high in England and Wales, the Netherlands and Denmark (higher than in Sweden).

Among the neoplasms showing increasing rates, cancer of the lung, bronchus and trachea is by far the most important subgroup. From an aetiological point of view the small rise in the relatively low death rates for neoplasm of the pancreas, prostate, bladder and ovaries, and last but not least of (a)leukaemia, may also be of great importance. Because of its dominant role in epidemiology and prevention, only the pattern of lung cancer will be summarized by sex, age and country (Figs. 7–11).

In practically all countries the death rates for cancer of the lung in men are rising rather rapidly, as shown for the Netherlands in Fig. 14. The rates

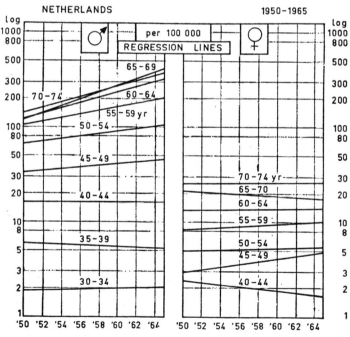

FIG. 14. Mortality from malignant neoplasm of lung, bronchus and trachea (162–165).

in women are nearly negligible compared to those in men—the sex ratio being as high as 5 to 20—but the differences by country and the slow but sure rise of female rates in some countries are important epidemiological symptoms. This increase in women will show an acceleration in coming decades, being the price the weaker sex pays for her emancipation as a smoker.

Mortality from lung cancer in males begins at the age of 25–30 and from ischaemic heart disease at about 20. The death rates for lung cancer increase with age, reaching their maximum at 65–75, while ischaemic heart disease continues to rise, even sharply, in the oldest age groups.

England & Wales and Scotland have, for both sexes, the highest death rates for lung cancer, closely followed (for men) by Finland. The USA and Australia have lower rates than Czechoslovakia and the Netherlands. In Sweden and Norway the rates are very low, much lower than in Denmark. The death rates for lung cancer are lowest in Norway and Japan for both sexes.

Two British surveys[2, 19] on the accuracy of certification of cause of death, comparing clinical and post-mortem diagnoses in hospitals, bring to light a considerable underdiagnosis of malignant disease of the lung (16 per cent), unaffected by age. If the same holds true for other countries lung cancer is occurring more frequently than mortality statistics suggest.

The broad range of death rates for lung cancer in men makes it understandable that the proportion of deaths from neoplasm of the lung to total deaths from neoplasms shows great variations in different countries: from 8 per cent in Japan to 37 per cent in Britain. The proportion for stomach cancer varies in men from 10 per cent in the USA to 23 per cent in Finland, while in Japan half of total deaths from neoplasms in men originate from stomach cancer and in women nearly 40 per cent.

Finland carries a threefold burden of high death rates for cardiovascular diseases, lung cancer and stomach cancer. From the age of 30 onwards age-specific mortality rates in Finland are much higher than in other European countries.

DISCUSSION

The uninterrupted decline of mortality in childhood and the triumphs of modern medicine make it difficult to realize that prevention is more or less powerless against the two major killing disorders in industrialized countries —cardiovascular diseases and neoplasms—and the third main killer: accidents. It is true that for women of all age groups mortality keeps falling, but mortality in men is increasing from the age of 40 onwards, or at least it is not decreasing.

It is also true that medical or surgical treatment may prolong life for a few years, but this success hardly diminishes the increasing excess male mortality in adults and the aged, mainly caused by ischaemic heart disease and lung cancer.

Excess male mortality has profound demographic and social implications. With ascending age the weaker sex is outnumbering the stronger sex more and more. The number of widows and fatherless children is steadily increasing and society loses people during the most productive ages of life. We are urgently in need of preventive measures—be they non-specific—to stem the flood.

Do we know enough of the aetiological factors in relation to ischaemic heart disease and lung cancer to organize prevention? Yes and no. Lung cancer is causally linked with cigarette smoking and with air pollution as a superimposed factor. Mortality from ischaemic heart disease is associated with cigarette smoking[12, 13]. Lack of physical activity causes an increased incidence and a higher fatality rate from ischaemic heart disease[14, 15, 16].

If half of all adolescents, young adults and middle-aged men would become non-smokers and physically active, total mortality in men could be reduced in a relatively short time by ten per cent, saving annually about one thousand men per million male inhabitants. Therapeutic trials aiming at lowering blood pressure or cholesterol content of the blood belong to curative and not to preventive medicine, but the borderline between primary and secondary prevention is not very sharp.

Do we need further research to fight the two major killing diseases in industrialized countries? Of course we do. Few pertinent facts are known about (specific) aetiological factors in the pathogenesis of atherosclerosis and neoplasms, except about lung cancer and some other neoplasms caused by environmental factors. Extensive laboratory studies remain indispensable.

But meanwhile epidemiological studies must be strengthened, especially epidemiological surveys which try to clarify differences and similarities between (neighbouring) countries, as discussed in this paper.

Why does the Japanese mortality pattern for cardiovascular diseases and neoplasms differ so much from those of western countries? Why are the death rates for ischaemic heart disease, lung cancer and stomach cancer much higher in Finland than in other Scandinavian countries? Why is mortality from lung cancer extremely high in Britain, high in

Czechoslovakia and the Netherlands, lower in the USA and Australia, and as low in Sweden as in Japan? Why is mortality from ischaemic heart disease as high in the USA as in Australia (and as high as in Finland)? Why has Sweden a relatively low increase in mortality from ischaemic heart disease, compared with the other countries? These questions could easily be extended.

The answers may be detected by carefully analysing smoking habits, (in)activity patterns and food customs in men and women, in different countries, preferably using standardized methods. As smoking, activity and diet patterns are changing rapidly, they must be analysed periodically. If we neglect this part of public health research it will be as difficult to analyse the trend in the decisive decade 1965–1975 as it is at present to analyse the trend during the past decades. Previous habits can hardly be taken into account.

National or regional morbidity surveys of ischaemic heart disease have proved to be important in complementing mortality analyses, but they are only practised in a few countries as they are difficult to carry out, especially longitudinal studies.

The broad range of death rates for lung cancer—from Japan via Sweden, Australia, the USA and the Netherlands to Finland and Britain—suggests that cigarette smoking (and air pollution) differs widely in these countries. As lung cancer has an induction period of two or more decades, smoking habits over a period of 20–30 years must be compared, not only quantitatively but also in relation to methods of smoking, such as inhaling and the proportion of the cigarette smoked.

Methods of smoking in the USA and England & Wales have been studied in both countries to explain the contradiction of lung cancer death rates in England being twice as high as in the USA, while cigarette consumption in the USA has been higher than in England & Wales over a long period of time[17, 18]. In the late fifties the length of cigarette ends that the smoker discards were measured in the USA, England & Wales, and in a small sample in the Netherlands. The butts in England and Holland are 1 cm. shorter than in the USA. "Quite a small difference in butt length might result in a substantial difference in the amount of carcinogen inspired."[14]

A similar paradox in the epidemiology of lung cancer as observed between the USA and England & Wales exists between the USA and the Netherlands. Although since the thirties cigarette consumption per person has been more than twice as high in the USA as in the Netherlands (after World War II even three times as high), mortality from lung cancer in the

USA is lower than in the Netherlands. During World War II cigarette smoking was a luxury in the Netherlands. Between 1950 and 1965 cigarette consumption per head doubled, but it is still half of the cigarette consumption in the USA.

For at least 20 years cigarette smoking per head has been about 25 per cent lower in Sweden than in Holland. Does this difference explain why mortality from lung cancer is much lower in Sweden than in the Netherlands? Cigarette consumption per head in Czechoslovakia and Holland has been about the same during the last decade. Both countries have nearly the same mortality from lung cancer.

Our knowledge about the prevention of cancer and cardiovascular diseases is regrettably incomplete, but we know enough of the high risk factors to start or to intensify prevention by health education. Cigarette smoking, physical inactivity and inadequate diet are personal factors, difficult to modify. Health education must be willing to agitate for unpopular reforms and doctors must give non-verbal education by personal example. Health education, based on explanation and aiming to reach primary prevention, must start in adolescence in order to get lasting results.

If we want to improve the health of mankind in industrialized countries we have to fight the major killing disorders: cancer and cardiovascular diseases. This fight is not spectacular and not popular and therefore not attractive, but it will bear fruit in a relatively short time. Pushing back the unfavourable change in morbidity and mortality in men admits of no delay.

SUMMARY

In industrialized countries cardiovascular diseases and cancer account for two-thirds of total mortality in both sexes (in Japan for 50 per cent). In men ischaemic heart disease accounts for two-thirds of mortality from all cardiovascular diseases, and lung cancer accounts for 20–40 per cent of mortality from all neoplasms.

The mortality pattern differs greatly from country to country, but also shows striking similarities. In both sexes the death rates for cardiovascular disease and neoplasms increase with age. The rates in men (for ischaemic heart diseases and lung cancer) continue to rise and in women to fall. Excess male mortality, ascending with age, has profound demographic and social implications.

In nearly all countries death rates for ischaemic heart disease are much higher than for cerebrovascular and hypertensive disease, especially in men. In Japan the reverse holds true for both sexes: death rates for ischaemic heart disease are extremely low and for hypertensive diseases extremely high.

In public health research, priority should be given to epidemiological surveys trying to clarify differences and similarities in mortality from ischaemic heart disease and lung cancer in various countries.

Notwithstanding our incomplete knowledge, enough is known of the high-risk factors to intensify the prevention of ischaemic heart disease and lung cancer by propagating non-smoking, physical activity and adequate diet among young and middle-aged men.

DISCUSSION

Fanconi: Emmett Holt has demonstrated[20] that the consumption of animal proteins parallels the frequency of mortality from degenerative heart diseases at the age of 55–59 years. However, it is very important not to jump to conclusions about causality from the parallelism of two separate facts. The cause of the high mortality may not be the animal protein intake but, as we heard just now, the amount of cholesterol, the increase of calories and fat in the food, or smoking or the sedentary life, and so on.

Pincus: The correlation of figures which happen to be popular at the moment, e.g. the number of cigarettes smoked or perhaps the amount of protein in a diet, must of course be done with great care and related to what one might call fundamental psychological factors governing the way cells function within people.

Evang: The comparative study of lung cancer supports very strongly the contention that the correlation between lung cancer and cigarette smoking is very high.

Garcia: In the fight against these diseases doctors must not only be good professionally but they must also be good educators and use their skills to influence others. Patients have to be trained to avoid the stresses of life—not to smoke, to diet, and a lot of other things—and of course they don't want to be changed. The doctor should therefore give a very clear explanation to the patient or somebody in his family and try to establish the good relationship which is so necessary. At the same time he must encourage patients to live their lives within certain limitations. When we try to apply health education we mostly concentrate on preventive measures and do not deal with medical problems. But to adapt a person to his new life as a chronic patient is a very difficult task and has to be accomplished in a very skilful way.

Burkitt: Cancer is a killing disease in developed countries, but I believe it is in the developing countries that we are going to discover causative environmental factors. In developed countries we cannot easily relate disease to environment, because people move and the environment changes, whereas in developing countries people live in a relatively static environment. If we are going to make a rational approach to the opportunities presented in countries like Africa for studies in geographical pathology we must be prepared to modify or abandon certain previously accepted concepts on which studies of geographical pathology have been built.

The tendency has been to assume that within an individual country the pattern of disease is uniform and that at the customs barrier the pattern changes. We must get away from this concept and look instead for the local patterns which may cross political boundaries and show wide variations in incidence within relatively short distances. If we can compare these local patterns, as we are doing in Africa, I believe we shall be able to relate environment to cancer.

Furthermore, if one assumes that a collection of slides in a central laboratory gives a picture of the pathology of cancer in a country, one is neglecting clinical diagnosis and building the whole structure on faulty foundations. As every up-country medical officer knows (and I have been one), whatever is sent to the laboratory is sent because one needs an answer. The tumour seen every day is not sent, because diagnosis is easy. Again, the pattern shown by analysis of histological material overlooks the inevitable biopsy selection which varies according to the particular skills of the men in the field: for example, in one East African country no oesophageal cancer biopsies are obtained except from the hospital in which one particular surgeon is working at the time, because he is one of the few men in the country who can take a biopsy through an oesophagoscope.

Evang: I agree with you in general, Mr. Burkitt, but there is a difference between these two main groups of diseases. As far as heart and circulatory diseases are concerned the developing countries are changing their life patterns more rapidly than the developed countries. In the developing countries we also have the difficulty of getting figures.

Eisenberg has listed the factors in heart and circulatory diseases under the initials SSHOHAD, which stand for smoking, stress, hypertension, obesity, heredity, activity and diet. The problem for epidemiologists is to quantitate and give priority to these factors.

Pincus: Consideration of what might be called genetic and other regulatory factors should not be overlooked. Longevity is associated with the genetic constitution and this is something which has been largely ignored in our haste to accuse cigarette smoking of every disease to which man now succumbs in his later years.

Secondly, the regulatory systems of the body, the endocrine systems, demonstrably play a role in both cancer and heart disease. This role is not too easy to define and it requires intensive study, but it is perhaps dangerous to accept uncritically the purely nutritive and other environmental causes of these diseases. Modern research is concerned largely with basic cellular mechanisms and also with the influence of smoking and diet upon these mechanisms, but it is only by understanding the basic mechanisms that we are going to be able to understand the diseases. I think Professor de Haas would agree with that.

de Haas: I do agree but these genetic factors do not explain the large differences between the sexes.

Pincus: That is where the hormones come in!

de Haas: The genetic factors are not very different in Finland and Sweden. The same differences in mortality from ischaemic heart disease and neoplasm of the lung that exist between countries may exist between different regions in the same country, where the genetic factors are considered to be more or less the same.

The epidemiological patterns in developing countries can certainly teach us a lot about the causes of cancer as well as about other medical problems, although the patterns of disease are completely different in developing countries and in industrialized countries.

It is true of course that autopsies don't reflect the situation of the whole population but on the other hand if they are carried out systematically for a long period of time what emerges, as has been shown in Japan, is more or less the same ratio between ischaemic heart disease and cerebrovascular disease as is found by clinicians in patients.

Lambo: If the genetic distribution could be assumed to be the same in a radically homogeneous group in a developing country, then we would be able to test the hypotheses concerning the effect of social variables on diseases such as cardiovascular disease. Social mobility is often very high within the same family in developing countries, and such activity may again be related to socioeconomic levels. This may be a way of arriving at a more precise definition of aetiological factors.

Querido: I support Professor Lambo's remark: in the western countries where these diseases account for two-thirds of the mortality rate, we are not making progress because the diseases we are studying are multifactorial, as has now been pointed out several times. But the problem becomes even worse because hypertension, for example, is a mixture of diseases, and then another factor comes in. In Japan, for example, is pyelonephritis a highly prevalent disease? Could it be a factor leading to the high incidence of hypertension in Japan?

de Haas: In some European countries mortality rates of chronic nephritis are given separately and therefore can be added to mortality from hypertensive diseases. It is impossible to make this comparison for all countries. Indeed in WHO statistics chronic nephritis as a cause of death is not a separate item. The proportion of mortality from chronic nephritis in mortality from all hypertensive diseases is small—in the Netherlands it is less than 2 per cent in both sexes.

Pequignot: In the developed countries, when we do a necropsy on an old person we often find that he was killed primarily by acute cardiovascular disease or cerebrovascular disease, but then we also find neoplasms, and I think that the part of neoplasms is undervalued in the mortality rates. Also, in these old age groups when we speak of accidental death it is not simply an accident but is due to osteoporosis.

de Haas: In our mortality analyses we usually exclude figures of people over 75, because in old age people may die from many causes and we often don't know the underlying cause. Mortality from accidents is much higher in men than in women. In both sexes mortality from accidents in old age is relatively small compared to other causes, but the rate is high compared to that in younger age groups.

Johnson-Marshall: The diseases you have described are really the product of contemporary living conditions. Commuting in urban settlements inevitably causes unnecessary nervous strain, and the physical planners could try to reduce the sources of tensions. The size of cities, the factors involved in large-scale commuting, the concentration of populations and the lack of recreational activities are common features associated with a large metropolitan city. Are they a cause or a contributory factor in these diseases?

de Haas: The mortality rate from cardiovascular diseases in rural and urban areas differs from country to country. Mental stress may be a factor contributing to mortality from ischaemic heart disease, but the concept of managerial disease, in vogue a few years ago, is not in conformity with the facts. In some factories with thousands of workers mortality from ischaemic heart disease has been analysed by profession: it is highest in the middle classes of workers and lower in the managerial group.

Dogramaci: Have you attempted to break down these statistics into age groups in developed and developing countries?

de Haas: For industrialized countries I have given age-specific rates by sex. These rates do not exist for developing countries.

Kaprio: In WHO's Eastern Mediterranean Region some cancer problems developing mainly in city populations have been studied. Some of the research workers had the impression that in the younger age groups there was a cancer pattern behind the infectious diseases that was higher than was originally expected. There was a feeling that cancer was there in various forms, but since the basic statistics were inadequate it was difficult to give the rates. But there are some publications relating to such information, especially from Iran (Cancer Institute of Iran). There were slightly different forms, for instance skin cancer was higher.

de Haas: Cancer of the liver (after chronic protein malnutrition) is more frequent in developing than in industrialized countries.

Candau: It is extremely important in epidemiological investigations to take into consideration not the political boundaries but the ethnic groups. Africa today has completely different population groups in neighbouring countries and even in the same country. One has to know exactly what type of population one is studying in order to see the differences from the epidemiological point of view in the incidence of different types of disease.

Mr. Burkitt mentioned also that the clinical aspect should not be forgotten. This is very true. The problem is made worse because pathologists all speak different languages!

Pincus: In Japan the incidence of cancer of the breast is extremely low, while in the United States it is probably the most frequent form of cancer in women. There is no doubt that there is an endocrine difference between these two groups of women and our figures show this. Similarly, we have a survey going on in a community in Massachusetts in which patients at high risk are contrasted with patients at low risk by some of the criteria that have been mentioned, namely smoking and so on. An endocrine difference between them clearly exists and we have figures which support this. These endogenous differences exist even in closely integrated communities and within a single community. The genetic factors are unfortunately more vague and can't be measured so well, but Dr. Candau is quite right: one must be very careful about the subgroups which one studies.

Banks: I am glad that Dr. Pincus and Dr. Candau have stressed the matter of genetics. It would be wrong at this stage to be too dogmatic about three factors: (1) the genetic aspects, about which comparatively little is known; (2) statistics, on which we perhaps tend to rely too much; and (3) comparative pathology, since ischaemic heart disease, neoplasms and so on also occur in animals, particularly in domestic animals.

Wolman: At the meeting of the Advisory Committee on Medical Research of WHO in 1966, studies on London bus drivers and bus conductors in the age group 35–45 years were reported[21]. This seemed to disclose certain hard facts which might be used for a mass approach to the education of people susceptible to coronaries. Do those studies strike you as having a bearing on future conclusions, Professor de Haas?

de Haas: The study on London bus drivers and conductors and other surveys strongly suggest that physical activity is an important factor in preventing mortality from ischaemic heart disease.

Kaprio: In that report[21] the groups at highest risk were pointed out, but it was acknowledged that they were already selected groups who had gone through a certain disease course. The Regional Office for Europe of WHO is now planning to develop a preventive programme in relationship to cardiovascular diseases. This may not be an easy task as in certain aspects not enough is known to justify public health programmes and one has to continue to pay attention to research both in the laboratory and epidemiologically.

With reference to the genetic aspects, my own country, Finland, has been mentioned. In Finland there are big differences in diseases between various territories and we are awaiting with great interest the results of epidemiological studies being done in the USSR, because we have some genetic links there.

REFERENCES

1. Haas, J. H. de (1954). Geographical pediatrics. *Acta Paediatrica*, **43**, suppl. 100, 374–381.
2. Heasman, M. A., and Lipworth, L. (1966). Accuracy of certification of cause of death. In *Studies on Medical Population Subjects*, No. 20. London: H.M.S.O.
3. Jablon, S., Angevine, D. M., Matsumoto, Y. S., and Ishida, M. (1966). On the significance of cause of death as recorded on death certificates in Hiroshima and Nagasaki, Japan. In *Epidemiological Study of Cancer and other Chronic Diseases*, pp. 445–465. Bethesda: National Cancer Institute Monograph No. 19.
4. World Health Organization (1966). *Studies on the Accuracy and Comparability of Statistics on Causes of Death; Final Report*. Geneva: WHO, EURO–215. 1/16.
5. World Health Organization. *Annual Epidemiological and Vital Statistics*, 1953–1961; World Health Statistics Annual, 1962–1963. Geneva: WHO.
6. Takahashi, E., Sasaki, N., Takeda, J. and Ito, H. (1957). The geographic distribution of cerebral hemorrhage and hypertension in Japan. *Human Biology*, **29**, 139–166.
7. Härö, A. S. (1966). Mortality in Finland versus other Scandinavian countries [in Finnish]. *Duodecim*, **82**, 1136–1151.
8. Haas, J. H. de (1964). *Changing Mortality Patterns and Cardiovascular Disease*. Haarlem: Bohn.
9. Padmavati, S. (1962). Epidemiology of cardiovascular disease in India; II, Ischemic heart disease. *Circulation*, **25**, 711–717.

REFERENCES

10. Kyu Taik Lee, Davies, J. N. P., and Florentin, R. A. (1966). Geographic studies of atherosclerosis. *Geriatrics*, **21**, 166–182.
11. Segi, M., and Kurihara, M. (1966). *Cancer Mortality for Selected Sites in 24 Countries*, No. 4. Sendai, Japan: Department of Public Health, Tohoku University School of Medicine.
12. James, G., and Rosenthal, T. (eds.) (1962). *Tobacco and Health*. Springfield: Thomas.
13. Advisory Committee to the Surgeon General of the Public Health Service. (1964). *Report on Smoking and Health*. Princeton, N.J.: Van Nostrand.
14. Fox, S. M., and Haskell, W. L. (1966). Physical activity and health maintenance. *Journal of Rehabilitation*.
15. Frank, C. W., Weinblatt, E., Shapiro, S., and Sager, R. V. (1966). Myocardial infarction in men. *Journal of the American Medical Association*, **198**, 1241–1245.
16. Katz, L. N. (1967). Physical fitness and coronary heart disease. *Circulation*, **35**, 405–414.
17. Hammond, E. C. (1958). Lung cancer death rates in England and Wales compared with those in the U.S.A. *British Medical Journal*, **2**, 649–654.
18. Doll, R., Hill, A. B., Gray, P. G., and Parr, E. A. (1959). Lung cancer mortality and the length of cigarette ends. *British Medical Journal*, **1**, 322–325.
19. Alderson, M. R., and Meade, T. W. (1967). Accuracy of diagnosis on death certificates compared with that in hospital records. *British Journal of Preventive and Social Medicine*, **21**, 22–29.
20. Holt, L. E., Jr. (1960). Protein economy in the growing child. *Postgraduate Medicine*, **27**, 783–798.
21. Advisory Committee on Medical Research. (1966). 8th session, Geneva, 20–24th June. Report to the Director-General. Restricted document ACMR 8/66. 21, pp. 9–11.

5

MENTAL AND BEHAVIOURAL DISORDERS

T. Adeoye Lambo

Department of Psychiatry and Neurology, University of Ibadan,
Nigeria

Cicely Williams has aptly observed that "The indices of health are not only rates of mortality and morbidity but also the incidence of violence, crime, alcoholism, delinquency and inadequacy."[1] Therefore, in any realistic attempt to assess the "health of mankind", mental and behavioural disorders are of such critical proportion and have such a tragic impact on the community that it would seem of great importance to identify, describe and assess the effect on society as a whole. Since one of the most spectacular features of developing countries is rapid social and cultural change, we have found that these disorders have not spared young developing countries. The concept of the "happy savage", free from the inhibitions and anxiety which characterize western civilizations, continues to remain a fascinating myth which satisfied the imagination of early field workers.

What are the common mental and behavioural disorders of our time? The well-known mental disorders are known to occur in all societies but some are peculiar to certain cultures[2]. Of particular relevance and importance here are the new patterns and distributions of mental and behavioural disorders consequent upon the aggravation of the inherent instability of modern societies by the strains and pressures characteristic of our time. Since a genuinely stable society is a fiction, social change is almost universal and makes the same recurring demands on human adaptiveness and human capacity to fashion a new and living way of life from old and superseded ones.

The major psychoses, especially the schizophrenias, continue to strike and disable individuals at the height of their expectations and potentiality. Organic psychoses and psychiatric disorders associated with endemic infections account for a high proportion of the psychiatric disorders in the tropics. Mental health of children continues to be a source of anxiety in many of these countries because of poor public health facilities, including maternal and child care clinics. Out of every ten children in need of psychiatric care in Nigeria, seven have had demonstrable organic impairment or physical damage due to infections, obstetric complications or severe malnutrition.

These health problems seem to occur with greater frequency nowadays; they affect greater numbers of people, require protracted therapeutic management, and cause untold suffering to the patients and their families alike. Especially in developing countries, they devastate human resources and lead to severe financial drain upon the nation and upon the individuals. The chronic disability which is associated with certain mental diseases, especially the psychoses, severely damages the victim's social relationships.

In many so-called affluent countries mental and behavioural disorders are of such importance that special programmes at national level have been called for to deal with them. Here I refer to the message from the President of the United States of America to the House of Representatives on the subject of mental illness and mental retardation, on February 5, 1963. In proposing a bold national mental health programme ''to assist in the inauguration of a wholly new emphasis and approach to care for the mentally ill'', the President showed that a period of inactivity had been tolerated for far too long. ''It has troubled our national conscience'' he said ''but only as a problem unpleasant to mention, easy to postpone and despairing in solution.''

Although we are still ignorant of the aetiological and other mitigating factors in many of these disorders, many studies have shown that the frequency of some of them depends upon the social setting and the way other people and social institutions respond to these disorders.

INCIDENCE AND PREVALENCE OF MENTAL AND BEHAVIOURAL DISORDERS

Several studies during the past two decades have suggested that the incidence and/or prevalence of mental illness is rising and seems to bear an inverse relationship to the socioeconomic structure. Accurate assessment of the amount of mental and behavioural disorder is difficult, partly because of the lack of reliable statistical data in many countries, and partly because the inherent nature of these disorders makes diagnosis difficult. Behavioural and psychological disorders of the kind we are examining here also tend to be culture-bound and this makes comparison at international level a difficult task. The rates of admission to mental hospitals which are often used are equally unreliable. The social forces which influence our case-finding are particularly intractable in international comparisons. Actually, such comparisons are hardly valid if the two populations to be compared differ in social and medical development. This means that epidemiological data from West European or North American countries are not of immediate use to us in Africa. However, the methods and the principles are the same.

In some technologically advanced countries, it has been stated that nearly 50 per cent of the hospital beds are occupied by the mentally ill, and some national surveys have suggested that as many as 10 per 1,000 of the population are suffering from severe mental disorders. The late Sir David Henderson wrote in 1955 that "psychiatry constitutes the other half of medicine" and stated that out of every 100 children born, eight would have a nervous breakdown and three would spend part of their lives in a mental hospital[3]. There is ample evidence to show that the position has not changed significantly for the better. Many observers in the field have stated that the tendency is towards a rising incidence.

In a recent lecture in London on psychosomatic diseases Denis Leigh[4] remarked that about 20 per cent of people were going to suffer from migraine some time during their life, 7 per cent would have asthma, 10 per cent peptic ulcer, and about the same number eczema. It would be quite permissible to compare these figures with what we have obtained from African material. The result would give an undistorted picture of the influence of different patterns of social development.

FACTORS ASSOCIATED WITH, OR LEADING TO AN INCREASE IN, MENTAL AND BEHAVIOURAL DISORDERS

Wherever social, economic and cultural conditions are changing rapidly, there are usually suggestions of an alarming increase in mental and behavioural disorders. They are very rarely supported by valid statistical information. However, in many developing countries which are undergoing rapid technological and social change more disorders are being seen. In part, this may in fact reflect a simple demographic phenomenon. For example, about 30 to 35 per cent of the population of emergent nations of Africa are under 15 years of age; many of them are under social and economic stress of one kind or another and tend to develop neurotic illness much earlier than is found in western countries. Certain social forces have been identified as acting as stress factors, thereby becoming part of the pathogenetic factors in mental disorder.

(i) *Urban ecology*

Many studies have shown that some relationship exists between urban environment and incidence and/or prevalence of mental illness and behavioural disorders. Faris and Dunham conducted a classic study to demonstrate this relationship between urban ecology and psychosis[5]. Ødegaard in his careful study has found the incidence of schizophrenia to be higher among Norwegian immigrants in America than in the corresponding population at home[6]. Eitinger's study[7] of displaced persons in Norway showed that mental morbidity was five times as high as in the native population.

Scotch in his study of the sociocultural factors in the epidemiology of Zulu hypertension found urban Zulu to have significantly higher mean blood pressures than rural Zulu[8]. Leighton, Lambo and others in their study among the Yoruba of Western Nigeria found a greater incidence of neurosis and psychosomatic disorders in urban populations than in rural areas[9].

Alcoholism, crime, delinquency, prostitution, suicide and other deviant behaviour patterns have been found to be more frequently associated with an urban environment, although this association in many cases has little or no aetiological significance. Inherent in this position is the acceptance of the unproven hypothesis of disorganization—isolation. Kennedy in his critical appraisal of the ecological approach has admitted the fact that it "...does yield a point of departure for other types of inquiry which show greater promise aetiologically."[10]

(ii) *Social and economic factors*

Environmental changes are known to have resulted in changes in the incidence and clinical picture of mental and behavioural disorders. The disturbances in which the influence of social development is most evident are the neuroses and the "socio-pathic" behaviour disorders. In this connexion it can be said that social development is, apparently, often a stress-producing factor and, as such, provokes anxiety and unhealthy psychological reactions. It constitutes, indeed, a menace to physical or mental stability, particularly for people who are physically or emotionally unstable because of malnutrition, chronic disease, or through unhealthy emotional experiences in infancy.

In western countries mental morbidity is found to be four times higher in the single than in the married. It is well-known, for instance, that schizophrenia is more common in the single than in the married. The high incidence of this disorder in the single is not an isolated phenomenon in its epidemiology, but it is part of a pattern. Sometimes it seems as if schizo-phrenia is most common in social groups which are somehow under-privileged and associated with a certain lack of skill, higher training and competitive abilities. We have seen that some of these social forces are to some extent selective. Selective social forces are very common in human societies. They push or pull the individuals towards certain groups and away from others. In spite of the difficulties in the interpretation of these social forces, sometimes the morbidity of a social group is so high and the social stress so evident that causal connexion is the unavoidable conclusion.

Roth (1959), writing on mental health problems of ageing and the aged, has observed "Mental illness among the aged presents one of the clear examples of social stress, a new and significant theme in medicine". He continues "In particular 'social isolation', which often recurs in the field of psychiatry in other contexts, offers a challenge for more precise defini-tion and practical action. Here the aged pose the problem of loneliness—a major cause of unhappiness and ill-health in modern society."[11]

In conclusion, I should like to stress the obvious fact that the field of mental and behavioural disorder is one which lies on the frontiers of many disciplines which have a right to share a lively interest in any form of con-certed action on the problems. Sociologists, cultural anthropologists, psychiatrists, demographers, and public health experts should ideally work in close collaboration in any research endeavour to obtain more scientific information on the physical and social hazards which continue to plague human societies in modern times.

DISCUSSION

Adrian: What is the incidence of epilepsy in Nigeria?

Lambo: It is unduly high among children up to 15 years of age. In fact about 40 per cent of our patients are children up to ten years of age. We feel that these diseases arise from infections, bad prenatal facilities and so on. Some are the result of physical hazards but many cases are due to prenatal damage.

le Riche: You have studied detribalized Scotsmen in Nova Scotia and compared them with detribalized Yorubas, Professor Lambo. Schizo-phrenia appears to be the major psychosis in these two groups.

Lambo: In 1965 we sent a questionnaire to psychiatric institutions in tropical countries ranging from South America to South-East Asia. The replies indicated that over 60 per cent of mental hospital beds are occupied by schizophrenics, in spite of the differences in the style of diagnosis. We felt that this was a field in which the international agencies might like to make a frontal attack and we are especially pleased to know that WHO has now started an international pilot study of schizophrenia in four developed countries and four developing countries—Nigeria being one of them. The study which compared the inhabitants of Nova Scotia with Yorubas in Nigeria[9] revealed some differences in the types of neurotic diseases from which both populations suffered. But on the whole these disorders in rural Nova Scotia, as compared with those in urban North American areas, showed the same relationship as we found between the mental diseases in Yoruba patients living in rural areas and those in urban areas.

Pequignot: In Paris between 20 and 30 per cent of patients entering the medical wards of a general hospital have psychiatric disorders[12, 13], though they may have other illnesses too. In the polyclinic (or outpatients department) only 10 per cent have psychiatric disorders, but these may not be quite so thoroughly examined. These figures are for obvious and severe psychiatric disorders and do not include psychosomatic disorders.

Paris, like all big cities, has many people who come from all over the country and from the developing countries. It is often very difficult to treat these people if they have psychiatric problems, because we may not know their cultural background or their language. Perhaps in the future each embassy will have a clinic for its own nationals.

Pincus: How extensively are psychoactive drugs used in developing countries? Is their effectiveness the same in these countries as in the western countries? In the western world their use is so enormous and so astounding that there may be a drug basis for contemporary behaviour patterns.

Some of our hospitals for juvenile delinquents are emptying rapidly because of the use of anticonvulsive drugs. People who had severe behavioural problems are reacting remarkably to their use. If anticonvulsive drugs are used to treat epilepsy in Nigeria do any behavioural changes result?

Lambo: Psychotropic drugs are used in some of the modern clinics, especially among the professional and sophisticated westernized Africans, although their use in Africa is not as widespread as in Manhattan, say. Of course these drugs are very expensive; most of the young countries cannot afford them so we have to find other curative and preventive measures.

Up to 40 per cent of the people who attend clinics have behavioural disorders as well as epilepsy and in some cases overt psychiatric disorders. We are now thinking on the same lines as in North America, that some behavioural disorders may be due to brain damage in children.

de Haas: The high proportion of schizophrenia in mental institutions may be a reflection of the demographic situation in developing countries. If the expectation of life is less than 50 years, illnesses of old age do not exist. In mental institutions for children in developed countries the mortality rate used to be very high—up to 30 per cent or even higher. This is no longer the case, but if the mortality among mentally disabled children in developing countries is similarly high then they do not become adults, and this indirectly influences the frequency of schizophrenia compared with other disorders.

Lambo: There is certainly a tendency for us to see more schizophrenics in the peak age group of 15—30 years. The disorders of old age were once unknown in most African countries, but we are beginning to see these too, as social and demographic changes take place. We are even beginning to admit some old people to hospital because young people now frequently move to other areas, leaving their aged parents behind. Of course some of these old people also have severe physical disorders associated with old age, so there is a combination of factors rather than the single factor of social isolation.

Candau: You mentioned the question of the common language of psychiatry, Professor Lambo. Are you satisfied with the definition of certain diseases like schizophrenia? Psychiatrists need a profound knowledge of the community where the patient lives, especially for an epidemiological study. For these comparative studies in eight countries, are you satisfied that you have a common language and common guide lines that will permit the conclusions to be generally comparable?

Lambo: Especially in Nigeria, we feel that for any such study to be valid it should be done within the national framework, i.e. cross-cultural comparison within the same national group. In Nigeria and other developing countries where things are changing very rapidly, for example, traditional, transitional and westernized groups of communities could be identified. A sample survey could be taken from these three types of community for valid comparison. The eight-country comparison would seem to be a scientific exercise of an ambitious type. At the same time in this international study we try to cut down the margin of diagnostic error by using standardized schedules. The narrowness of the terms of reference which we have now accepted from WHO means that we may have to exclude quite a number of people who might have been classified as schizophrenic according to our local standard. The cross-national comparison has its difficulties, but it may lead to more valid and refined methods of assessing mental disorders within various cultures.

Garcia: Dr. Candau's question is very important. How are we to define a normal person? How are we to define a mature person? We haven't enough specialists in this field to agree on the exact classification of mental and psychiatric disorders. In many countries the health services are so devoted to the fight against the physical disorders that mental disorders are overlooked, although the doctors are aware, from research, that perhaps 20–24 per cent of neurotics exist in the population. We have 5 per cent of alcoholics in our country; we are producers of good wine but we are consumers too and this is often the background to many illnesses—tuberculosis, diabetes, heart conditions. All the doctors are aware that it is a factor causing illness, but because of the cultural aspect they take no notice and look upon this in the same way as whether a person is small or tall!

Lambo: It is a universal problem, but if we are going to wait until we can standardize every aspect of human behaviour, we shall have to wait a thousand years! What we can do is to consider, within the particular cultural framework, what is abnormal at that particular time. The question of standardization is a real problem, but it should not deter us from trying to produce results, especially in the field of research on mental disorders. Within the national framework in most of the developing countries a great deal could be done to compare, isolate and identify social, cultural and genetic factors by population studies, but very little work is being done at present. I would like to emphasize the tremendous need for research, not isolated research but research spread over a wide field, implicating all the relevant disciplines. Without demographers and sociologists to carry out population analyses we can't really make any headway.

Evang: In the economically and technically advanced countries in the west the established number of beds needed for chronic psychotics is around 30 per 10,000 people, and for mentally retarded cases it is about 20 per 10,000. With chemotherapy these figures for psychotics are being reduced a little, not because the patients are cured but because the turnover is quicker. Have you established your own estimated needs in Nigeria? I ask because in the USSR, for example, only 7–10 beds per 10,000 were said to be needed for chronic psychotics and in China (mainland) the figures were even lower.

Lambo: We have tried to determine these needs, but social attitudes have to be considered here—in other words, the degree of tolerance towards mental illness within a community. For example we now see neuroses and various psychosomatic disorders in children in urban areas. From a small enquiry in rural areas we have discovered that children there also had neuroses in the past, but their parents did not complain about these symptoms and did not bring the children for psychiatric help. We have tried to estimate the increasing number in the light of social and cultural changes, because as developing countries become more and more industrialized, the tendency will be to see and treat more such people.

Kaprio: There has been a lot of talk about integration of treatment in general hospitals and in psychiatric hospitals. In many countries attempts have been made to reorganize psychiatric treatment and to create a new administrative pattern. In many parts of the United States, however, there is a complete separation between the mental health and physical health organizations. Have you any comments on the benefits of integration? In certain countries it is claimed that if old people are provided with really good medical care for their physical conditions and have their nutritional standards improved, then the number entering mental hospitals can be cut considerably. This might enable some countries which have large older populations to keep down the number of beds needed in mental hospitals.

Lambo: The advantages to be gained from such integration are great, especially in countries where trained staff are scarce and where we have to rely on general medical officers to carry out specific psychiatric tasks. Because of the obvious association between physical illnesses and some psychiatric disorders in tropical countries, we think that the incidence of mental illness could be cut by at least 40 per cent if active public health measures could be taken. The developing countries should not make the mistake of concentrating all their efforts on the eradication of physical illnesses and communicable diseases, while forgetting the social and cultural needs of the community.

REFERENCES

1. Williams, C. D. (1958). Social medicine in developing countries. *Lancet*, **1**, 919.
2. Yap, P. M. (1951). Mental diseases peculiar to certain cultures: a survey of comparative psychiatry. *Journal of Mental Science*, **97**, 313.
3. Henderson, D. (1955). Why psychiatry? *British Medical Journal*, **2**, 519.
4. Leigh, D. (1966). Psychosomatics today. *Lancet*, **2**, 1064.
5. Faris, R., and Dunham, H. W. (1939). *Mental Disorders in Urban Areas: An Ecological Study of Schizophrenia and other Psychoses.* Chicago: University of Chicago Press.
6. Ødegaard, O. (1932). Emigration and insanity: a study of mental disease among the Norwegian-born population of Minnesota. *Acta Psychiatrica et Neurologica*, suppl. 4.
7. Eitinger, L. (1959). The incidence of mental disease among refugees in Norway. *Journal of Mental Science*, **105**, 326.
8. Scotch, N. A. (1963). Sociocultural factors in epidemiology of Zulu hypertension. *American Journal of Public Health*, **53**, 1205.
9. Leighton, A. H., Lambo, T. A., Hughes, C. C., Leighton, D. C., Murphy, J. M., and Macklin, D. B. (1963). *Psychiatric Disorders among the Yoruba.* Ithaca, N.Y.: Cornell University Press.

REFERENCES

10. Kennedy, M. C. (1964). Is there an ecology of mental illness? *International Journal of Social Psychiatry*, 10, no. 2, p. 119.
11. Roth, M. (1959). Mental health problems of ageing and the aged. *Bulletin of the World Health Organization*, 21, 527.
12. Justin-Besançon, L., Pequignot, H., and Paillerets, F. de (1961). Les problèmes psychiatriques d'un service de médecine générale. *Semaine des hôpitaux de Paris*, 37, 831–845.
13. Pequignot, H., Guerre, J., Portos, J. L., and Perrier, F. J. (1965). Les problèmes psychiatriques du consultant de médecine générale. *Entretiens de Bichat*.

6

OCCUPATIONAL HEALTH
AND ITS ASSESSMENT

HARUO KATSUNUMA
*Department of Public Health, Faculty of Medicine,
University of Tokyo, Japan*

OCCUPATIONAL health services are essentially *preventive* in nature, although they include first-aid treatment for occupational accidents or illness. Rapid industrialization has meant that occupational health services have become more comprehensive than before. Occupational health, including industrial health, began in some countries by dealing with occupational diseases such as pneumoconiosis and poisonings from metals and chemicals or radiation hazards; in other countries more attention was paid to illnesses causing sick absenteeism.

Comprehensive health care, with special reference to mental health, has also been encouraged by the increased respect for human dignity in modern society. Recent advances in the social sciences and economics have shown that a not inconsiderable part of the rise in the gross national product and income is due to improvements in the level of health, and economic growth is closely related to the better health of the general population.

This fact has led to the concept of *health investment* which is supported by data reported by Mushkin[1] from the United States.

Occupational *safety* has been strongly stressed in all countries for many years, but more attention should be paid to rehabilitation after accidents. Safety programmes should therefore be considered as a part of the health programme. A safety programme requires some specific technology of its own, but improvements are more likely when it is run as part of the comprehensive health care programme.

Control measures directed against occupational *poisonings* or intoxications are also a major task of occupational health services, together with the prevention of occupational injuries. Environmental factors need to be further studied so that biological criteria for health and safety control can be established. "Fitting the environment to the man" is to be emphasized in this respect, and much research is still needed on the so-called "maximum allowable limit" for existing and potentially deleterious environmental factors.

A CONTRIBUTION TO THE ANALYSIS OF INDUSTRIAL SICK ABSENCE

Statistics for industrial sick absence consist principally of analyses of prevalence and incidence. The Sick Absence Statistics of the Permanent Committee and International Association on Occupational Health[2] in 1957 recommended that the period covered by these analyses should be the calendar days of one full year.

In Japanese industries, however, sick absence is recorded only for working days, and only when absence is for more than three days. Since industrial sick absence is directly connected to the loss of actual working days, the analysis given here is based on work days and not on calendar days.

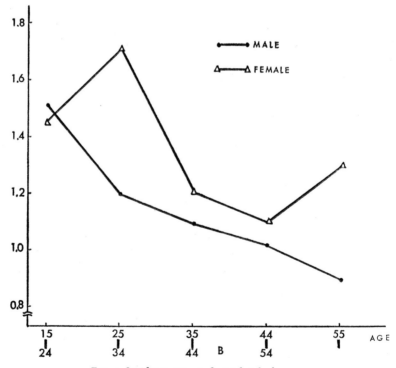

FIG. 1. Incidence rate, industrial sick absence.

A country-wide study was performed in 1964–65 to record all the sick absences in the year in terms of full calendar days and of working days. The study covered 42,000 workers in the steel, electrical, automobile, shipbuilding, chemical, textile, metal refinery, mining, electric power, transportation and communication industries.

The incidence rate was high among younger workers and remarkably high in females of 25–34 years old (Fig. 1). This was considered to be due to the potential health problems of young married female workers. On the other hand, the disability rate was high among older workers (Fig. 2), and it was again high in female workers in the age group 25–34, the curve of the disability rate being bimodal (Fig. 2). This suggested that the same conditions applied as in the incidence analysis.

The severity rate was low among younger workers and gradually increased with age (Fig. 3). However, the figures for those aged 55 or more are exceptional and this may be due to the small number observed. The number of days of absence was about 2 per cent in both males and females.

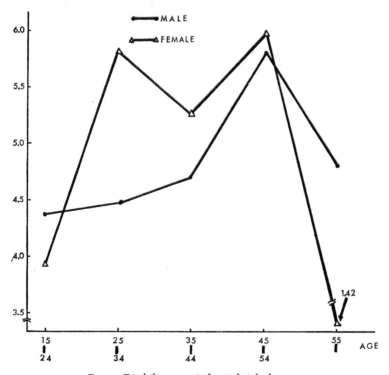

FIG. 2. Disability rate, industrial sick absence.

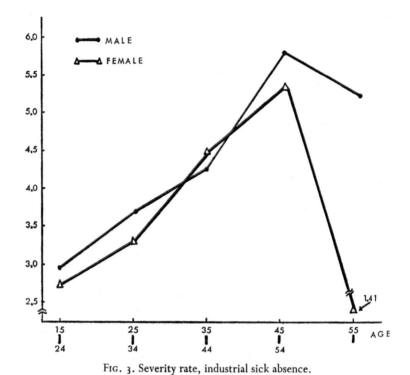

FIG. 3. Severity rate, industrial sick absence.

TOXICOLOGICAL TESTING FOR OCCUPATIONAL HEALTH AND SAFETY

(1) *Recent trends in industrial toxicological testing*

Industrial toxicology originally aimed to develop preventive and curative measures for industrial poisoning. Therefore, testing was concentrated on the materials considered as important causative agents in industrial poisoning. A new and wide spectrum of industrial toxicological testing, however, has resulted from the enlargement of public responsibility. Industry has to offer toxicologically safe products to the lay public, and should prevent both its manufacturing activities and the use of its products from causing public nuisance problems. The toxicity of trace amounts of any chemical substances involved in the products must be tested.

Frequently, the precise nature of the chemical substance cannot be identified before testing must take place. Occasionally it happens that both the toxicological and chemical investigations are successful, but in most cases it is essential to assess toxicological safety more speedily than is practicable for full chemical identification.

In addition to the extension of industrial toxicology into the field of production, the situation in industrial toxicology appears to be changing, that is, chronic insidious cases of poisoning are increasing as compared with acute severe cases.

Some new system of toxicological testing, especially for long-term testing, is therefore needed. What problems are included in toxicological testing? The first and most essential problem is the gap between man and experimental animals. The second problem is to find an indicator by which the toxicity can be evaluated. The third problem is the cost of testing, which, especially in chronic testing, is very time-consuming and expensive. Efforts to overcome these problems are being made by toxicologists in many countries, but their results have not so far been very effective. We must find a way out of these difficulties.

(2) *Extrapolation from animal experiments to man*

Two approaches are usually adopted. One is to use as many species of experimental animals as possible, and the other is to adopt a "safety factor" when the actual decision is made about the safety or otherwise of a particular substance. Both these approaches are considered reasonable and acceptable, and a well-matched combination of the two may be the best method. An essential criticism, however, remains concerning materials of which the toxicity in human beings is not known and cannot be assumed from the known toxicity of analogous materials. The most sensible way to avoid risk is to have full knowledge of comparative biological details for each strain and species of experimental animals used.

(3) *What indicators are necessary and appropriate in judging toxicity?*

The number of indicators used as criteria has continued to increase. In addition to the usual criteria, such as changes in body weight, food and water intake, mortality, organ to body weight ratio, and haematological, histological and biochemical changes, functional tests on the liver, kidney and respiratory function are also carried out in routine toxicological testing. Any metabolic change in the living organism of the referred material must be analysed, especially in material of unknown toxicity. Carcinogenicity, embryopathic activity and sensitizing activity must also be considered for testing, however difficult, costly and time-consuming.

To carry out this huge task, a variety of specialists should co-operate in a specific organization with good facilities. As an example, the British Industrial Biological Research Association (BIBRA)[3] is of special interest. This association is financed by subscription fees from industries and grants from government, and it has two main departments, Information and Research. The staff of the research department includes pathologists, histochemists, biochemists, toxicologists, analytical chemists and animal technicians.

Comprehensive testing is not always necessary but new material of unknown toxicity should of course be tested with the utmost comprehensiveness. However, often relatively simple criteria would be adequate to assess whether the material should be rejected.

The answer to the question of what indicators are necessary can be obtained only from an understanding of the full context of a toxicological testing system.

(4) *How to finance toxicological testing*

The financial problem is a common difficulty, seen at every level concerned with toxicological testing. The levels are those of government, associations of industries, and individual industries. BIBRA is in this respect an exemplary model for the solution of the great burden of finance in an industrialized country.

The cost of toxicological testing is closely connected to the system of testing. The Fison Pest Control Company, for example, has developed a system of toxicological testing in its procedure for the development of new products. In this, a substance is assessed simultaneously for its pesticidal and toxicological activity. In the early stage of development of new pesticides, many materials are screened out by the tests for acute toxicity. Toxicological rejection is the main purpose of the testing. Later, the few selected materials are toxicologically tested.

To satisfy the contradictory demands for speed, low cost, and safety, a particular system of testing adapted to the particular conditions at each level is required.

(5) *Toxicological testing system for unidentified materials*[4]

A different system of testing is needed for unidentified material because of the danger of unexpected *toxicity in the final products*. For instance, food additives frequently change when they react with food or in food processing. In these cases, toxicological testing of the final products is essential, whatever the results of testing the food additive itself.

In collaboration with a chemical company we have been carrying out toxicological testing on plastic film used for food packaging. A variety of chemicals, such as an initiator, plasticizer, stabilizer, antioxidant, and others, are used in the manufacture of this film. To determine what combination of these chemicals should be rejected or adopted from the view-point of toxicological safety, acute and 90-day feeding tests have been carried out. When the results were compared with previous results of toxicological tests on the individual chemicals, it was possible to decide which chemical or combination of chemicals should be rejected. Chronic tests have been programmed to discover which combinations are safe.

CONCEPT OF PHYSIOLOGICAL VALUES IN RELATION TO HEALTH AND MEDICAL PRACTICE

A feature of medical progress in recent decades is that laboratory tests are of increasing importance not only in clinical diagnosis but also in general health examinations.

When a test result is obtained in either clinical diagnosis or health examination, its normality or abnormality has to be assessed and a decision made as to whether the examinee is diseased or healthy. For this purpose, a set of values with an upper and a lower limit is empirically determined for each particular test item. If the value found is outside the normal range, the usual decision is simply that it is a morbid finding. However, this kind of checking procedure is not generally acceptable because these empirically known ''normal'' ranges are not always the product of well-planned surveys and are not based on a firm concept of normality.

Over 15 years ago, during the post-war period when the nutritional level was comparatively low in our country, we observed some ''improvement'' in normal values in accumulated data on the specific gravity of whole blood (Fig. 4). Repeated observations of the total leucocyte count for a group of

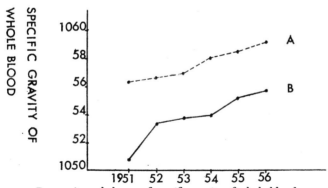

FIG. 4. Annual change of specific gravity of whole blood.
A. In research workers (Dept. of Public Health, University of Tokyo).
B. In workers in a chemical industry handling nitrobenzene.

119

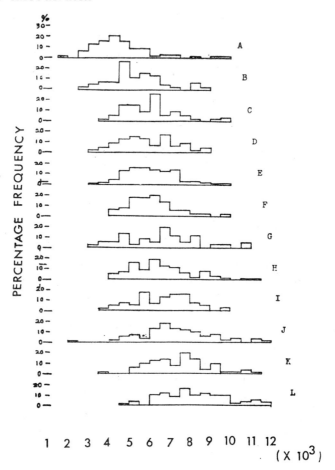

FIG. 5. Individual differences in total leucocyte count.

healthy individuals revealed that certain variations exist which can be statistically analysed for their variances. Consequently, remarkable individual differences have been recognized[5] (Table I; Fig. 5).

These features were also seen in data other than the leucocyte count, for instance in the specific gravity of whole blood, the erythrocyte count, haemoglobin level, haematocrit, body temperature, pulse rate, bodyweight, blood pressure and so on[6]. The results indicate that certain fluctuations in so-called normal values can be expressed as within-individual and between-individual variances. Both are considered to be related to biological information processing. The within-individual variation is, presumably, an aspect of homeostasis or the feedback mechanism in the body,

Table I

FREQUENCY DISTRIBUTION OF TOTAL LEUCOCYTE COUNT

Individual count (10^3)	A	B	C	D	E	F	G	H	I	J	K	L	Total
1·5–1·9	1												1
2·0–2·4										1			1
2·5–2·9	7	1											8
3·0–3·4	14	2		1	1		1						19
3·5–3·9	18	3	1	2	2		2	1			1		30
4·0–4·4	24	3	3	4	5	3	2	6	2	1			53
4·5–4·9	18	12	8	6	14	4	5	8	3	3		1	82
5·0–5·4	10	5	8	7	18	9	1	18	2	4	6	2	90
5·5–5·9	10	7	5	6	18	9	3	11	8	2	10		89
6·0–6·4	2	6	14	3	16	10	2	21	3	8	12	6	103
6·5–6·9	3	2	3	8	14	7	7	15	6	11	14	7	97
7·0–7·4	3	1	5	3	16	3	4	13	7	8	8	5	76
7·5–7·9			3	4	3	3	2	7	7	7	21	10	67
8·0–8·4	1	3	1	1	3	1	4	1	3	6	15	6	45
8·5–8·9		1		2	2	1		9	2	3	4	7	31
9·0–9·4	1		1		1			1	2	4	10	6	26
9·5–9·9	1		2		1	1	1	1	1	1	1	6	16
10·0–10·4										2	1	1	4
10·5–10·9							2	1			4	2	9
11·0–11·4								1		2	1	3	7
11·5–11·9										1		2	3
13·5–13·9							1						1
Total	113	46	54	47	114	51	37	114	46	64	108	64	858
Average	4·5	5·4	6·1	5·9	6·1	6·1	6·6	6·5	6·8	7·3	7·5	8·2	6·4
Standard deviation	1·31	1·33	1·32	1·34	1·16	1·14	1·85	1·41	1·67	1·73	1·42	1·62	1·74

and some of the between-individual variance is assumed to follow genetic and/or individually accumulated biological information.

From present knowledge it seems that the level used for evaluation, whether a given value is normal or not, should be settled, not in general terms but from the operational standpoint of a particular health programme.

SUGGESTION FOR AN INTERNATIONAL OCCUPATIONAL HEALTH CENTRE USING A COMPUTER SYSTEM (IOHACS)

For the administration of occupational health services, a computer network system as shown in Fig. 6 is recommended, on the following lines:

(1) In-put or accumulation of information

Information will be collected from various sources, domestic or international, and governmental or private, etc. This information must be classified through theme-analysis, and then compared with an information-need.

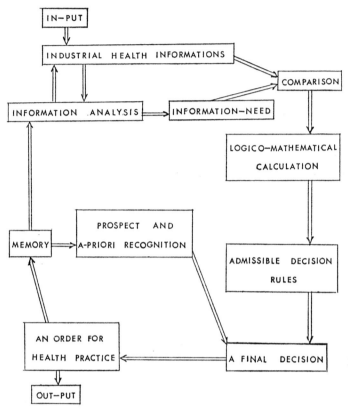

FIG. 6. Suggested network system for IOHACS.

(2) *Information treatment*

Through the process of comparison, the data are treated logico-mathematically to get admissible decision rules. The most suitable rule can be selected out of the admissible decision rules. After the forecast or the prospect has been examined and established, the decision-making can be carried out. An order concerning the administration of occupational health and safety can be given to the line.

(3) *Out-put or health action*

When an order is issued or an out-put given, it must be remembered and recognized. *A priori* recognition is connected with the prospective view on the one hand, and with our next information-need on the other hand, through information analysis. Thus, the network system is completed.

(4) Preventive maintenance

It would be important to keep the network system active at all times, and the direction of preventive measures should be under central control. I would like to call the system "International Occupational Health Administration by Computer System" (IOHACS). The classification, listing and retrieval system of information should be done at an international administrative centre. Subcentres in respective countries could get any necessary information in some tabulated form or in a classified form from the centre by an on-line connexion, even through artificial satellite, if necessary.

For listing and retrieval, a coding technique must be internationally applied in some language or in a computer language such as Algol or Fortran. The information treatment is fairly easy when decision-making models are given for particular cases.

SUMMARY

Some basic problems in occupational health and safety are reported briefly. The proper assessment of industrial sick absence and toxicological testing of identified and unidentified substances would improve the present situation in occupational health and safety as well as in general public health. Physiological values must be intensively studied, not only for health and medical science in general terms but also for occupational health and safety, in which their assessment is very important and indeed indispensable.

A method of computerized treatment of all toxicological information covering common and rare poisons, and including massive evidence of the normality of many physiological parameters, is discussed which can be applied to groups of any size within industry or in the community, at national or international levels. There is a great need for world co-operation in the handling of information about the interrelationship of industrialization and health.

DISCUSSION

Wolman: The whole problem of measuring the toxicity of known and unknown chemicals is a characteristic one for the industrially-developed countries. Literally thousands of new compounds now exist, many of which are unidentifiable by the very people who produce them, and the toxicity problem runs through all the uses to which they may be put. A simple example is the use of plastic materials for the protection of food-stuffs or for plastic pipes. In the United States the National Research Council was last year assigned the task of developing a simpler approach to the measurement particularly of chronic toxicity. In a company producing complex organics the number of animals used for toxicological purposes becomes astronomical, as do the cost and the difficulties of interpreting masses of data. However, the transfer of that kind of problem to the developing countries is unwarranted at the moment. The problems in those countries, as I shall describe in my paper, are not yet microchemical in nature, but microbiological. These areas are still plagued with the communicable diseases which Professor le Riche listed earlier.

Lindop: I don't quite agree that these problems do not occur in developing countries. At the moment some countries know that a particular industrial process is harmful to health, but they need the commodities in their economy. They therefore farm out the project to another country, perhaps to a developing country, which will then be exposed to this particular health hazard. Additives for the rubber industry and radio-isotopes for the clock and watch-making industry are two examples. The computer centre Professor Katsunuma described could very well be used to exchange information about the reasons for national industrial precautions, so that the people who need the work, but who perhaps have not got these safety precautions in their national legislation, would not be exploited.

Katsunuma: I am very interested in steps of that kind but the fact that health precautions are often closely connected with commercial secrets can sometimes be a barrier. I am at present thinking of how we can overcome this barrier.

Wolman: In all public health activity one must have priorities, one must have selectivity, and one must decide among a series of choices what one can do in a developing country. This is not to disagree with the comment that you made, Dr. Lindop: developing countries certainly have innumerable areas of industrial development that pose the issues Professor Katsunuma has just been discussing. In those cases I would hope that the best of modern knowledge and understanding would be applied, but the great problems of the developing countries do not really lie in the manufacture of radioactive watch dials or of additives for rubber and the like, although I am perfectly aware that such problems exist.

Candau: I think what Dr. Lindop said is a little different, and that it is an extremely important problem. It is exactly what happened earlier with drugs: drugs whose use was proscribed within a country were nevertheless still manufactured in that country for export. We had this problem with the quality of penicillin in certain countries until 1952, and even now some countries produce drugs only for export. The reason for this is not so bad as it might appear; but the people of the developing countries naturally start worrying why these drugs are thought good enough for them and not good enough for the people in the countries which manufacture them.

Professor Katsunuma, two things especially worry me about studies of toxicological problems and accidents in industry. The first is that there is a group of workers subject to occupational diseases which is completely outside industry and which receives no attention—the agricultural workers. The second is that the industrial health people worry too much about the situation in factories and forget the problem of effluents from those factories and their effect on the community.

Katsunuma: I agree. These are important world-wide problems.

Garcia: To what extent can one depend on legal measures and on educational efforts to prevent or control the occupational diseases?

Katsunuma: Health statistics in civilized countries are quite reliable at present, except for occupational injuries, and this defect is closely connected to the closed-shop system of industry. In Japan, for example, about twenty cases of lead poisoning are reported annually, but I cannot believe this is the true number! So I can't say how well the regulations or laws work at present.

Evang: Accidents in industry and, later, occupational diseases in industry were the first groups of diseases to be covered by any type of social insurance. This special type of social legislation was originally established in continental Europe (Bismarck) and repeated all over the world. The result is that many of the advanced industrial countries have two sets of health services, two sets of health control under different ministries and with different constitutional responsibilities. Is the time now ripe for applying one and the same principle to a disease or an accident, regardless of whether it happens to occur within a factory or outside? It seems to me to be ridiculous to have two such sets of standards.

Katsunuma: In Japan we are facing exactly this problem. A heated discussion is going on about how we can deal with it.

Pequignot: France is one of the countries with a special social insurance scheme for industrial accidents and occupational diseases. A few years ago this was extended to cover accidents occurring between the home and the place of work. This scheme is certainly better for the worker, but from the statistical and epidemiological point of view it is bad. The statistics of industrial accidents in France also cover many traffic accidents which are in

5*

fact not related to the person's occupation. Prevention of industrial accidents and traffic accidents are two separate problems, not necessarily linked.

Banks: Integration in a comprehensive health programme is one of the greatest problems which we have to face, whether we are an old industrial country or in the fortunate state of being able to start afresh. Professor Katsunuma, how far has Japan already gone in the setting up of a toxicological service on the lines which you described to us?

Katsunuma: We ourselves have been helping some of the industries, and also agriculture in a rural community. We are recommending an integrated approach to the health authorities, who should work together with people from the Ministry of Agriculture and Forestry and with the Labour Ministry, to solve toxicological problems with our help. This system is getting on well now. However, toxicological problems in agriculture are quite complicated ones.

Johnson-Marshall: The whole tradition of rice production leads to a basic occupational hazard. I would have thought that great efforts might have been made to change the traditional methods of transplantation of rice and to change the methods of culture at present used in large parts of the world.

In complete contrast, we also need changes in building industry techniques: for instance, the inclement weather of northern Europe when experienced during large-scale operations on building sites can have a serious effect on health. Industrial prefabrication would benefit not only efficiency but also the health of the building workers.

REFERENCES

1. Mushkin, S. J. (1962). Health as an investment. *Journal of Political Economy*, **70**, suppl. no. 5 (part 2), 129–157.
2. Sick Absence Statistics Committee (1957). *Report of the Sick Absence Statistics Committee of the Permanent Committee and International Association on Occupational Health*, 40–56.
3. British Industrial Biological Research Association (1965). *Annual Report, 1965*, 3–41. Carshalton, Surrey: BIBRA.
4. Katsunuma, H., and Suzuki, T. (1966). On the toxicity of unidentified chemical substances. *Igaku no Ayumi* [Progress in Medicine], **56**, 581–584.
5. Katsunuma, H., and Akira Koizumi (1962). A contribution to the knowledge of normal variation in total leucocyte count. *Japanese Journal of Physiology*, **12**, 251–256.
6. Katsunuma, H. (1965). A contribution to the knowledge of normal variation in several haematological data. *XXIII International Congress of Physiological Sciences*, Abstracts of Papers, 98.

7

POPULATION GROWTH AND AGE COMPOSITION

GREGORY PINCUS
Worcester Foundation for Experimental Biology,
Shrewsbury, Massachusetts

THE PRESENT AND THE FUTURE

E XCESSIVE fertility in natural populations has been overcome by a variety of selective mechanisms in which mortality is generally the decisive equilibrating factor. Even in the growth of the human family high death rates were held accountable for the relatively slow rate of increase to modern times. That rate of increase is illustrated by the data of Fig. 1, which also projects future growth to the year 2000. The remarkable acceleration postulated from 1960 onwards appears justified by the world total of 3,350 million attained by mid-1966. Certainly, if one regards the changes during recent years in mortality and birth rates in a number of countries (Table I), the remarkable drop in the former and the lack of any such decrease in the latter (except for Japan which undertook a positive programme of birth control) must obviously lead to a significant population increase.

Table I

CHANGES IN BIRTH AND MORTALITY RATES IN SELECTED COUNTRIES

	Birth rates per 1,000		Death rates per 1,000	
Country	1940	1960	1940	1960
Mexico	44·3	45·0	23·2	11·4
Costa Rica	44·6	42·9	17·3	8·6
Chile	33·4	35·4	21·6	11·9
Venezuela	36·0	49·6	16·6	8·0
Ceylon	35·8	37·0	20·6	9·1
Malaya	40·7	37·7	20·1	9·5
Singapore	45·0	38·0	20·9	6·3
Japan	29·4	17·2	16·8	7·6

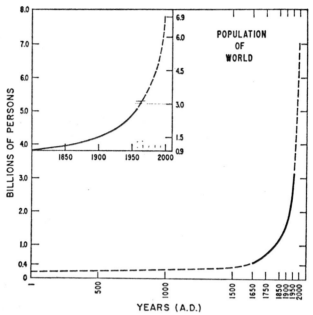

FIG. 1. Estimated population of the world from A.D. 1 to A.D. 1960
and the projected population A.D. 2000.

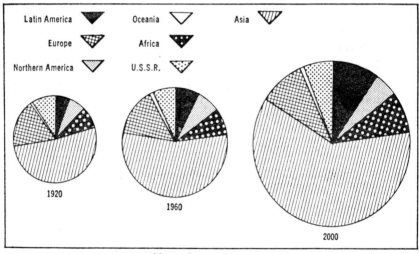

FIG. 2. World population changes, 1920 to 2000.

When we examine the rate of population increase projected by the
United Nations for various areas of the world[1], we arrive at the data presented in Fig. 2, which indicate that Asia's proportion of the world's

population will rise from 55 per cent in 1950 to 62 per cent in 2000, Latin America's will rise from 6·5 per cent to over 9 per cent, Africa's will remain constant at 8 per cent, Europe's (including the USSR) will drop from 23 to 15 per cent, and North America's will decline from nearly 7 to about 5 per cent. These projections postulate fertility continuing at the present rate to 1975 and then declining. On any of a number of fairly reasonable bases the general outcome appears to involve greatest increases both relative and absolute in the regions of the world with the lowest incomes per head. This may be deduced from the United Nations projections shown in Fig. 32.

Furthermore, the increase in food supplies necessary to maintain the population at a minimum adequate nutritional standard is greatest in the less developed regions of the world, as may be seen in the United Nations estimates of needed resources shown in Table II. The underdeveloped countries are increasing in population much faster than they are increasing food production.

Table II

PERCENTAGE INCREASES OF FOOD SUPPLY NEEDED DURING 1958–1980
TO MEET ANTICIPATED REQUIREMENTS IN VARIOUS REGIONS OF THE WORLD

REGIONS	Projected population growth 1958–1980*	Increase of food supply per head at present required to meet target	Total increase of food supply, 1958–1980 required to meet target and population growth	Rate of annual increase needed 1958–1980	Recent annual rate of increase in food supply†
Underdeveloped countries	56	33	107	3·4	2·7
Latin America	85‡	5‡	94‡	3·1‡	2·5§
Far East	55	41	86	2·9	3·0¶
Near East	62	17	90	3·0	3·1
Africa	36	28	55	2·0	1·3
Developed countries	28	—	28	1·2	3·6
World	48	14	69	2·4	2·9

* Based on United Nations "Medium" projections[3].
† Computed from averages of food production in 1952/53 and 1959/60, FAO[4,5].
‡ Excluding River Plate countries.
§ Including River Plate countries.
¶ Excluding mainland China.

But these are the simple requirements of maintenance and they fail to take into account goals for improvement. Hauser[6] has demonstrated the enormous increases in aggregate income that Asia, Africa and Latin

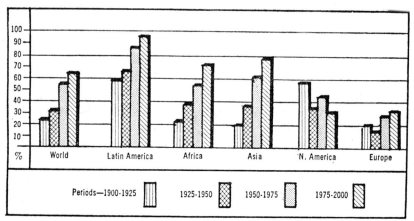

FIG. 3. Percentage population increases by major regions, 1900 to 2000[2]. The United Nations projections to the year 2000 show a relatively small increase in population in western Europe and North America and the greatest increases in Latin America and Asia.

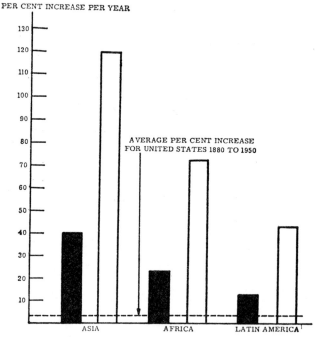

FIG. 4. Increases in aggregate income necessary to match 1950 European and North American incomes per head by 2000, with projected populations (calculated from United Nations data).

■ Necessary to match Europe.
□ Necessary to match North America.

America must attain by the year 2000 in order to equal those which existed in Europe and North America in 1950 (Fig. 4). This goal is utterly impossible if even medium projected population increases occur. Asia would have to increase income per head 62-fold, Africa 38-fold and Latin America 23-fold by the year 2000 to equal North American 1950 standards; annual increases in income of 40 per cent for Asia, 24 per cent for Africa and 14 per cent for Latin America would be needed to equal Europe's 1950 level.

Finally, present-day population increases will tend to cause in the less developed regions an increasing proportion of younger persons. Table III shows United Nations data in 1966 for the proportion of persons under 15 years of age in various regions of the world. It is clear that the less developed regions have a much larger proportion than the other regions. A vivid contrast may be seen in the 1955 data for age distributions of men and women in Costa Rica and the 1956 data for Sweden, presented graphically in Fig. 5; Costa Rica is increasing its population at the rate of about 3 per cent per year, Sweden at the rate of 0·6 per cent per year. Table IV shows the projected population increases by age groups for selected rapidly growing countries. Here it is evident that by 1975 the proportion of persons aged 15 to 19 will be greater than that of older persons. The pressures exerted upon emerging countries by this sort of age composition are great and

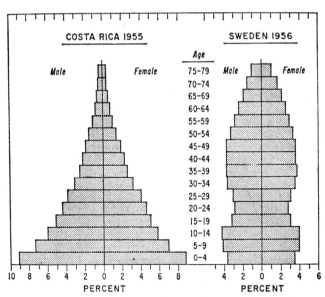

FIG. 5. Percentage distribution by age of the population of Costa Rica in 1955 and of the population of Sweden in 1956.

various. There is not only the obvious reproductive potential of younger persons. There are demands for the adequate nutrition of younger and presumably more calorie-consuming groups. There are problems of education and training, and in this area the less developed countries seem to retrogress—in the period 1960 to 1966 200 million illiterates were added, chiefly by these countries. Even now only 30 per cent of the children of these countries are in school, and the average duration of schooling is less than three years. There are problems of employment and family structure, of aspirations and ideologies. Will this lead to rigid minimal imposed incomes, limited occupation and unrequitable hope?

Table III

POPULATION UNDER 15 YEARS OF AGE IN VARIOUS
REGIONS OF THE WORLD—1966

	Per cent
Africa	43
Asia	39
South America	41
Middle America	44
United States and Canada	31
Europe (except USSR)	25
USSR	31

Table IV

PROJECTED POPULATION INCREASES (%) 1960–1975

Countries	Total*	Ages 15–59	Ages 15–19
Mexico	60	57	66
Brazil	49	45	54
Indonesia	47	40	70
Pakistan	53	48	58
India	42	36	45
Mainland China	52	46	83

* Developed countries = 21%

FERTILITY CONTROL

Since all the nations of the world are agreed upon the desirability of employing the many health measures that reduce the death rate, there is no likelihood of an increase in mortality to offset continuing high fertility.

Therefore, the recourse must be to reducing the birth rate. This truism has been demonstrated and repeated many times[6, 7, 8, 9]. The low birth rates of the more developed countries presumably reflect the use of birth control methods. Thus, it has been calculated by Whelpton, Campbell and Patterson[10] that contraception is used in the United States at one time or another in approximately 87 per cent of the marriages of white married women aged 18 to 39 years. In contrast, Agarwala[11] reports that of 84,000,000 couples of reproductive age in India 1·1 million have been sterilized, 0·4 million have used intrauterine devices and 0·5 million used other contraceptives. This is 2·4 per cent of the reproductive couples, and it has been calculated that 65 per cent of the fertile couples should be using antifertility measures to bring the Indian birth rate down by 1975 from 40 per 1,000 to the 25 per 1,000 calculated as necessary to maintain present living standards. In a recent comprehensive review of world developments in family planning[12] country after country is reported as endorsing mass use of contraceptives, but the actual rates of participation appear to be most meagre in the less developed countries. Perhaps the best record is that of Hong Kong which reports visits to contraceptive clinics of as many as 7 per cent of married couples. It is obvious that such visits do not necessarily guarantee efficient contraception. However, data on birth rates indicate a drop from rates varying from 34 to 40 per 1,000 before 1958 to 29 to 32 per 1,000 since 1961. Fig. 6 presents data on births in Hong Kong and the number estimated as prevented by contraception during the period 1951

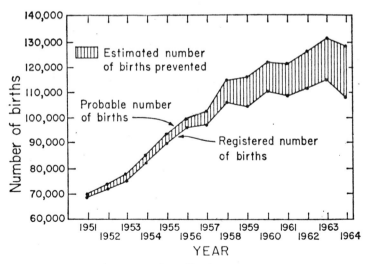

FIG. 6. Number of births in Hong Kong.

133

to 1964. It is clear that increase by birth has been slowed down in a city area long exposed to birth control propaganda and methods under a government that has, if anything, promoted contraceptives.

The outstanding example of a country that has faced the fact of excess population increase and met it with an action programme is Japan, which has had a remarkable post-war decline in the birth rate (see Table I). By establishing the legality of induced abortions and encouraging propaganda for family limitation by this method, Japan has reduced its birth rate to the level of European and Northern American countries. Data on morbidity and mortality due to the use of induced abortion in Japan are difficult to find, but Koya and co-workers[13] report "serious" complications in 5 per cent of the Japanese after the first abortion and 54 per cent with no complaints at all; death rates have been calculated at seven to eight per 100,000. It is notable that in recent years government efforts in Japan have been directed to reducing the abortion rate and introducing contraception as a means of family limitation. In the 1960's one conception in every ten ended in induced abortion. According to Muramatsu[14] the proportion of contraceptive users among wives under 50 years of age in Japan rose from 19·5 per cent in 1950 to 51·9 per cent in 1965.

In many countries provoked abortion, though illegal, is widely practised. In a sample studied in Santiago, Chile, 29 per cent of women of reproductive age admitted to one or more provoked abortions; the average number was 2·8 per woman. The ratio of abortions to births is given in the data[15] of Table V. Over 40 per cent of the abortion cases were hospitalized. The cost in terms of hospital and medical expense, of time lost to productive employment, of mortality and consequent family burden has not been calculated. But the statistics cited in Table VI indicate some of the medical burden. Armijo and Monreal[15] conclude from the Santiago data that "...economic reasons and ignorance of birth control methods appear to be the basic explanations for the alarming upward trend of provoked abortion."

Table V

NUMBER OF BIRTHS, ALL ABORTIONS, PROVOKED ABORTIONS,
AND RATIOS OF ABORTIONS TO BIRTHS FOUND IN THE SAMPLE,
SANTIAGO, 1952–61 and 1961

	1952–61	1961
Births	3,267	362
All abortions	1,310	165
Provoked abortions	762	82
Ratios per 100 live births:		
All abortions	40·1	45·6
Provoked abortions	23·3	22·6

Table VI

STATISTICS OF ABORTION IN SANTIAGO[15]

(1) Abortion accounted for 8·1 per cent of all admissions to hospitals run by the National Health Service.

(2) For each 100 deliveries, 24·3 abortion cases were admitted in Santiago and 34·3 to the provincial hospitals. This shows the number of obstetrical beds which are being occupied by abortion cases.

(3) Abortion alone accounted for 35 per cent of all surgical operations performed in some of the Emergency Departments surveyed. (In one case, 78 per cent of all surgical operations consisted of uterine curettage.)

(4) Abortion accounted for 17·7 per cent of all blood transfusions and 26·7 per cent of the total blood volume dispensed in Emergency Departments in Santiago.

The prevention of excess fertility by the use of effective and simple methods of contraception clearly appears to be the desideratum. The pregnancy rates with the various methods that have had experimental study are presented in Table VII. Clearly pregnancy prevention is optimally accomplished by the use of the oral contraceptives in which an oestrogen and a progestin are combined ("combined steroids" of Table VII) to form the components of what has come to be known as "the pill" which is taken for 20 or 21 days of a 28-day month. The use of the same (or similar) steroids in which the regimen of oral use during a 28-day month is a sequence of oestrogen alone (for 10 or 15 days of a 20-day cycle of use) followed by progestin plus oestrogen (for 10 or 5 days) appears to be less effective and about as efficient as the insertion of a plastic intrauterine device.

Table VII

NUMBER OF PREGNANCIES PER 100 YEARS OF EXPOSURE
FOR VARIOUS METHODS OF CONTRACEPTION

Method	Pregnancy rate
Douche	31*
Rhythm	24*
Jelly alone	20*
Withdrawal	18*
Condom	14*
Diaphragm	12*
Intrauterine devices	5†
Sequential steroids	5‡
Combined steroids	0·1 to 0·3§

* From Venning[16].
† Estimated from data summarized by Pincus[17].
‡ Data of Mears[18].
§ Venning[19].

These data are for fertility while the contraceptors are supposed to be using the method indicated. The data include "patient error" as well as possible deficiencies of the method itself. Obviously, with the more modern methods contraceptive efficiency is adequate for formidable inroads into human fertility provided they are widely accepted and used. Data on acceptance of contraception in less developed countries are hard to come by. One either finds "preliminary" accounts of undocumented enthusiasm (cf. ref. 12) or evasion of statistics. The data of Agarwala[11] represent the outcome of many years of family planning programmes of official government health agencies with some voluntary group effort—the record is one of dismal inadequacy. When they offered for use primarily intravaginal foam tablets having relatively poor contraceptive efficiency, Wyon and Gordon[20] found after four years of study in the Punjab that of the eligible fertile women in a group of villages of about 16,000 population, 39 per cent at one time or another used the method but 17 per cent emerged as fairly regular users. This was inadequate for any useful effect on the birth rate. A project on a tea plantation in Ceylon where a pill was offered[21] resulted in accessions of 159 women in 1963 which rose to 290 in early 1965. The birth rate in the fertile community in which pill users were a minority fell from 29·0 per 1,000 at the beginning of the study to 21·1 at the end—a significant drop. In a village on the Nile delta in Egypt 524 families were questioned about family planning in 1962. By 1966 57 per cent were using contraceptive methods: 220 accepted the use of oral contraceptives and 79 other methods. After one year of an action programme in Taichung City, Taiwan[22], 13 per cent of all married women aged 20 to 29 became contraceptors, about 80 per cent of these choosing intrauterine devices; the total choosing contraception amounts to 20–25 per cent of those considered "eligible", i.e. not already using contraceptives, pregnant or sterile. Instances could be multiplied with considerable variations from locality to locality.

More pertinent to the problem is the question of consistency of use of any method. It is all very well to enlist couples as contraceptors, but how long do they remain as users? Fig. 7 shows data from three projects in which oral contraceptives were offered and three in which the intrauterine device known as the "loop" was used[23]. It may be seen that for Slough the data indicate that after four years over 60 per cent of the women starting on oral contraceptives remain as users whereas in Bombay only 30 per cent remained after about the same period of time. For the intrauterine device experience is less, but after two years in a study in the United States 60 per cent remained as users and after only one and a half years in Taiwan about

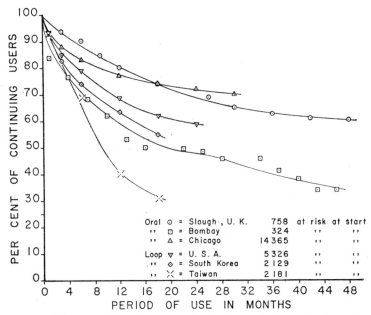

FIG. 7. All drop-outs for all reasons, including loss to follow-up, in six studies of contraceptive use.

30 per cent remained. Depending on the locality the rates of drop-out may obviously vary considerably.

Some years ago we initiated a project in Puerto Rico and Haiti in which women volunteering for study were assigned in a random fashion either to an oral contraceptive (Enovid, 5 mg.) or a vaginal foam or jelly. This was called the Maternal Health Study and involved regular follow-up of the volunteers with annual physical examinations, various laboratory tests, careful medical histories, and so on. Tallies were kept of women leaving the projects and their reasons for so doing. Table VIII presents the data collected on these drop-outs, with 16 categories of their reasons for leaving and the percentages of those leaving assignable to each category. The Puerto Rico clinics were at Rio Piedras, which is a lower-class section of metropolitan San Juan, Caguas, which is a town approximately 25 miles from San Juan, and Ponce, the second city of Puerto Rico. The Haiti clinic is in the capital city, Port-au-Prince.

The data of Table VIII have several noteworthy features, but first some characteristics of the communities involved should be noted. Puerto Rico, with a population of 2·7 million, has had a rather lengthy history of action programmes for birth control under a law which sanctions contraceptive advice and makes legal voluntary sterilization in either sex; there has also been propaganda and campaigning against birth control by various Catholic organizations. Haiti, with a population of 4· 8 million, has had no organized family planning or governmental sanction until very recently; sterilization is not legal and information on birth control has been limited for various reasons.

Taking the various categories in order, we observe: (1) leaving due to lack of interest is small and about the same in all clinics; (2) changing to another contraceptive method consistently occurs most frequently in vaginal contraceptive users in all clinics; (3) sterilization of the wife accounts for a small but significant percentage in Puerto Rico and occurs most frequently among vaginal contraceptive users; (4) sterilization of or separation from the husband is obviously more frequent in the Puerto Rico clinics, and in fact all of those leaving in Haiti did so because of loss of or separation from a husband; (5) the husband's opposition to the method used is somewhat more frequent in the Puerto Rico groups, but in both Puerto Rico and Haiti the vaginal method is regularly considered less desirable; (6) illness is a minor cause for leaving in all groups; (7) complaints of undesirable effects of use are much more frequent among oral contraceptive users and account for about one-fifth of the drop-outs among the users in Rio Piedras and Caguas; (8) propaganda against oral contraceptives is primarily responsible for the leavers in this category in Puerto Rico; (9) and (10) are categories with relatively minor occurrences and roughly similar in frequencies throughout; (11) is the major cause for leaving among oral contraceptive users in Haiti and presumably reflects lack of understanding or carelessness in a relatively illiterate group of volunteers under rather strict supervision—it is possible that the degree of permissiveness or compulsion on the part of the supervisors concerned may play a role at all the clinics; (12) and (13) represent women lost to supervision—here it would appear that the Haitian users of vaginal contraceptives tend by moving to be lost to follow-up most frequently, but we suspect this loss is due to dissatisfaction with the method and often deliberate evasion of attempts to find the subjects; (14) is a minor but significant cause for leaving in Puerto Rico but negligible in Haiti; (15) reflects failure to follow directions in oral contraceptive users and the known deficiencies of vaginal contraception; (16) is a category which includes primarily those for whom no reason for leaving has been obtained.

Among the major features of these data are the marked differences in reasons for leaving collected in Haiti and in Puerto Rico. Attitudes of the subjects and of the project supervisors may be responsible for these dif-

Table VIII

PATIENTS LOST TO MATERNAL HEALTH STUDY AT FOUR CLINICS (% OF TOTAL LEAVING)

Category no.	Reason for discontinuance	Rio Piedras		Caguas		Ponce		Haiti	
		Oral	Other	Oral	Other	Oral	Other	Oral	Other
1	Not interested	2·9	1·5	2·1	0·4	4·2	4·5	1·3	0·6
2	Changed to another contraceptive method	12·9	22·4	6·8	16·5	1·8	8·8	0·0	5·5
3	Sterilized or hysterectomized	3·1	4·7	3·1	6·7	1·1	1·3	0·2	0·1
4	Separated or husband sterilized	9·1	7·6	22·5	8·9	9·3	13·2	5·0	3·7
5	Husband opposed	3·8	5·8	4·2	9·8	3·2	3·9	0·6	3·5
6	Illness	3·3	0·9	2·1	0·9	3·4	0·4	1·3	0·1
7	Complaints	22·3	2·3	19·4	0·9	6·3	0·2	6·4	2·9
8	Fear, adverse conflict, propaganda or religion	5·9	0·6	8·9	0·4	2·1	0·2	0·2	0·1
9	Refused physical check-up	4·0	5·1	3·1	1·3	0·3	0·4	1·0	1·0
10	Private doctor's orders	2·7	0·2	0·0	0·0	0·0	0·2	0·1	0·0
11	Did not follow instructions	6·4	7·2	2·1	1·3	0·0	1·1	59·0	16·5
12	Moved away	11·0	10·0	9·9	12·5	14·0	10·3	20·6	49·5
13	Deceased	0·0	0·2	0·6	0·4	0·3	0·2	0·3	0·2
14	Wanted another child	2·1	2·3	3·1	2·2	1·1	1·7	0·5	0·0
15	Pregnancy	8·2	28·7	8·4	36·2	15·0	46·6	2·8	15·1
16	Miscellaneous, usually unspecified	2·4	1·1	4·3	1·3	28·0	6·9	0·8	1·2
	Total numbers of women	1,424	1,754	191	224	379	466	1,189	1,041

ferences in category assignment and should be regarded with some caution. Another feature which is clear is the preference for the oral contraceptive reflected in the proportions wishing to change method or to be sterilized (categories 2 and 3), in the alleged opposition of the husband (category 5), and in the occurrence of pregnancy in users (category 15). Undesired side effects and adverse propaganda (categories 7 and 8) are between them significant and perhaps related causes for oral contraceptive rejection. Failure to use the oral contraceptive method properly (categories 11 and 15) accounts for another significant group of leavers.

Table IX

PROPORTION OF PATIENTS LEAVING EXPOSED TO RISK OF CONCEPTION

(Categories 1, 5, 7, 8, 9, 11, 14 and 16)

Clinic	Per cent exposed	
	Oral	Other
Rio Piedras	49·8	25·9
Caguas	47·1	7·6
Ponce	43·2	18·9
Haiti	69·8	25·8

If we attempt to calculate the proportions of subjects leaving the project who then become exposed to the risk of conception, we arrive, using some obvious assumptions, at the data of Table IX. Superficially it would appear that the vaginal contraceptors may quit with less risk, but it is obvious that a high proportion become pregnant during use (category 15) compared to the oral contraceptive users. If we add the data of this category to those of Table IX, we emerge with figures of 43 to 65 per cent for vaginal contraceptors and 55 to 72 per cent for oral contraceptors. If this were to occur in a single year, marked effects upon the birth rate would not be likely. However, when we calculate annual rates of leaving (Table X), we observe in the various groups percentages varying from 8·9 to 40 per cent in any one year (or portion thereof). These data indicate also the consistent tendency in 1965 and 1966 for a greater proportion of drop-outs in vaginal contraceptors in all clinics.

From the percentages leaving listed in Table X it might be deduced that the study populations have declined over the years. Since a recruitment programme has been followed in each study centre, there has in fact been an increase from year to year in the number of cases listed as active (Table XI). The sources of additions were new cases recruited at hospitals *post partum* or through neighbours or friends or by visit in certain areas, but

POPULATION GROWTH AND AGE COMPOSITION

Table X

PERCENTAGES OF STUDY POPULATION LISTED AS INACTIVATED, DISCONTINUED, LOST TO FOLLOW-UP OR DEAD

Clinic	1963		1964		1965		1966	
	Oral	Other	Oral	Other	Oral	Other	Oral	Other
Rio Piedras	15·2*	12·8*	21·8	31·8	31·6	43·2	19·3†	29·2†
Caguas	13·4‡	25·2‡	18·8	17·1	18·2	22·1	12·4§	13·1§
Ponce	—	—	13·1¶	8·9¶	22·8	26·1	18·5§	24·2§
Haiti	18·0¶	30·9¶	37·7	27·1	30·9	40·0	34·7§	37·5§

* Period of 3 months.
† Period of 10 months
‡ Period of 4 months
§ Period of 11 months.
¶ Period of 5 months.

quite interesting were those who returned after leaving and who were listed as reactivated. The proportion so listed are presented in Table XII, which indicates that after the initial year of recruitment drop-outs tend to return in significant ratio to the total study population. Furthermore, they return to the use of the contraceptive originally assigned and with no clearly pre-ferential return to one type over the other.

Table XI

ACTIVE CASES IN THE MATERNAL HEALTH STUDY

Clinic	1963		1964		1965		1966	
	Oral	Other	Oral	Other	Oral	Other	Oral	Other
Rio Piedras	569*	588*	969	869	1,015	798	1,095	824†
Caguas	123‡	98‡	239	223	329	303	353§	324§
Ponce	—	—	299¶	306¶	640	592	905§	814§
Haiti	441‡	264‡	519	471	715	568	735§	605§

* 4 months.
† 10 months
‡ 5 months.
§ 11 months.
¶ 6 months.

Since these are primarily populations recruited for study and research, it is difficult to draw conclusions that may be significant for public health or hospital clinics. Moreover, we have no good means of determining accurately either the composition or nature of the base population drawn upon and the authentic effects on birth rates. Our data do show, however, that family limitation involves a population in flux, that regular increase in recruitment may occur over a number of years, that return to

Table XII

PERCENTAGES OF ACTIVE CASES LISTED AS REACTIVATED

Clinic	1963		1964		1965		1966	
	Oral	Other	Oral	Other	Oral	Other	Oral	Other
Rio Piedras	4·6*	4·1*	12·0	13·7	11·7	18·4	8·7	12·6†
Caguas	4·9‡	5·1‡	4·2	5·3	7·9	8·8	7·9§	5·9§
Ponce	—	—	0·7¶	0·7¶	15·2	8·4	15·6§	16·2§
Haiti	12·9‡	26·9‡	15·4	15·7	19·0	17·8	14·1§	20·7§

* 4 months.
† 10 months.
‡ 5 months
§ 11 months.
¶ 6 months.

contraception is a ponderable phenomenon among leavers, and that either of the methods employed may initially be accepted equally and the ratio of users of both may be rather well maintained over several years.

Considerations of population pressures and birth rates often lead to the benefits of fertility control to mother, children and family being ignored. Guttmacher[24] has summarized some of these benefits. Contraception has value: (a) in early marriage during the period of mutual adjustment, (b) in preventing some of the undesirable phenomena attendant upon too-frequent pregnancy, (c) in preventing the morbidity and mortality attendant upon late birth order among both mothers and children, (d) in preventing aggravation of illness and disease in the many conditions in which pregnancy is contraindicated, (e) in preventing inherited disease, (f) in preventing the many consequences of pregnancy occurring out of wedlock. The particular values of contraception to families of lower economic status have been studied intensively by Rainwater and Weinstein[25], and the social consequences of ethical and value judgments affected by responsible parenthood have been many times discussed, e.g. by Fagley[26]. The general judgment is clear that both physical and mental health may be promoted by judicious family planning.

CONCLUSIONS

The foregoing discussion has involved a set of fairly simple propositions: (a) world population increase rates are accelerating to a point of over-population unless control is exercised, (b) population increase is outstripping resources, particularly in less developed countries, (c) a major source of the increase is a maintenance of birth rates in the face of declining death rates, (d) this leads to an excess of young individuals of reproductive age, thus enhancing population increase potential, (e) reduction in birth rates would appear to be the most practical means of checking excess population increase, (f) among methods which have been employed, abortion as a public policy has worked effectively, particularly in Japan, (g) in most countries the use of contraceptives would appear to be more acceptable, (h) extremely efficient contraceptive methods have been developed in recent years and two of them, the oral ovulation-inhibiting steroid preparations and the intrauterine devices, appear to have an excellent potential for widespread use, (i) large-scale experience with these methods is still in process, but the available data suggest fair acceptance and maintenance of use with considerable variation from country to country, and (j) the contribution to maternal and child health through contraception of spaced childbirths and birth limitation with the attendant hygienic measures requires elaboration.

DISCUSSION

Florey : This is what has been called the age of rising expectations. Everybody expects the quality of their life to get better, but in fact some things may well get worse, and in many parts of the world there is not much hope of improvement for, say, the rest of this century. Dr. Pincus mentioned motivation and I believe that this is very important, particularly in countries where the problems are not obvious. For example, in this country projections that were made in 1955 on the basis of current trends showed that the net reproduction rate would fall to less than one by 1975. Then for some completely unknown reason the birth rate started to rise and it went on rising until last year. Why this happened nobody knows. Perfectly good birth control methods and propaganda were available, and there was no inhibition of discussion.

The theme of this session is the major factors aggravating world health problems, and the increase in population is unquestionably one of those factors.

Wright: Can the population figures at the end of this century be reduced below the UN median forecast, which is of the order of 6,000 million people? There are difficulties, I think, in feeling that anything substantial can be done before the end of the century. Firstly, the UN median forecast is already well below the figures based on the continuation of the present trends, as Dr. Pincus has pointed out; on present trends the world population would go up to 7,000 million or more by A.D. 2000. Secondly, the longer expectation of life automatically increases the total population. Thirdly, the reduction in child death rates means that an increasing number of women reach child-bearing age, so that even if the size of the family is reduced the number of the families is likely to be increased. In Great Britain it took 60 years for the number of live births per family to fall from just under six to just over two. This was in a country where we had reasonable communications during the period accompanying the industrial revolution. We are now expecting the problem to be solved within 33 years in the underdeveloped countries, where communications, treatment and so on are still lacking. It is very important to remember this, certainly from the point of view of food supplies between now and the end of the century.

Wolman: The statistical prophecies appear to take no account of any of the anticipated and hopeful economic changes in any of the countries we are discussing. This troubles me a great deal, especially as the statistical prophecies of the last 40–50 years have been distinguished largely by their errors and not by their accuracies. All the statistical prophets in the 1930's were completely wrong. A secondary point is that the rise in the standard of living may possibly result in an automatic change in birth rates.

Fanconi: In Manila in 1965 I had a long discussion with a paediatrician, Miss Fe del Mundo, on the question of birth control in the Philippines. The rate of increase in the population there is very high, and it is very difficult to have birth control because it is a primitive Catholic country. When I asked her if she thought it was right to help parents to have very large families in such poor conditions, Miss Fe del Mundo said simply that it was her duty. Later a well-known phrase of Kant's came to my mind: "Two things impress my soul more and more—the stars in the sky and the moral law in me". Changing this phrase a little, I could say: "Two things impress my soul as a physician and as a paediatrician—the enormous progress of medical science going on around me, and inside me the need to help and to conserve the life of people even if they are poor, retarded and abnormal."

Pincus: I would be even more frank than you, Professor Fanconi: I would say that the Catholic Church is the biggest impediment that I know of to the spread of adequate means of birth control and its use throughout the world. Fortunately it is not a very great impediment. In Puerto Rico, where we conducted our experiments, religious objections to the use of oral contraceptives accounted for the refusal of only about one woman in a hundred, in a fairly good survey of possible long-term use. In terms of practical application, I suspect that it isn't as difficult as might have been implied by what your Philippine doctor said. The difficulty probably lies in getting the medical profession to realize its duty, because people turn to them for advice. In Puerto Rico the response of the medical profession was at first so unanimously disapproving that we were only able to recruit one doctor to help us. Now the situation has changed: the island is dotted with clinics to which Catholic physicians come to give advice on contraceptives. The same thing is now happening throughout Chile and in many other Latin American countries. The trend is definitely there but whether it will be adequately upsurging remains to be seen.

Candau: What was a religious problem will very soon become a political problem unless we can stop the pressure being brought to bear by foreigners on other countries. The great obstacles to birth control in many countries are: (1) the existence of minority groups anxious to increase their numbers and their political influence. This, with all the implications involved, deters a government from advocating a family planning programme, though for obvious reasons it is not publicized; (2) the desire of white populations not to give the impression that they are afraid of being numerically overwhelmed by populations of other colours. These observations arise from my experience in dealing with many countries.

I think the figures for the cost of the control of abortion refer to illegal abortion, and have nothing to do with legal abortion as a method of birth control. We should keep this in mind because the cost of the complications of illegal abortion is completely different. To apply birth control to large numbers we need still simpler methods. If we could find a pill that we could give once a month, it could be used for populations with very low levels of education. I think this is an important point. Again, the intra-uterine device will have to be better than the one we have today, with which the failure rate is about 25 per cent. Medical research could do a lot for us public health people by finding a better birth control method.

Evang: Dr. Pincus showed that the increase in population started in Europe about 300 years ago, around 1650. In India or any similar country exactly the same thing occurred, except that the turning point came 100 years later, in 1750. This is why the so-called white races have increased much more rapidly than all the coloured races of the world so far. As Dr. Candau pointed out, it is therefore highly provocative if the white races, who have already had all the opportunities to increase, approach in a tactless way the question of increase of the coloured races, especially in Africa, where these feelings are very strong. So far I know of only one African country where the government has overcome this point and specifically asked for assistance in population control.

I agree that none of the existing methods of contraception is satisfactory and here of course the relationship between motivation and method comes in. Dr. Pincus referred to the experiment in the Punjab, where the people were given the choice between five different types of contraceptives. The foam tablet was chosen and the acceptance rate was very high during the pilot period but then it just petered out, for the simple reason that the method was not safe. Women are the same all over the world—they do not produce children on the basis of world statistics but on the basis of their personal situation. In Norway we thought we saw the victory at El Alamein reflected nine months later by an increase in the birth rate. Similarly the cold war was reflected in 1948 by a decreased birth rate, in spite of the fact that the economic boom worked the other way. The sociologists would have to be brought in here.

Florey: The point has been made that this is no longer a religious but a political problem. Are we to infer that we should fold our hands and do absolutely nothing, letting these people starve to death if that is what they want to do?

Candau: No; I think that the pressure of foreigners alone will not solve the problem. Pressure cannot be brought to bear from outside; one has to create a motivation within the population itself. $10 invested in birth control is said to be worth more than $100,000 invested in economic development, but no country is going to accept this. The position is very clear—we have to educate the people of the country in this respect. No method of birth control can be effective without a minimum of health services and this is where the problem lies. From the point of view of safety and efficacy, we are discrediting the present methods by the way we are using them; we are discrediting the intrauterine device by the way we are using it—it is a reasonably good method and quite cheap if it is used in the correct way, but it cannot be used as it has been in several countries of the world today. We are already disillusioned with it.

Florey: By "we" in this context I suppose that white people are meant. Do you propose to leave it entirely to the Indians or the Africans to solve their own problems? Or if "we" take a hand are we going to be accused of trying to reduce their populations by back-door methods?

Candau: I don't think it is such a difficult problem, because in all these countries there are leaders who can shoulder their own responsibilities. We must be able to show the leaders of these countries what the needs are and their importance in relation to the development of the country. What we need to know is how a particular country is going to develop economically, and what manpower it needs. Pressure cannot be exerted from outside. Motivation inside a country has to be created to get the right results.

REFERENCES

1. Freedom from Hunger Campaign, Basic Study No. 7. (1962). *Population and Food Supply*. New York: UN Office of Public Information, Sales No. 62.1.22.
2. Population Reference Bureau. (1959). *Population Bulletin*, **15,** 28.
3. Population Studies, No. 28. (1958). *The Future Growth of World Population*. New York: UN Dept. of Economic and Social Affairs, Sales No. 58. XIII. 2.
4. Food and Agriculture Organization. (1960). *The State of Food and Agriculture*. Rome: FAO.
5. See ref. 1.
6. Hauser, P. M. (1960). *Population Perspectives*. New Brunswick, New Jersey: Rutgers University Press.
7. Mudd, S. (ed.) (1964). *The Population Crisis and the Use of World Resources*. The Hague: Junk.
8. Kiser, C. V. (ed.) (1962). *Research in Family Planning*. Princeton, New Jersey: Princeton University Press.
9. Greep, R. O. (ed.) (1963). *Human Fertility and Population Problems*. Cambridge, Massachusetts: Schenkman.
10. Whelpton, P. K., Campbell, A. A., and Patterson, J. E. (1965). *Fertility and Family Planning in the United States*. Princeton, New Jersey: Princeton University Press.
11. Agarwala, S. N. (1966). Some aspects of the family planning programme. *Journal of Family Welfare*, **12,** no. 4, p. 1.
12. Berelson, B., Anderson, R. X., Harkavy, O., Maier, J., Mauldin, W. P., and Segal, S. J. (eds.) (1966). *Family Planning and Population Programs*. Chicago, Illinois: University of Chicago Press.
13. Koya, Y., Muramatsu, M., Agata, S., and Koya, T. (1953). Preliminary report of a survey of health and demographic aspects of induced abortion in Japan. *Archives of the Population Association of Japan*, **2,** 1–9.
14. Muramatsu, M. (1966). Japan. In *Family Planning and Population Programs*, pp. 7–19, ed. Berelson, B., Anderson, R. K., Harkavy, O., Maier, J., Mauldin, W. P., and Segal, S. J. Chicago, Illinois: University of Chicago Press.
15. Armijo, R., and Monreal, T. (1965). Epidemiology of provoked abortion in Santiago, Chile. In *Population Dynamics*, pp. 137–160, ed. Muramatsu, M., and Harper, P. A. Baltimore, Maryland: Johns Hopkins Press.
16. Venning, G. R. (1965). The influence of contraceptive practice upon maternal and child health. *Metabolism* **14,** 457.
17. Pincus, G. (1965). *The Control of Fertility*. New York: Academic Press.
18. Mears, E. (1965). Clinical application of oral contraceptives. In *Agents Affecting Fertility*, pp. 211–243, eds. Austin, C. G. and Perry, J. S. London: J. and A. Churchill.
19. Venning, G. R. (1965). Contraception and world population. In *Ovulation*, pp. 178–199, ed. Greenblatt, R. B. Philadelphia: J. B. Lippincott.
20. Wyon, J. B., and Gordon, J. E. (1962). In *Research in Family Planning*, pp. 17–65, ed. Kiser, C. V. Princeton, New Jersey: Princeton University Press.
21. Venning, G. R. (1966). Reduction in the birthrate in a community associated with the administration of oral contraceptives. *Research on Steroids*, **2,** 435–438.

147

22. Berelson, B. (1965). Family planning programs in Taiwan. In *Population Dynamics*, pp. 87–97, eds. Muramatsu, M., and Harper, P. A. Baltimore, Maryland: Johns Hopkins Press.
23. Venning, G. R. Unpublished data.
24. Guttmacher, A. (1959). *Babies by Choice or by Chance*. Garden City, New York: Doubleday.
25. Rainwater, L., and Weinstein, K. K. (1960). *And the Poor Get Children*. Chicago, Illinois: Quadrangle Books.
26. Fagley, R. M. (1960). *The Population Explosion and Christian Responsibility*. New York: Oxford University Press.

8

FAULTY NUTRITION: FAILURES IN FOOD SUPPLY, VARIETY AND DISTRIBUTION

Sir Norman Wright

British Association for the Advancement of Science

I N considering how far faulty nutrition should be classed as one of the
major factors aggravating world health problems I have assumed that
my task is twofold: first, to indicate what proportion of the world's
population is affected by such faulty nutrition and what are its consequences in relation to world health, and second, to assess the extent to
which either present or improved health services could be expected to
ameliorate the resulting aggravation. For this purpose it will be desirable
to deal with the subject under two major heads: the effect of failures in the
total supplies of food, which lead primarily to *undernutrition*, and the
effect of *lack of variety in the food supplies*, which is the primary cause
of *malnutrition*, and therefore of the incidence of specific deficiency
diseases.

UNDERNUTRITION

Turning first to undernutrition, namely the extent to which people have
insufficient to eat in terms of their total energy or calorie requirements, the
facts are, I think, undisputed. It is, of course, true that the *per caput* energy
requirements of the less developed countries, which are chiefly located in
the tropics or sub-tropics, are generally smaller than those of the developed
countries in temperate areas such as ours. Thus, with higher environmental
temperatures the energy requirement is lowered, and the smaller body size
and lower body weight of most tropical inhabitants further reduce their
food needs. Moreover the relatively lower level of working activity which
is typical of many underdeveloped areas also reduces the need for food.

On the other hand, it must equally be recognized that, apart from the environmental temperatures, the other two variables are themselves affected by the level of food intake; low supplies of calories due to poverty are important contributory causes both of reduced body size and lower body weight, and of reduced working activity. In this sense food requirement figures must surely always be considered from a dynamic rather than a static aspect, otherwise man will find himself in a vicious circle of poverty leading to low food intake; low food intake leading to reduced body-weight and low levels of activity; low levels of activity leading to decreased productivity; and decreased productivity leading to still greater poverty.

Moreover, a deficiency in the total food supplies of a country, when expressed in terms of an average figure, fails to reveal differences between different areas and different social groups within that country, and therefore fails to give a true measure of the degree of undernutrition of the poorer-fed sections of the population. Further, a country whose population lives at a subsistence level, with no possibility of building up local reserves and with no adequate communications for the distribution of relief supplies, is particularly vulnerable to seasonal changes in food production, and catastrophically vulnerable to crop failures, which can rapidly produce famine conditions.

Quantitatively the most recent and authoritative estimate of the extent of undernutrition is that published by FAO in its *Third World Food Survey*[1]. Briefly the survey shows that the proportion of undernourished people would seem to lie between 10 and 15 per cent. Expressed in this way the proportion may not appear very striking. But if the percentages are converted into absolute figures, they indicate that *no less than 300 to 500 million people in the world are actually hungry and underfed* in terms of their total calorie intake.

I cannot emphasize too strongly the adverse effects of such undernutrition on the health of any population. As most of you will know, observations in countries where there have been degrees of undernutrition varying from severe though temporary food shortages (as in the two world wars) to semi-starvation (as in many natural famines) indicate that under such conditions there is not only weight loss and reduction in physical activity, but also characteristic behavioural symptoms. These are seen as lack of mental alertness and coherent and creative thinking, apathy, depression and irritability—leading in extreme instances to an increasing loss of moral standards and social ties. There is, too, clear evidence that such undernutrition is one of the most potent factors in lowering resistance to disease.

Unfortunately this is a field in which even the most efficient health services can do little to alleviate the position, since the problem is essentially one of providing more adequate total supplies of food—a responsibility which rests primarily on those concerned with agricultural production or with the alternative means (provided foreign currency is available) of increasing food supplies by importation.

In most of the less developed countries, there are, however, inadequacies not only in the quantity of food, but also in its quality—leading to malnutrition as well as to undernutrition. In the developed countries the diet is commonly drawn from a wide variety of sources, and staple cereals and starchy roots do not constitute an abnormally high proportion of the total food intake. The reverse is true of the less developed countries[2]. Thus, whereas the proportion of staple cereals and starchy roots in the North American diet is estimated to be only 25 per cent, and in the British diet less than 30 per cent, in Latin America it is 54 per cent, in Africa 66, in the Near East 71 and in the Far East over 73 per cent. Conversely, while the proportion of animal products—milk, meat, eggs and fish—in the North American diet reaches the exceptionally high figure of 40 per cent, and in the British diet nearly 30 per cent, the figure for Latin America is only 17 per cent, for Africa 11, for the Near East 9, and for the Far East 5 per cent. These differences are reflected in a shortage of protein, and particularly of animal protein, in the diets of the less developed countries. Simultaneously, owing to the lack of variety, such diets also tend to lack adequate quantities of vitamins and essential mineral constituents. This in turn leads to the incidence of specific deficiency diseases—diseases which are now seldom encountered in the more developed countries.

Of these diseases, probably the most widespread in its incidence and the most damaging in its effects, particularly with children, is *kwashiorkor*, which is due primarily to protein-calorie deficiencies. The typical symptoms of the acute form of this disease are oedema and skin sores, accompanied by liver degeneration; unless promptly treated by the administration of supplementary protein the child usually dies.

Acute cases of this nature form, however, only a small part of the total problem of protein-calorie deficiencies in children. Less acute cases are widely prevalent, and may not only result in lasting though concealed damage but frequently intensify the effects of diseases such as measles or dysentery, with a resulting high death rate not found among better-fed populations.

Side by side with kwashiorkor I should also mention *marasmus*, characterized by wasting in place of oedema and associated less with specific protein deficiency than with a diet generally unsatisfactory in both quantity and quality—yet no less fatal to the young child. There is accumulating evidence that both these conditions are common not only in Africa, but also in many parts of Central and Latin America, and in Asia and the Far East.

Kwashiorkor is, however, not the only deficiency disease attributable to malnutrition in the less developed countries. In many Eastern countries *avitaminosis A* is stated to be at least as potent as smallpox and venereal disease in destroying children's sight, and it is still prevalent in certain areas of Africa, of Asia and of Latin America. *Pellagra* is still endemic among populations which subsist largely on a maize diet; it is found in areas of Africa and the Near East and, sporadically, in Latin America. *Rickets*, normally rare in tropical countries, exists nevertheless in Africa, in parts of Asia and in the Near East. Finally, *nutritional anaemia*, associated with iron deficiency, still constitutes a serious health hazard, especially among expectant mothers and young children, and is the principal factor affecting maternal death rate in a number of the less developed countries.

On a world scale the extent of malnutrition is difficult to assess, since there are few reliable figures either to indicate the incidence of the deficiency diseases which I have mentioned, or to gauge the extent of increased susceptibility to infectious conditions and of lack of full health and vigour which result from diets which are inadequate in either quantity or quality.

The unreliability of mortality statistics is incidentally well illustrated in a comparison made between figures taken from the civil register in one Latin-American country with those obtained in a special study undertaken by the Nutrition Institute of Central America and Panama (INCAP)[3] where, out of 109 deaths in children aged one to four years, the study revealed that 40 occurred in those with signs and symptoms of severe malnutrition, though only *one* was listed in the civil register as "death resulting from malnutrition". As has recently been stated in a WHO publication[4] (which also provides a useful summary of existing knowledge of malnutrition and disease) "...unless a country possesses a good system of communications, a literate population, the means whereby sick people can be efficiently examined by medically qualified persons, and accurate records of the number and causes of disease and death, there will be little or no sound knowledge on which to base an idea of the extent of disease and the level of health. In few places do such conditions exist."

Nevertheless, by using a less direct method of assessment, i.e. by combining such evidence as is available on the extent of malnutrition in individual less developed countries with an estimate of its incidence in well-developed countries enjoying high nutritional standards, FAO's *Third World Food Survey* has concluded that up to half of the world's population, or *between 1,000 and 1,500 million people, suffer today from either undernutrition or malnutrition or both.*

I have already referred to the fact that even the most efficient health services can do little to alleviate the problem of undernutrition; the same difficulty arises in relation to malnutrition, since the provision of an adequately varied diet depends primarily on a country's food production and on its food import policies. Nevertheless there are directions in which the health services can play a valuable part. The passage which I have already quoted from the WHO publication[4] clearly indicates the need for more thorough studies of the incidence of deficiency diseases in the less developed countries—an obvious responsibility of the health services. With the help of such studies these services could provide valuable guidance as to the directions in which the production of specific protective foods should be encouraged. Moreover, some of the deficiency diseases, once identified, can be alleviated by specific supplements to the diet, while nutrition education, leading to a better appreciation of the need for dietary improvements, is also a field in which the health services should be clearly and closely concerned. But at best these can only be considered as steps in the right direction; as with undernutrition, the alleviation of malnutrition must primarily be the responsibility of those concerned with a country's agricultural production or with the extent of its food imports.

FUTURE FOOD NEEDS

I have so far only dealt with the problems of undernutrition and malnutrition as they exist today. In the preceding paper Dr. Pincus indicated the far greater problem with which we are likely to be faced in the future as a result of the increase in the rate of population growth. If we are to appreciate the extent to which the failures in food supply, variety and distribution are likely to aggravate world health problems during the remainder of the century, it would seem desirable to determine what these combined problems of present malnutrition and of future population growth will mean in terms of the world's future food needs, and whether these needs are likely to be met.

As regards the world's future food needs, I propose to confine my estimates to two main groups of foods, namely cereals and animal products (in which I include milk, meat, eggs and of course fish). Briefly, based on the existing dietary levels in the developed countries, and on reasonably

153

SIR NORMAN WRIGHT

improved levels in the less developed countries, it appears that by 1975—
only eight years hence—we shall have to increase the world's cereal production by over one-third, and the world's output of animal products by
nearly two-thirds. By the year A.D. 2000, only 33 years from now, we
shall have to have doubled the world's cereal production and trebled its
output of animal products. Indeed, for some of the less developed countries
to achieve fully adequate dietary levels by this date in order to avoid the
risks of malnutrition, their outputs of animal products will have to be increased by from fourfold to sixfold over the present levels. Can this be done?

The possibility of increasing food supplies

The answer is, in theory, "yes". Recent careful studies[5] of the potentialities of the world's agriculture and fisheries indicate that, provided the
less developed countries can and will adopt modern production techniques
—for example, the provision of irrigation, the application of artificial
fertilizers, the breeding of better seeds, the adoption of mechanized agricultural techniques, the utilization of plant pesticides, and the control of
animal diseases, as well as the improvement of fishing methods and the
adoption of fish culture (to mention some of the main requirements)—
provided the less developed countries can and will adopt these techniques, we can
foresee the possibility of increasing food production on a sufficiently large
scale to meet the world's food needs up to the end of the century.

It will, however, also be essential to dovetail these improved techniques
with increased capital investment, with improvements in economic incentives, with structural improvements in such basic factors as land tenure,
with organizational improvements in the agricultural and related services
and with increases in the purchasing power of the consumer.

I have said that the answer *in theory* is that the needed increases could be
achieved. It is likely, however, that achievement *in practice* will be far
more open to question, hedged in as it is with so many provisos and so many
imponderables. Certainly FAO's latest estimates of world food production[6] provide no grounds for optimism. As its Director-General states in
his foreword to these estimates: "Any remaining complacency about the
food and agriculture situation must surely have been dispelled by the events
of the past year. As a result of widespread drought world food production
...was no larger in 1965/66 than the year before, when there were 70
million less people to feed." And, after referring to the depletion in the
world's food stocks, he adds "*Thus the world food situation is now more pre-
carious than at any time since the period of acute shortage immediately after the
second world war.*"

CONCLUSIONS

The conclusions of the present paper seem obvious. The shortage in the world's food supply, as well as the defects in its variety and distribution, already represents a major factor aggravating world health problems and, save for a miracle of organization and will-power on the part of developed and developing countries alike, will remain such a major aggravating factor within the foreseeable future—an aggravating factor which, alas, even the provision of the most adequate health services can do little to alleviate.

Nevertheless it would seem to me only fair to add (though I have not dealt specifically with this aspect of the subject in my paper) that health improvement, in so far as it leads to greatly accelerated population increase, is as aggravating a factor in tackling the world's food problem as is food shortage and lack of variety an aggravating factor in hindering health improvement. This can hardly be termed a vicious circle, for the factors involved are contradictory and not supplementary. It does represent, however, a baffling paradox which must be as much the concern of those responsible for the world's health services as of those struggling to meet the world's food needs.

DISCUSSION

Florey: This is very like the situation in medicine: we are getting very good at diagnosis nowadays but the therapy is not quite so good. What therapy could be used to deal with the disease diagnosed by Sir Norman Wright?

Doxiadis: Sir Norman, you started by speaking of the dynamics of the situation. How does the percentage of underfed people today compare with that of any other period of the past?

Wright: No adequate international records were kept until FAO came into existence in 1945, when one of the first things it did was to assess the position. Dr. Sen's statement which I quoted indicates that there cannot have been much improvement since the war years.

Doxiadis: Greece is a poor country, yet the population is probably much better fed now than at any other time in its history. This has happened in several countries, and so, although I recognize that speaking on a percentage basis is misleading, because we forget the hundreds of millions of people lying behind the percentages, I suspect that there has been a percentage improvement. Is this not a good sign?

Wright: Greece is one of the half-dozen developing countries where FAO has emphasized that food production has very substantially increased.

If this could be done by all the developing countries it would make an enormous difference to the world position; the trouble is that it is not being done, or in some countries it is only being done in certain areas. On a world basis total food production *per caput* has decreased. In the developing countries we have managed to make ends meet largely by using surpluses, notably those generously given by the United States, but the stocks are now going down and how they are going to be replaced we don't know.

le Riche: There are limits to the available arable land all over the world, even with the best use, and the costs of the utilization of this land are going up and up. In the underdeveloped countries the capital to buy the machines to do some of the reclamation work isn't there, the people to teach the farmers to do this are lacking, and it is often very difficult to change the agricultural methods. This is part of the problem. There are even countries whose food production has decreased. Since oil production has expanded in Libya less food has been grown and instead canned food is imported from the United States.

Doxiadis: But the additional oil produced in Libya has perhaps contributed to additional food production in other countries.

le Riche: Most of the oil is going to the developed countries which are already rich and not to the underdeveloped countries.

Doxiadis: Is there any hope that food production will increase if we are not forced to produce more by the need for more food? Is there any such parallel in our history or in the history of humanity as a whole?

le Riche: It is true that we will only produce more food if we are forced to do so, but the countries which can grow more food have possibly reached their maximum production on a sustained yield basis.

Evang: It is generally accepted, Dr. Doxiadis, that with the exception of some few underprivileged groups of people, on average the food status of the populations today is better than it has been before, as you said, with the exception again of some very few countries. On the other hand, to my mind, it is utterly impossible to use the experience of the past in a situation which is radically new: for the first time in the history of mankind quantitative problems turn up in the most awesome possible form, namely in the form of the size of the globe on which we live and the number of people and the amount of resources.

Querido: I would like to break down the problem into areas: China will look after itself, so that removes 800 million people. Are we therefore concerned mainly with Africa, India and Latin America? Were your figures based only on those areas, Sir Norman?

Wright: I purposely omitted any reference to regional differences. Walter Pawley[5] has shown that in North America and Europe food production should continue to be adequate. Latin America and Africa both have adequate natural resources, if properly developed, to produce enough food; the Near East could produce enough if the water problem could be solved—possibly by desalination if it could be made cheap enough. The real problem of the world is therefore the Far East, especially the Indian sub-continent. Here it is questionable whether the natural resources are sufficient to be able to produce sufficient food locally. In my view we have tended in our aid to underdeveloped countries to concentrate too much on Africa. The real problem area as far as food is concerned is Asia.

Beer: In some areas where there is semi-starvation or a grave shortage of food, sometimes up to 30 per cent of actual production is lost through inadequate storage and lack of knowledge about storage. Better internal local distribution could also greatly augment the supplies of food. On the question of regional distribution I don't think we should write off China— quite a lot of the Canadian surplus production has gone there. Chinese economists in China told me that their lack of adequate internal transport means that one area may have a surplus, while perhaps only 200 kilometres away there is starvation. I would agree that Asia is the vital area, but something could be done if one could do anything about storage, and also if one could, slowly, change some traditional food habits. The possibilities should also be considered of preserving fish or other protein sources by new freezing plants. How quickly do you think these factors can affect your figures?

Wright: There are perfectly good methods for improving storage, but they are just not adopted in the developing countries. One of the difficulties of getting them adopted is that the whole question of cost in relation to agricultural benefit has never been properly studied and stressed.

Candau: If one-third of the grain production of the world is destroyed by rats and other animals then in India about 50 per cent must be lost in this way. This is a cultural problem which is extremely difficult to solve. WHO has been fighting rats but only as vectors of plague, not as destroyers of food. FAO has done much more in the way of protection of food.

Kaprio: I was struck by the health education aspect when health was compared with the agricultural side. I visited a country where a heated discussion was going on about the rights of certain animals; at the same time that country had a crash programme for the intrauterine device. The development of rational thinking in these societies sometimes seems to be expected to happen much more quickly on the health side than in other fields. Perhaps we should have an international discussion about changing habits.

Evang: W. R. Aykroyd many years ago spoke of cassava as "the poor man's crop", and indicated that health education, even under the most difficult conditions, might change the type of crop produced. Secondly, mothers are strongly motivated to change their food habits if they see with their own eyes the improvement in the health of their children.

Banks: We have not really paid enough attention to the part that village women and women in general play in food education and health education, or to the influence that they can exert and can be persuaded to exert. Expectant mothers evacuated from London into rural regions during the Second World War at first refused to eat "rabbit food". But within a month or so they were very happily eating these "rabbit foods" because the midwives had good powers of persuasion and told them of the nutritional benefits to themselves and their children. Similarly the person who is going to persuade a woman not to have any more children is not the high-level bureaucrat, but the woman who has just delivered her, and who says: "Listen, my dear, you have had enough children. You must now stop."

Wolman: May I add a note of optimism? I have just come from Taiwan and land tenure has changed the whole agricultural situation in that country. There is a high degree of professional competence in agriculture, but this is accompanied by land banks, by co-operative credits, by the production of fertilizers, by what we would call the county farm agent, and so on. Coupled with that is the demonstration in India, for example, of the production of artificial fertilizers in the last few years. A recent review for the U.S. Agency for International Development indicated that India could within a period of 10—15 years become self-sustaining in food and it may be on the road to that goal by the combination of land tenure changes, the use of fertilizers, and more modern techniques. It is not quite true that one cannot transfer technology to a country with a great lack of sophistication. For example, transistor radios are used side by side with oxcarts on the same road into Calcutta; there is a tremendous production of transistor radios in an economy which is very backward in other directions. That kind of transfer of technology does take place even though we may be impatient with its rate of introduction.

Wright: The new techniques and fertilizers are certainly used to some extent. But land tenure in India is a very great problem. No government before or I believe after independence has dared to touch the system, which consists not only of the equal division of land between each son, but also the fragmentation of the good, the bad and the indifferent land, which goes equally to each—thereby reducing holdings to virtually uncultivable areas. The World Food Programme is providing food for certain areas where the land tenure system is being changed, a process which usually involves a temporary local food shortage, but the real difficulty is that the land tenure system is often so inborn in a country that it is very difficult to get rid of it.

de Haas: It is very difficult to separate malnutrition from diseases like malaria—malnutrition is much more serious if malaria is also present. After the war in many regions malaria was eradicated or partly eradicated and that gave the impression that the state of nutrition had been improved. On the other hand in the last few years malnutrition in Asia has apparently become even worse than previously. An optimistic element is our experience in 1964 in China, which was very impressive: we visited children's hospitals and departments in the big cities, we visited dozens of schools and crèches in towns and communes, and we walked through the streets, yet we did not see a single case of malnutrition. In a big Asian city like Shanghai, before 1950 notorious for its poverty, absence of malnutrition is a miracle.

One of the most shocking things about malnutrition in children is xerophthalmia, an eye disease caused by vitamin A deficiency which can be prevented by administering regularly a small dose of cod-liver oil or carotene. The protein problem is rather more difficult, especially from a world point of view, but xerophthalmia could be prevented more easily than rickets in European countries. As these toddlers usually suffer from general malnutrition death often has mercy on them before they become blind schoolchildren or adults.

Lambo: In the developing countries we have a large number of human problems peculiar to our environment. This discussion has stressed the interrelatedness of many factors: one cannot separate a segment of life from the others, and this is very important. Economic and political factors are interwoven and interrelated. Economic manipulation from other countries may spell disaster for young countries. For example, a country in Africa wanted to borrow money from a developed country but one of the conditions was that part of this money should be spent in the developed country and consequently disused war-planes were purchased! Similar conditions are often imposed, so dealings between nations do not seem to be as straightforward as one would wish.

Another point is that in developing countries it is often cheaper to import certain manufactured goods than to produce them locally.

Florey: In Japan we have an example of a country which is adapting itself with unbelievable speed to the condition known as modern civilization, although it has had very great problems to face.

Katsunuma: Our pattern of life is quite different from the western type and our nutritional problems are also somewhat different. The nutritional problems must be analysed locally if possible and the local problems must be considered when outside aid is given. Every inch of land is already fully cultivated in Japan, so the only thing we can do is to improve the methods of cultivation.

Florey: This necessity may be the spur that is needed everywhere.

Lindop: The natural resources and the time available are too small and too short for possible self-help in nutrition. The therapy we need is a technological breakthrough to tide us over until people could provide enough of the classical foodstuffs for themselves. The technical knowledge now exists for the production of high-quality protein by yeast from petroleum and crude oil[7] which could probably, if an all-out effort were made, cover this interim short-term period. But there are commercial interests vested in this particular technological breakthrough. When enquiries were made by a scientist in New Zealand for the particular strain of yeast which could enable developing countries to obtain such protein the oil companies were able to help neither with details of the method nor with the supply of a culture of the micro-organism[8].

It would be an extremely good thing if a group like ours, as well as making accurate diagnoses and assessments, could pinpoint the reasons why therapy for the state of the world is apparently failing at the moment. A lot of it is due to this problem of vested interests, even when the technological breakthrough is potentially there.

Pincus: The problem is the one that Dr. Candau pointed out, that is, the culture pattern of the country involved. We have the resources under our feet and out in the fields. The technology is not too difficult—the costs according to N. W. Pirie are certainly much less than the gains. When Pirie tried to introduce his protein-from-leaf-foliage method in several so-called underdeveloped countries, he met a solid wall of opposition, of the sort that people concerned with fertility control often meet. The culture pattern of a country is an important barrier.

Katsunuma: The protein content of our food in Japan is still low and we have been thinking about doing something with *Chlorella*, which can be used as a source of protein.

Evang: Norway has just been through a small political crisis because we stopped our fishermen taking from the ocean more of the extremely valuable fats and proteins, because there was no market for them, at the same time as we were discussing how we could assist developing countries to improve their nutrition. Is it really impossible to use all this beautiful protein, fats, and vitamins A and D, under the present circumstances?

Katsunuma: We eat a lot of fish, but the fishing industry is limited, for various reasons, and it is getting more expensive to buy fish. That is why I referred to the possibility of developing *Chlorella* in addition.

Cohen: Is kwashiorkor seen in Japan?

Katsunuma: I don't think so.

Cohen: That is very interesting in relationship to the percentage of proteins in cereals and animal products. We are apt to stress the animal proteins, but the cereal proteins can also make a significant contribution to the protein supply. This is particularly apparent in countries in which flour is an important constituent of the diet.

Querido: The WHO report in 1960 on endemic goitre[9] suggested that there are about 200 million goitrous people in the world. Adequate iodine prophylaxis can reduce this number to a small fraction. However, it is not easy to achieve this prophylaxis through salt enrichment in developing countries, because salt production and distribution may not be under government control. Another difficulty is the lack of roads to remote mountainous areas where generally the incidence of severe endemic goitre is the highest.

What I want to stress is not endemic goitre as such but the fact that it leads to a high incidence of endemic cretinism in severely affected areas, an incidence which is the same as it was when its existence was first reported centuries ago. I have had the doubtful privilege of seeing endemic cretinism in the classic areas such as the foothills of the Himalayas, the Andean mountains of Ecuador and the Highlands of New Guinea. This disease has a crippling effect on such communities—sometimes it affects up to 10 per cent of a community, and deaf-mutism alone can account for 5 per cent.

Endemic cretinism presents itself in a wide spectrum of irreversible physical and mental retardation, including partial-to-complete deafness and deaf-mutism, and neurological symptoms, sometimes combined with hypothyroidism, in all grades and all combinations. Nobody knows whether many more than the numbers actually recognized as abnormal are affected. In these areas there are only crude means of assessing the extent of the problem. The conditions for the community will change profoundly after adequate iodine prophylaxis, if only through the disappearance of those classified as cretins. (We should do away with the term "classical cretin" in this context as it only represents one end of the scale.)

If we wait until the developing countries have their roads and their salt legislation the birth of defective children in these areas will continue as before. J. B. Stanbury in Boston and I are both convinced that endemic cretinism should be attacked separately by methods other than salt iodization, for example by the parenteral administration of iodized oil (such as Ethiodol, May & Baker) and of long-acting iodine preparations. Although some progress with this technique has been made in goitre prophylaxis, detailed studies are required to assess its value for the prevention of cretinism.

This problem could then be tackled on the lines of, for example, the anti-yaws campaigns, with mobile units.

Candau: Great progress has been made in the last 15 years because before that potassium iodide could only be added to very refined salt. In 1950 studies[10] made here in London at the Chilean Iodine Educational Bureau showed the possibility of adding potassium iodate and this changed the whole question of goitre prophylaxis. As a result in Latin America the Institute of Nutrition of Central America and Panama set up several programmes and many countries like Peru, Colombia and Ecuador have established the required legislation. But there still remains the difficulty of reaching large groups of people living in areas of Brazil, for example, where it is practically impossible to control the commercial channels of salt. It is not really a question of legislation but of knowing where the salt comes from. This is one proof that the application of the results of research is not such a simple matter as we think. We have the answers to many things but we are not able to apply them to the people who need them.

Querido: But what I am concerned with is that so many cretins are born in the severely goitrous areas. My point is that we should leave the question of the goitre, because that will take another 30–40 years to solve, and attack the problem of cretinism separately, not by salt iodization but by other means. Cretinism is an irreversibly defective condition which exerts its social effects throughout the whole community. This is a clear example of a serious disease which could be effectively prevented by simple measures once an adequate level of health services, roads, etc., has been achieved.

REFERENCES

1. Food and Agriculture Organization. (1963). *Third World Food Survey.* Rome: FAO, FFHC Basic Study No. 11.

REFERENCES

2. Wright, N. C. (1961). The current food supply situation and present trends. In *Hunger: Can It Be Averted?* pp. 1–14. London: British Association for the Advancement of Science.
3. Scrimshaw, N. S., and Behar, M. (1959). World-wide occurrence of protein malnutrition. *Federation Proceedings* (Federation of American Societies for Experimental Biology), **18**, no. 2, 82.
4. World Health Organization. (1963). *Malnutrition and Disease*. Geneva: WHO, FFHC Basic Study No. 12.
5. Pawley, W. H. (1963). *Possibilities of Increasing World Food Production*. Rome: FAO, FFHC Basic Study No. 10.
6. Food and Agriculture Organization. (1966). *The State of Food and Agriculture*. Rome: FAO.
7. Champagnat, A. (1965). Protein from petroleum. *Scientific American*, **213**, no. 4, 13–17.
8. Read, J. (1967). Protein from petroleum. *Pugwash Newsletter*, 4, 81–82 (abstract).
9. Clements, F. W., and others. (1960). *Endemic Goitre*. Geneva: WHO Monograph Series, No. 44.
10. Kelly, F. C. (1953). Studies on stability of iodine compounds in iodized salt. *Bulletin of the World Health Organization*, 9, 217–230.

9

POLLUTION OF WATER, AIR AND FOOD

ABEL WOLMAN

The Johns Hopkins University, Baltimore, Maryland

THE term "environmental pollution" has been appropriately defined as: "...the unfavorable alteration of our surroundings wholly or largely as a by-product of man's actions, through direct or indirect effects of changes in energy patterns, radiation levels, chemical and physical constitution and abundances of organisms. These changes may affect man directly, or through his supplies of water and of agricultural and other biological products, his physical objects or possessions, or his opportunities for recreation and appreciation of nature."[1]

In simple terms, when man works, breathes, plays, fights or eats he creates environmental stresses and always has done so. In recent years the explosions of population, of urban societies and of industrialization have led us to realize that the quality of our environment needs to be restored and that the environmental factors determining community well-being need to be accurately assessed. These factors are, however, highly variable in their impact on health, economy or ecology. The battle to control or abate the pollution of water, air or food has many fronts and many logistical techniques, none of which follows the same formula.

Most recent reviews of these environmental issues reflect the conditions and the challenges of the so-called "developed" countries, which are characterized by major industrialization, old urban centres and long-forgotten victories over the communicable diseases. The expectation of life at birth of their people approaches the seventies and their disease spectra are aptly listed under the categories of "cancer, stroke and heart failure". In these societies, the problems of water, air and food are most often microchemical (e.g. surfactants, pesticides) rather than microbiological (typhoid, cholera bacilli) in origin.

Only a few documents of international origin (and not always these) take the precaution of pointing out that the world they describe is inhabited by

164

less than one-third of the people of the globe. The other two-thirds live under the circumstances and the environmental insults characteristic of over a half a century ago. Even in pollution, the East does not meet the West. The communicable diseases, accounts of which have almost vanished from western textbooks, are still the first or second causes of disability and death in this other world. And the vectors for transmission are predominantly the water and the food—where they are available. The enteric diseases, such as the infant diarrhoeas, the typhoid fevers, the choleras, and the diseases associated with degraded environments, wait to be eliminated in reality rather than only from the textbook of the western practitioner.

Expert committees tend to universalize the characteristics of the problems of the environment. The water pollution abatement necessities of the United States, England or the USSR and the air pollution warnings of Los Angeles, London, or Donora, Pennsylvania, have some counterparts developing in Asia, Africa and South America. But since resources for attack are inevitably limited, the prime necessity in public health is to select which battlegrounds have priority. As already noted, a large part of the world still suffers from the microbiological hazards of water and food. The problems of air pollution are episodic in incidence and by no means widespread, but they will undoubtedly mount if industrialization proceeds rapidly. The lessons of the industrialized countries, hopefully, will be used to the maximum when correctives are applied in the developing areas.

Fortunately, epidemiological findings are relatively clearer and more helpful in isolating methods of attack on disease in the less-favoured countries than in the western world. In the latter universe, with some major exceptions, one now searches for disease effects of subtle, long-term and chronic complexes due to environmental pollutants. A great deal of valuable statistical and laboratory effort has been expended in the last five or ten years in these arenas. The search for the impacts of carcinogens, pesticides, and other synthetic chemicals upon man is both difficult and frustrating. In any event, real progress in disclosures is being made. Of greater importance is the conclusion emerging from the Air Pollution Medical Research Conferences[2] held in Los Angeles in March, 1966, namely that "Despite the problems which hamper epidemiological and medical research, there was general agreement that control of air pollution should not be held up merely because certain questions were unresolved."

At the same conferences disappointment was expressed that the findings sometimes did not confirm what some believed should be the experimental result. The problem of differentiating in this area of inquiry between association and causation is perhaps more difficult than in many other more obvious fields of activity.[3]

From the U.S. congressional hearings[4] in the mid-summer of 1966 a similar conclusion might be gleaned regarding both air and water pollution abatement. It was abundantly clear that epidemiological support for many actions was less elaborate than were the technological tools for abatement. It was agreed by most witnesses that progress in correctives should be militantly pursued simultaneously with basic and applied research into disease manifestation and causation. Part of this emphasis upon *not* slowing up abatement stems from the fact that important considerations other than health—such as physical deterioration of materials, recreational debits, agricultural losses—dominated some of the hearings.

It is not an exaggeration to say that in much of the industrialized world, society has concluded that the quality of the environment needs to be restored. The decision is deliberate that such regulation is an appropriate and necessary function of a social system "seeking to reduce pollution or its effects". How to do this, how much money to spend and on what, what institutional machinery must be devised, what criteria and standards of attainment are appropriate, what functions and incentives motivate private enterprise—all these questions now confront governments and their constituents in the conscious intent to close the gap between the so-called "polluted" and the "desired" environment. For many of the countries in the more highly developed western world, therefore, the immediate future will undoubtedly be characterized by a drive towards correctives, economically devised, frequently re-directed and pushing towards newer social and political machinery. The returns in improved health of the individual should be predictably high, although the warrant for the predictions remains to be increasingly validated by medical and epidemiological inquiries of a complex and difficult nature.

THE OTHER WORLD

Let us turn now to the world of the other 2,000 million people. What are their environmental concerns? Are they the same as those just reviewed? If not, where does the student of world health problems centre his attack? Aside from the obvious obstacles to progress arising from unprecedented rates of population growth, the environmental stresses are different in kind from those of the industrially developed countries. They are reminiscent of late nineteenth and early twentieth century sanitary conditions or much worse.

In the first place, it is unrealistic to confront the citizen of Africa, Latin America, or Asia with programmes directed towards abatement of micro-chemical pollution of water and food—and in some instances, air—when in fact vast numbers of people have neither water, food nor industry. The minute quantities of water available are invariably microbiologically contaminated. In food preparation, the most elementary principles of hygiene are violated. In general, standards of personal hygiene are necessarily non-existent, because opportunities for cleanliness are distinguished by their absence. Pollution by bacteria, viruses, and other organisms is widespread. The diseases associated with these are almost ignored in the newer text-books of the western world. Yet cholera, typhoid fever, dysentery, bil-harziasis, filariasis, and trachoma reach the proportions characteristic of bygone ages.

If one had the power to select the public health action that would have the maximum impact upon the deleterious environment, the order of choice might well be as follows:

(1) *The provision of adequate quantities of safe water*

Such to be continuously available to all people, easily accessible, prefer-ably within the house. It is now abundantly clear that many significant returns in health come from the ability to keep clean. Sometimes even the simple liquid, not quite meeting the highest quality possible in the most sophisticated societies, has beneficent values in raising the level of personal hygiene—and on the reduction of disease.

How do the 2,000 million people fare in this feature of the environment? Detailed quantitative estimates of the adequacy and availability of water are unfortunately scarce. Sufficient information has been accumulated, how-ever, by the World Health Organization, the United States Agency for International Development, and others to disclose an appalling deficiency in either water service or water quality.

USAID recently reviewed this situation for urban population centres of more than 5,000 people[5], with the results shown in Table I. In the rural areas in all these countries, the people are even less favoured and the female carrier of water is almost the universal image.

In South Asia some 61 per cent of the urban population is not served from public piped supplies. In India alone over 52 million people await new services. In contrast, some 86 per cent of the urban population in Latin America is served from piped supplies. Even there, however, service is often only intermittent, due either to shortage of supply or inadequate facil-ities for distribution. Invariably, quality leaves something to be desired.

Table

WATER SUPPLIES AND WASTE DISPOSAL IN URBAN AREAS OF
DEVELOPING COUNTRIES*

	Water		Waste disposal		
	Nos. supplied by outside pipes (millions)	Nos. with no supply	Nos. with outside privies (millions)	Nos. without privies	Total estimated urban population (millions)
Latin America	30	15	32·2	26	101
Africa	12	11	10	16	35
Near East	9·5	6·5	{ 26	78	119
South Asia	25	58			
Far East	31	15	9	39	54
Total	107·5	105·5	77·2	159	309
% of urban population	(35%)	(34%)	(25%)	(51%)	

* Data taken from USAID, unpublished survey material.

This dismal picture of lack of water service, aggravated each day by population growth and by serious delays in remedial action, was confirmed in somewhat greater detail by the excellent WHO inventory carried out in 1963 by Dieterich and Henderson. [6] The urban* water supply conditions in 75 selected countries were reviewed. The conclusions of this analysis were as follows :

(a) Urban water supply conditions are unsatisfactory or grossly unsatisfactory in most of the selected 75 countries.

(b) Urban waterworks construction in almost all the 75 countries proceeds at too slow a rate to close existing gaps and to match future needs.

(c) Urban water supply conditions have reached a point where shortcomings are a potential danger to urban health and economic development.

Viewed from the vantage point of 1967, it is regrettably clear that the situation, with a few important exceptions, is worse today than when the above canvasses were made. Each year the gap has widened rather than closed, in spite of temporary surges in governmental interest. Today, that interest appears to be on the decline.

(2) *The removal of human excreta from continuous human contact*

One of the most important public health activities, since the days of Moses, has been the concern of man with the disposal of his wastes. For

---

* The urban population here considered was 320 million out of a total of 1,351 million.

almost a century this function has been recognized and reasonably implemented in most developed countries. In these latter, the issues of today are concerned, not so much with removal of excreta from the place of dwelling, as with their proper disposal or treatment at more remote points.

This second world of which we speak shows exactly contrary conditions. Here, in both urban and rural settings, man's wastes are in daily intimate contact with man. The public health sequels are manifest and great. As with water supply, the problems posed with human excreta are elementary. They have been largely resolved in the western world. They remain to be confronted in the rest of the world.

The magnitude of this environmental problem is shown in Table I, based on observations by USAID. [5] The findings, as one might expect, are more disheartening than those for water supplies, because waste disposal has always lagged behind community water service in every country in the world. Rarely was money simultaneously available for both installations.

In the regions surveyed only 24 per cent of the urban population is connected to sewers, 25 per cent have privies, and 51 per cent are not served at all.

These data are given here primarily to suggest that these people, and their counterparts elsewhere, await the elimination of primitive facilities and not the reduction of phosphates, nitrogen compounds, and exotic organic and inorganic complexes in the sewage. These latter are not yet the dominant issues in most of the countries. That they do occur in a few instances is of course true and they should be handled as practicably as possible.

(3) *Problems associated with water*

Cleanliness, if not exactly next to Godliness, has at least a close kinship on the public health front. It is only in recent years that it has become increasingly clear that the ability to wash prevents both water-associated and other diseases to a significant extent. Mills and Reincke noted that when ample quantities of good water were brought into a community, diseases other than water-borne fell markedly in incidence. More recently, Leslie Banks[7] has observed a similar situation in England, where dermatoses have declined with the rise in environmental cleanliness.

This general category of sanitary deficiencies prevailing in many developing countries and affecting many millions of people needs no further emphasis, but it is as well to record at least two examples of the scourges which no longer plague the industrialized world. These are trachoma and bilharziasis, in both of which the roles of personal hygiene, of available water and of sanitary handling of human excreta are of major importance.

While the search for vaccines, for specific therapeutic substances, and for molluscicides is diligently pursued, government policies in the stimulation of an improved environment are weak and reflect a perennial frustration.

(4) *Food*

In the midst of recurring food shortages, malnutrition and starvation, it might appear that reference to food sanitation is peculiarly inappropriate. It is true, however, that better sanitary management of food is not only possible, but essential, even under the stresses so frequent in low-income countries. Here, parallels between the practices of East and West are unfortunately far too common. Food-borne epidemics prevail in both regions and are often unreported though large in attack.

The same sanitary rules are applicable in both societies and are violated much too frequently in both. It is strange that unhygienic personal habits should persist to this day, both where water for washing hands is abundantly available and where it is at a severe premium. It is not an anachronism that in 1964 an editorial in the *Journal of the Royal Society of Health*[8] was entitled "Wash your Hands", and stated that, at least in England, the practice of hand-washing after toilet use is violated as often as it is honoured. The snail's pace of educating the food handler in the importance of fingers, flies and filth is one of the few debits universally shared!

DESPAIR OR OPTIMISM

Pollution of water, air and food means different things to different people in various parts of the world. In the developed or relatively high-income countries of the world the drive towards restoring the quality of the environment is strong. Public awareness of the need for correctives has been heavily stimulated by the emergence of industrial products which are potential or actual hazards to health, by economic loss or by aesthetic objection. Since these countries have long benefited from the elimination of much communicable disease, the public concerns itself with the improvement of the environment for other more subtle and long-range benefits. The pace with which these changes will proceed will depend upon public policy, budgets, manpower, and competitive necessities.

In the second world, the dominant necessities in environmental improvement are those familiar in the west fifty or a hundred years ago. The impact of environmental deficiencies upon obvious communicable disease is prompt, clear and ever present. The solutions, although obvious, are very difficult because of the absence of money, professional and skilled man-power, and institutional structure and management. None of these is to be overcome overnight. The distressing contrast between the developed and the developing countries is made even more formidable by the fact that, in the former, the birth rate averages 21, while in the latter it is 40 per 1,000 population. In these countries, the public health Alice in Wonderland must run far more rapidly than it is normally supposed to do in order to make any progress whatever.

THERAPY

I would like to add a word about therapy in relation to pollution of water, food and air. In water supply and waste disposal the restraints upon us lie in what I call the three ''M's'': money, management and professional man-power. The variations between countries and between regions in these three are tremendous. No small amount of their effort ought to be directed to the three ''M's'', at least in the environmental field. Our conversations should not be with each other, but with ministers of finance, and education, and with those who deal with administration and the provision of new insti-tutional structures. It is very difficult to work in a country to improve the environment when all three ''M's'' are lacking, when there are neither engineers nor artisans. The simple problem of having someone who knows how to repair a water main becomes more important than the philosophical question of whether that region should have a water system. An individual who knows how to change a valve is more necessary under some circum-stances than a highly skilled sanitary or civil engineer.

As to money, the investment needed in water systems for the 2,000 million people of the developing countries is great. It is so great that it intimidates every minister of health, because it outshines his total operating budget by many, many times. The opportunity for using large capital sums in these countries, repayable by their citizens, has been demonstrated increasingly in the last ten years. There is a successful way of doing this. One example comes from Central and South America. Ten years ago the total amount of money lent by international banks to South America for water supplies was less than US $100,000. In November, 1966 this figure had risen to nearly $600 million. This accounts for some of my optimism. It is true that, in South America, two of the ''M's'' already existed: man-power of high skill, and management structure of equally good potential. The problem is to create all three of the ''M's'' in other parts of the world as rapidly as possible.

Most of my own dealings are no longer with the technicians, the medical officers, or even the sanitary engineers, but with the bankers. The search for money is a major part of our obligation.

In summary, therefore, one may well look forward with optimism to an improved quality of environment in the more industrially advanced areas. In those regions less well favoured, the prospect is still gloomy. Although we should not despair, we cannot rest upon any past laurels, because they are in scarce supply!

DISCUSSION

Florey: When you have diagnosed the trouble and decided on the therapy who do you consider should carry it out, Professor Wolman?

Wolman: In general, if Dr. Candau will forgive me, it is not the Minister of Health, who is mostly intimidated by the Minister of Finance. One must turn to the economist, usually to the Director of Public Works. He is the contact with the Minister of Finance or, more important, with the congressional committee or its corresponding body. In the Philippines and Taiwan, from which I have just come, my contacts with the Ministry of Health were purely social. The day's work was with the congressional committees and with the bankers, because that's where the money is.

Candau: When you went to Latin America in 1943, Professor Wolman, the number of sanitary engineers could be counted on the fingers of one hand—there was in fact no such profession then. For me the most urgent of the three "M's" is manpower. The right therapy is impossible unless someone inside the country can do the nursing. An impossible situation is created when pressure comes from outside for a water supply to be installed if the government can't find one of its own nationals sufficiently qualified to advise it on what this entails. Yet once the manpower is available, money will be easier to obtain. The proposal, whatever it is, has to be acceptable to the bank, and no bank will give money unless certain conditions are met.

On the question of who should carry out the therapy, I don't disagree at all, Professor Wolman. I think the responsibility for the water supply belongs not to the Minister of Health but to the local authorities—to the mayor of the community or to the Minister of Public Works. However, it is also true that no one wants to take any responsibility for the small towns and rural areas except the Minister of Health.

Johnson-Marshall: Professor Wolman's points could be dealt with in a number of stages. First, one must insist on enclosed drainage systems and on a pure water supply—this does not necessarily mean adding chemicals to it, but ensuring that it is as pure as it comes out of the original catchment, and ensuring that water catchments are carefully safeguarded. It includes waste removal and air pollution controls, such as clean air legislation. Stage II is the environmental planning stage, where certain industrial sources of pollution are located, or relocated, away from living areas. Stage III is to regard waste as a potential resource instead of as a negative factor. After this one could go on to the basic problem of the effect of increases of all kinds. In water supply the population increase first leads to the Stage I water need, but then as the standard of living goes up so does the *per caput* demand for water. This leads to a re-examination of our attitude to the conservation of commodities. Whether it is water or anything else that human beings use, we need a completely new approach in terms of conservation—the opposite approach to that of conspicuous consumption.

Florey: That applies particularly to developed countries. Whenever I offer a guest a glass of water I warn them it has been used six times already, but it is still perfectly good water. I suppose this would be true over a lot of this country, and it is a miracle of water technology. Would you be satisfied with a good water-treatment plant, Professor Wolman, or would you insist on having a pure catchment?

Wolman: I would go even further, as I hinted. Our problem is really to provide people with the maximum possible use of a liquid with the minimum of energy loss in fetching and carrying water for long distances.

Doxiadis: To proceed on the basis of universal standards of requirements is, I think, very dangerous. We cannot say that we want a particular quantity of water, or a certain type of environment: we can only say that what we need is an improvement in conditions which leads to an upward curve. In developing countries, what we want is that the next stage be better than the present one, whatever this is. In areas without enough water, we need some water in the first stage. The desire of some authorities to have universally fixed and constant standards militates against the eventual solution of the problems. We don't live in a static world, and we must be able to think in terms of development. That is why I asked earlier whether the percentage of people who get proper food today is lower or higher than it was in earlier years. It is impossible for everybody on this earth to get the same amount of food overnight, and it may also not be necessary. We must have standards which will continuously improve for everyone. For those who suffer they must be improved at a higher speed than for the others. But we cannot hope to achieve progress by sudden jumps. Even if we had the economic means, are we allowed to feed an undernourished population tomorrow with the diet of the American citizen? In the post-war period in Greece people who received too much food too quickly had more diseases than during the occupation, simply because they were not accustomed to so much food, and they needed time to readjust themselves to the digestion of greater quantities.

Banks: When the era of sanitation began, a little more than 100 years ago, it was the medical profession that took the lead. Over the years the medical officer of health has grown away from this field and devoted himself largely to personal health services, while the man who was first called an inspector of nuisances became a sanitary inspector, and then a public health inspector. There has been an enormous development in public health engineering, to which the problems of big cities naturally lend themselves. But in the vast rural areas of the developing countries many of the people who should be leading the attack on environmental hazards have been trained wholly and solely to deal with personal medical problems and the cure of disease by the most modern clinical methods.

Wolman: When Dr. Candau referred to the development of manpower, he was referring to the whole scale of manpower development, not to this hierarchy of public health engineer or sanitary engineer alone, or even of medical doctors. I share Dr. Candau's view that in a country where professional manpower is at a high premium one works with what one has; that is, one develops the lower levels of technicians. In many instances, with some guidance, they can do a great many of the things which more highly trained people do elsewhere. The alternative to pursuing that route is to do nothing. Even the lowliest village artisan has a capacity for doing things in this field, for which he can be well trained. I do not wait for the millennium, either in manpower, management, or money, because in the impoverished developing country in many instances more than money is available: self-help is available, and village energy is available—village women can be used very effectively in the improvement of environmental sanitation. Where the hierarchy exists, that is fine. Where it does not exist, we shall begin to generate it, but in the meantime we must use the next 10, 20 or 30 years as effectively as possible.

Florey: Are demonstration areas with competent people, local or foreign, any use for showing that a system works?

Wolman: I am allergic to demonstration projects for sanitation purposes. My experience has been that they do not demonstrate, because they are insulated or isolated from the surrounding areas. They may be better used for agricultural demonstration, although I am not too sure of that.

Florey: How would you set about getting the ladies of the village to help? *Wolman*: One talks with the people, intriguing them with the principles that are to be adopted. When they return to their areas, having accepted the principles, they then interest the leaders of the village, or even the leaders of the great urban centres. This is a time-consuming but successful approach.

Dr. Candau observed that some time has to be devoted to the rural areas. In England, the United States, and a good deal of the rest of Europe, environmental practices of sound nature went from the urban areas to the village rather than the other way around. Yet the general emphasis every-where, particularly by people running for office, is that something has to be done in the villages. Is that a sound principle? I would not forget the villages, but I would not, as is done in many countries, devote 99 per cent of my energy to running around them. When I am all finished, I have not accomplished much.

Garcia: Community organization is a good method of organizing local resources when it is done by local leaders, or by health leaders such as sanitary inspectors or health educators. I agree with Professor Wolman that demonstration areas are not generally useful, but they may be useful just to establish confidence. When we improve something in one village, the women and the authorities of the next village always look to see what is happening and then they try to surpass that.

Kaprio: There have certainly been many unsuccessful demonstrations and WHO terminology has changed from "demonstration area" to "pilot area". One has to start somewhere and "pilot area" implies that the situation is ready and the motivation exists to start some scheme. A water supply programme in one city may be a pilot for another, which will again be taken up in a third place. Local as well as international experts can still assist a country to locate the place where a movement may start, and even though it may not succeed this is a different approach. Hundreds of demon-stration programmes have not spread, but I hope that the next generation of pilot programmes will spread a little bit better.

Wolman: The environmental protective services in the developed countries were not spontaneously generated: they were slow, progressive developments. The 20,000 community water services in the United States are looked upon by many people in underdeveloped countries as having suddenly been there. As one who worked with them for decades, I can assure you they were not suddenly there. We had to take exactly the same steps of stimulation, of ingenious approaches, and imaginative institutions, as I am talking about in the developing countries. This lesson has to be learned; these services were not there from time immemorial London's water supply was a long time coming!

Evang: This has also to do with the question of centralization or decentralization of health services. In the developed countries this started out around 1840–1860. Much of the responsibility for health was turned over to the municipalities, and while they couldn't do much in other fields of health, what they could do was to provide water and later on also to deal with sewage disposal. This holds true still for many areas of the world. We have to organize the demand. In some Indian villages, for example, we found that it did not work to tell people this was to protect their health. However, the latrines became a status symbol. If you could offer your guests a glass of water, and also a latrine, that was something. On that basis, progress came from below, not from above.

Bankers, of course, are people who invest money, but they want to get money back. Is it your suggestion, Professor Wolman, that the poor peoples of the world should buy their water commercially?

Wolman: Without question. They will never get it otherwise, but they are able to get it in this way. We have demonstrated this not once but a dozen times. At least in the United States, it was not the vital statistics tables that convinced the mayors and civic councils to buy water—it was fire protection: we sold it on fire insurance premiums, not on the typhoid fever death rate. Incidentally, in our early days typhoid fever provided a very salutary death rate—it was high, and we have lost that great advantage of misfortune!

Lindop: The developing countries, as well as looking at the ways that the others have got over some of their water and drainage problems, should also look at the reasons why we are failing in our own countries. In this country we still have rural areas with open drainage. If we could discover how to convince our own rural areas that they should do something about this, we might be able to help the developing countries better.

Wolman: I always find myself in a position of being more optimistic than you sense. Great Britain has done more in the provision of rural water supplies than almost any other country in the world; you have every reason to be proud of it. You may not have accomplished all that you might do in rural areas for drainage, but in rural water supply you have done really great things over the last ten years. As Dr. Doxiadis pointed out, one does not provide everything for everybody simultaneously. That millennium is still round the corner.

Lindop: Surely the principle is that one learns more from the experiment that fails than from the experiment that succeeds?

Wolman: I do not think the experiment has failed.

Lindop: But the causes of the failure to complete the project here might be useful in principle for detecting why other areas fail even to start the project.

Wolman: My diagnosis is that people behave pretty much the same everywhere. They do not all buy water, sewerage and drainage as promptly as we would like, and in that respect I think the Indian village has counterparts in Great Britain and in the United States and elsewhere.

le Riche: I have been visiting London for 20 years or so and I wish to compliment all the people concerned who have very nearly cleaned up this city with regard to air pollution. I have no scientific evidence for this, but I think London is much cleaner now than either Toronto or New York.

Wolman: London, like Los Angeles and New York, is the victim of its topography and meteorology!

REFERENCES

1. Environmental Pollution Panel, President's Science Advisory Committee (November, 1965). *Report on Restoring the Quality of Our Environment.* Washington, D.C.
2. Goldsmith, J. R. (1966). Air Pollution Medical Research (report on A.M.A. conferences). *Science,* **154,** 1588–1591.
3. Hill, A. B. (1965). The Environment and Disease: Association or Causation? *Proceedings of the Royal Society of Medicine,* **58,** 295–300.
4. Hearings before the Subcommittee on Science, Research and Development. (1966). *The Adequacy of Technology for Pollution Abatement,* Vol. 1. U.S. House of Representatives, 89th Congress, Second Session.
5. United States Agency for International Development. Unpublished information.
6. Dieterich, B. H., and Henderson, J. M. (1963). *Urban Water Supply Conditions and Needs in Seventy-Five Developing Countries.* Geneva: WHO, Public Health Papers No. 23.
7. Banks, A. L. (1954). Ecology in relation to dermatology. In *Modern Trends in Dermatology,* Vol. 2. London: Butterworth & Co.
8. Editorial (1964). Wash your hands. *Journal of the Royal Society of Health,* **84,** 179.

10

THE INHUMAN CITY

C. A. DOXIADIS
Doxiadis Associates, Athens

To deal with the city of man in a symposium dedicated to the health of mankind is very natural; it is in the city that one-third of mankind lives today and this proportion is increasing at such a rate that in the second half of the next century, three generations from now, more than 95 per cent of mankind will be living in cities.

It is for this reason that when I speak of the "city of man" I mean the large contemporary urban human settlements; it is to them that the additional millions will be added. Minor centres cannot grow easily unless they become parts of greater urban concentrations; and even so they present the same type of problems as the major areas—only the scale is different. Every era has one type of settlement which corresponds to its civilization; this type imposes its characteristics even on the pre-existing settlements.

I find it very difficult to make a direct relationship between the health of mankind and the city. I could certainly mention the fact that in the cities man is breathing contaminated air and consequently developing cancer of the lungs more easily than he would be in the open countryside, but I could also answer that the city provides him with pure water which is very rare in villages. I could certainly mention many diseases generated in the city, but I could also answer that the city developed medicine and only the big city can afford the great hospitals which support research and provide different specialized services for different kinds of diseases and people.

The definition of the relationship of the health of mankind and the city is even more difficult if we do not limit health to the body of man only, but consider the total man. What can we say in answer to the fact that while the city provides a better water supply and a sewerage system more of its inhabitants suffer from nervous complaints?

Many statistics which attempt to relate diseases to cities and villages are quite misleading because they do not succeed in defining two important aspects: the question of where a disease really belongs (in the city where it was diagnosed or the countryside where it was caused?), and that of the real nature of the area where it was diagnosed. Is, for example, a small suburb of a great metropolitan area a village or garden-city, or is it actually a part of the metropolis? On the one hand, it breathes the metropolitan area's fumes, and on the other its people are forced to commute over even longer distances than those of the metropolis.

I do not believe that I am entitled to relate the health of mankind to the city and express any opinion about whether it leads to better or worse health conditions for man. In order to make any such attempt one must study this very serious subject much more carefully. I think however that I am entitled to speak about the inhuman city since it is apparent that conditions in the larger cities are becoming less and less suitable for man as we know him today.

This is the first point that I want to make: our diagnosis is that our present-day city is inhuman and that it is becoming more so with every day that passes. If it is inhuman, it cannot be better for the health of mankind; it creates grave problems for man.

We now have to conceive a therapy. If the city is inhuman and becoming increasingly so, should we not eliminate it, or turn it into a better city? Or perhaps we should devise new ways of living in new types of human settlements. It is necessary to tackle this problem afresh, which brings me to my second point: we must set new goals for the city and find new solutions for our problems. To achieve this we need the development of a systematic method of approach.

It is not reasonable to imagine that we can eliminate the present-day city or even limit its growth to any great extent—its dimensions will necessarily remain inhuman. Our real challenge is to create human conditions within the inhuman frame of the city; and this is my third and last point: our task is the conception and creation of the human city within an inhuman frame.

THE CITY IS INHUMAN

Our present-day city is becoming more inhuman than the city of the past. We can understand this if we look at it in several ways. The very fact that although in the past man could walk from one end of his city to the other, he cannot do so today, shows the inhuman dimensions of the city. Of course he can use an automobile to achieve his end, but he must be able to pay for it and, if he cannot drive, pay someone to drive it; and the risks on the road are many.

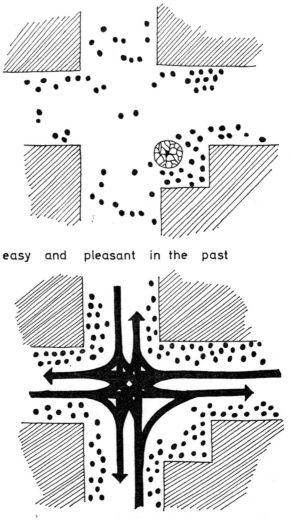

easy   and   pleasant   in   the   past

very difficult and dangerous at present

Fig. 1. Contacts between people in public space.

The air we breathe is not suitable for man, neither is the water we drink. We have to purify them both, but even so the danger will not be eliminated, since while we purify the air inside the buildings we throw the contaminated air outdoors and breathe it when we go out for some fresh air. In the same way we are spoiling many other natural resources—spoiling land and destroying beautiful landscapes, flowers and birds, which Aldous Huxley called "half the subject matter of English poetry".[1]

In this city man is no longer free to move; he may have gained large dimensions by high speeds but he has lost his freedom to move in the micro-space around him. Our children are not free to run across the street. We are not yet in a position to know how many of our phobias and nervous diseases are caused by the fact that man is not free to move in his city—he has been gradually squeezed out of his squares and streets (Fig. 1).

Human society does not operate properly in our cities. In spite of the myth that we are now living at higher densities, the truth is that density is now two and a half times lower than at the beginning of our century, before the influx of the automobile; it has gone down from 80 persons per acre in 1900 to 30 persons per acre, or 2·5 times less, in the major cities of the world today. Such lower densities may mean larger building plots but they also mean larger distances between people, fewer services available to them and fewer contacts between them.

We try to ameliorate conditions in this inhuman city in several ways, but we do not manage to satisfy man. We build, for example, new housing schemes for the slum dwellers; they are not satisfied when they move into them and we wonder why, forgetting that we may have moved them into an area with purer air but we have deprived them of their friends and have increased their commuting time by two hours a day, that is by one-third of their free time during which they could see their children and wives, enjoy themselves, relax, read or think. By our action we concentrated on one aspect of man alone, and we have asked people to move to get better houses where there is pure air which can now be contaminated.

We fail to satisfy man and to turn our city into a more human one and this is true for the city in its details and in its total structure and function. We even still fail to see this failure of ours and therefore the situation gets worse—we are actually building the inhuman city—and we are getting more and more confused within it.

The basic reason behind our failure to understand and to build the human city is that we fail to understand two basic facts. First, man should not be seen as body only, but also as senses, mind and soul, which create different requirements for him. We are dealing with total man. His relationship to his environment, his habitat, his settlements is a very complex one which cannot be faced by an isolated action, such as the building of houses or the opening of highways (Fig. 2). As an example I mention that it is wrong to deal with ''housing'' as a separate problem. Nobody wants to be ''housed'' only, or in some way ''shelved'' somewhere. Everybody wants to live and we must find ways to satisfy the life of the total man. If we speak of the health of mankind we must think of the health of the total man.

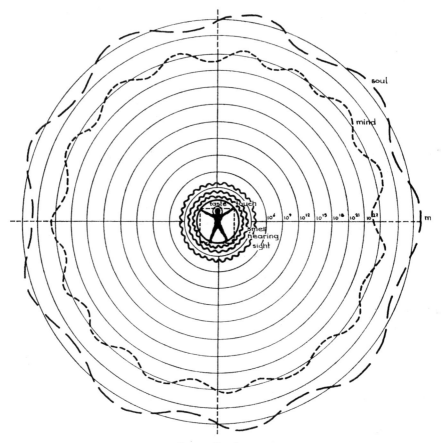

FIG. 2. Total man.

Second, the city does not consist only of buildings, as it was fashionable to think two generations ago, or of traffic lines, as it became more fashionable to think after the war, or of social or racial problems, as is becoming fashionable today. The city consists of five elements born in this order: Nature, Man, Society, Shells (buildings of all kinds) and Networks (roads and railroads, water and power, etc.) (Fig. 3).

Because we fail to understand these two facts we have upset the balance between man and his city, and, as a consequence, man is suffering in the city which has become inhuman.

It may be asked at this point why we are building an inhuman city, and the answer is that that is not our purpose, but the multitude of new functions, opportunities and choices add up to an inhuman whole. The purpose of the new city is to offer a wider range of choices to man; as a result of this man

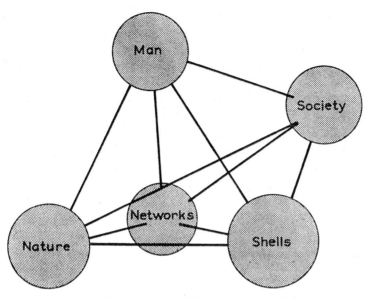

FIG. 3. The city consists of five interconnected elements.

has more choices, but he is suffering within an inhuman structure which results in the inhuman functioning of the city.

This inhuman city is by necessity one in which the health of man, regardless of the additional amenities available, is being threatened more and more. We know that modern man has greater longevity than at any time before, and the fact that longevity increases with urbanization would contradict any opposite statement. But we cannot claim that man is happier in this city—this longevity may show its cost in the quality of his life—and quality is an ultimate goal.

I do not know whether a recent statement by Dr. René Dubos that if these conditions continue " . . . eventually half the population would have to be doctors, nurses, or psychiatrists tending to the physical ailments and neuroses of the other half"[2] is true, but I do not see any trend which might prove the opposite. There is a great danger that the inhuman city might be leading man to disaster.

NEW GOALS FOR THE CITY

Since the city of man is becoming inhuman and this is caused by the absence of balance between man and his city we must try and create a new balance. Some people have come up with an easy but also, in many respects, naive answer: to eliminate the city. These are Utopian thoughts. Others are proud of man's ability to adapt himself and foresee his complete adaptation —but I ask, what will be the goal of this adaptation?

It is not wise to think of changing man. Together with Nature, Man is the oldest element of the city. Society is younger but still much older than Shells, while Networks are the youngest element of all. It is only reasonable to start changing the system by changing the one product which did not have the time to develop enough by trial and error, that is the Networks. We can then try to change the next element in age, the Shells.

In order to achieve any change, however, we must understand the situation as clearly as possible and develop a systematic method of approach. We must understand man and set goals for him, we must understand the city and set goals for it; we must achieve this both for the system as a whole and for all its parts. We must then try and organize all relationships into a system which minimizes the inhuman conditions and maximizes the services provided by it.

In order to be able to proceed in this way we must first manage to understand man and his relationship to his environment; and to do so we must develop an ability to measure the phenomena of interrelationships. Man is

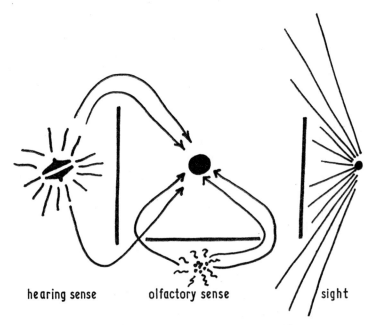

hearing sense   olfactory sense   sight

FIG. 4. Man is connected with space in several ways.

the recipient of many influences from his surroundings. These influences can be positive or negative, they can have beneficial or destructive effects on him. In a very simplified way we can understand that while his body is physically defined and limited, his senses, his "hidden dimensions" as Edward Hall aptly named them[3], allow him to reach far beyond his body, and this in different ways. His taste is very limited in space; his touch does not go beyond the body; his olfactory sense does not reach far, but goes around objects; his hearing operates in a similar way; and his sight, which reaches far out, is limited by any non-diaphanous obstruction (Fig. 4).

Mind and psyche reach far beyond the spheres of body and senses and open new horizons which later are, or may be, conquered by man physically. Total man has therefore to be considered as consisting of one area which he occupies physically, and of much greater areas with which he is connected in several ways (Fig. 5).

On the basis of such methods we can then proceed and measure the inter-relationship between man and his environment, thinking in terms of time and influences. We have first to measure the time of man's exposure to different conditions. This can be done on an Ekistic Logarithmic Scale, showing all types of space units to which man belongs, as in Fig. 6, which presents the amount of time spent by one male and one female in a big city.

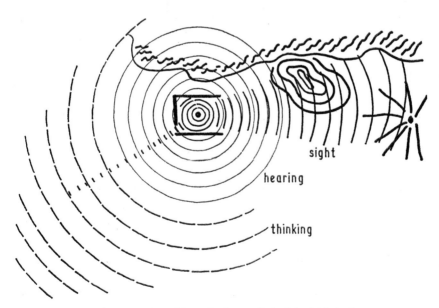

sight

hearing

thinking

FIG. 5. Total man consists of several spheres of which his body is the centre.

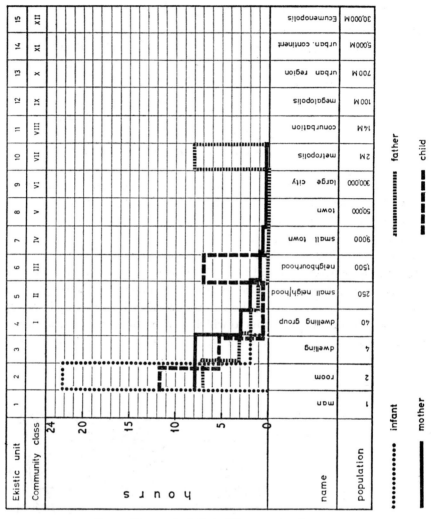

FIG. 6. Time spent daily in different units of space.

For every such position in space, or for every set of conditions in every such position, we can measure the satisfaction derived because of the environment. This satisfaction can be represented separately for body (Sb), senses (Ss), mind (Sm) and psyche (Sp) (Fig. 7), and then these divisions can be added to find the total satisfaction for a given condition at a given space (St = Sb + Ss + Sm + Sp).

We can then proceed to compare the actual satisfaction with the expected normal one (so much clean air versus so much expected, so much

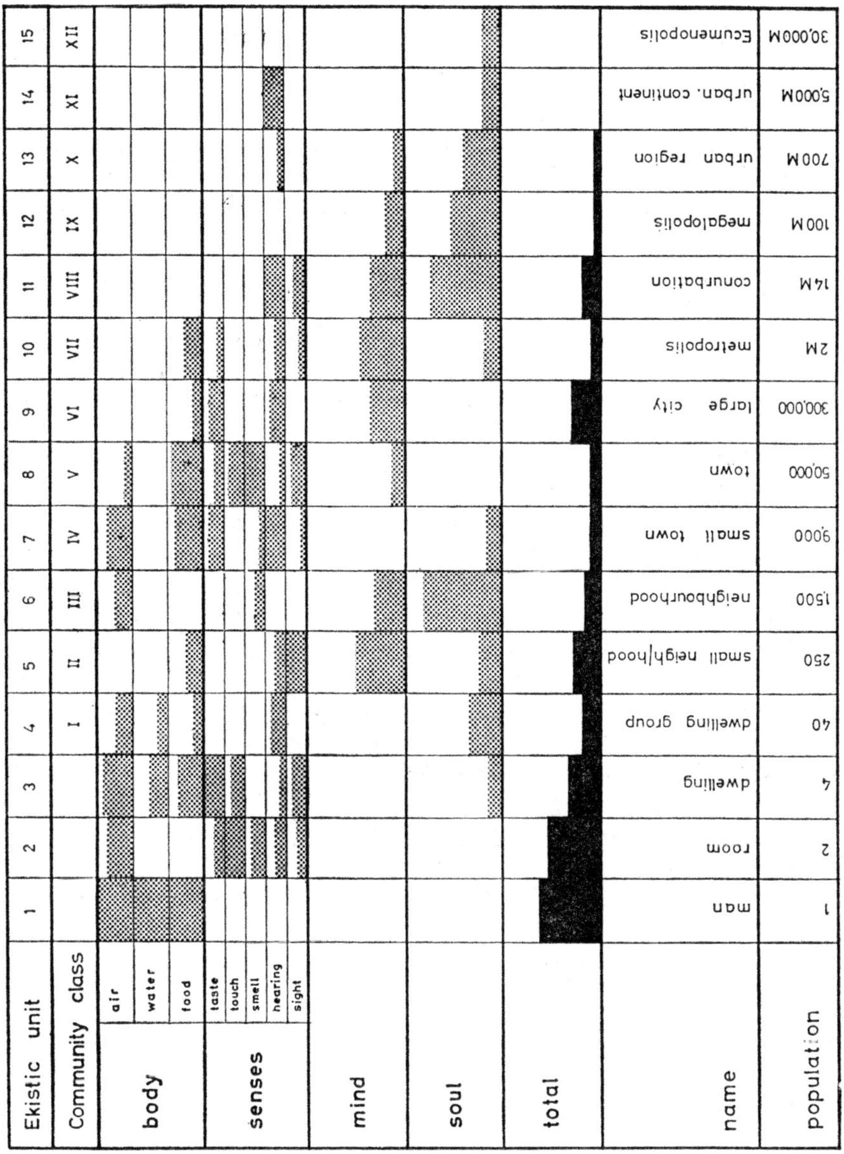

Ekistic unit	Community class	body (air, water, food)	senses (taste, touch, smell, hearing, sight)	mind	soul	total	name	population
1							man	1
2							room	2
3							dwelling	4
4	I						dwelling group	40
5	II						small neighbourhood	250
6	III						neighbourhood	1500
7	IV						small town	9000
8	V						town	50,000
9	VI						large city	300,000
10	VII						metropolis	2 M
11	VIII						conurbation	14 M
12	IX						megalopolis	100 M
13	X						urban region	700 M
14	XI						urban. continent	5,000 M
15	XII						Ecumenopolis	30,000 M

FIG. 7. Satisfaction of several needs of man (illustrative case).

temperature, aesthetic satisfaction, etc.) and present the total satisfaction per unit of space and condition in relation to time spent (Fig. 8). Such a presentation alone can lead to conclusions about the importance of each unit of the total settlement, for each individual or family or group, and conclusions about the changes which are necessary.

187

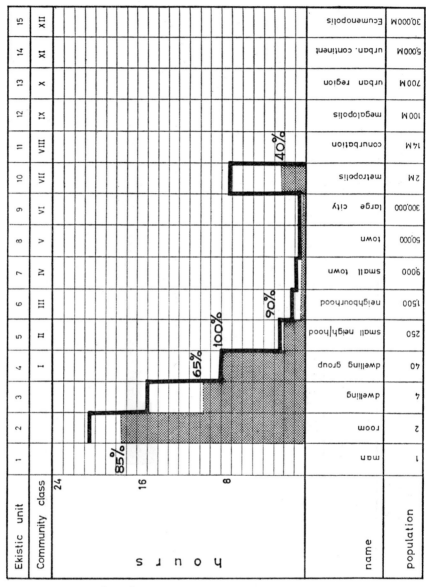

FIG. 8. Total satisfaction expressed as a percentage of time of exposure.

I am not saying that we can achieve this easily or immediately, but unless we do it we cannot hope for rational decisions on the interrelationships of man and his city; if we cannot do so by measurements then at least we must try to do so by feeling the situation, even by using our intuition, just as the first doctors had to do before they measured any of the conditions of the human body or psyche.

Such considerations lead to the conception of normal conditions as a basis for comparisons, and to the criteria to be used and the goals to be attained. What kind of conditions do we consider normal for which kind of man? Speaking to doctors, I do not need to say that there are no diseases, only patients—but now we are dealing with diseases and we need to define the average normal conditions.

At this point we must admit that today we lack the courage to act in a normative way and arrive at solutions. Do we want people, for example, to live in a city with contaminated air and be protected in their rooms by the purification of the air? Do we prefer them to live part of their time in air-conditioned rooms, or also in houses or streets? And how about the noise, and all the other external influences? We must acquire the knowledge and courage to define human goals, and to do this we need a new field of knowledge and action, which I tentatively name *Anthropics*, concerned with man in terrestrial space, and the existing and desirable conditions for him. Unless we start in this way our efforts for our cities will be in vain.

If we achieve this, we can turn our attention to the city. Its goal is to make man happy and safe. This has to be achieved by bringing people as close together as possible in order to serve each other, and by keeping them apart so that they cannot hurt each other. The one condition contradicts the other; we have, therefore, to find the solution which maximizes the services and minimizes the inconveniences. This can be achieved by the proper creation of Shells and Networks (Fig. 9) which is the role of *Ekistics*, the science of human settlements.

In the past, we could do without Anthropics and Ekistics because all dimensions were human, or—because man uses animals—nearly human. Man learned by trial and error to deal with small-size problems. Now the forces are great and inhuman and the danger, because of the cohabitation of man with them, in the same space, is great. Our action has to be based on scientific knowledge; and towards this end we must mobilize all our resources.

THE HUMAN CITY

We have now to turn our attention to the city which serves human goals, happiness and safety, and try to conceive and build it. Unlike the inhuman city of the present in which we deal with what we have—and fail, we must now start from our goals and try to create the human city.

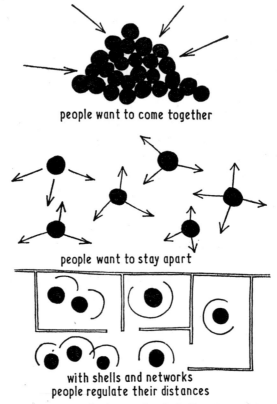

people want to come together

people want to stay apart

with shells and networks
people regulate their distances

FIG. 9. People alone and with shells and networks.

With this we have to pose the question of how it is possible to create a human city out of an inhuman one. The dimensions of the city of the present and future are inhuman and we have already admitted that to think of eliminating the city of these dimensions is Utopian. It is at this point, however, that mankind has made a grave mistake; we have assumed that because the dimensions and forces are inhuman, we must either change them, or become resigned to an inhuman city. This is wrong! The dimensions and forces within the city are going to become even more inhuman, but the city can become human.

We can see how this is possible from the example of a modern jet-plane; its speed is inhuman, so is its frame, but inside it man lives in a human scale, he can walk, sit and sleep. It is interesting that at low marginal speeds, when the wind is moving the aeroplane, this becomes more difficult. Man had to run beside the first aeroplanes until they could develop their take-off speed, and he was uncomfortable inside them; now their frame is completely incompatible with man, but their interior preserves his scale.

If this has been proved in one case, there is no reason why it should not be successful in the case of the city. The question is how we can translate the goals which we set for man—happiness and safety and his satisfaction—into a city structure and function. I can neither enter into the details of this problem, nor build the overall system of the city of the future; the subject is too big and I would have to become too technical. I could, however, mention some principles which are indispensable to the solution of our problem and give some idea of the road we should follow.

Since we want to create a human city we must define the limits of the natural human scale and build a unit of the city corresponding to this scale. We must then build the city of inhuman dimensions by the repetition of the human unit, in the same way in which nature builds living organisms by a repetition of cells. This unit then becomes the cell of the human city and corresponds to the human community in the human scale. Since a major city will grow and expand over increasingly larger areas, we have to devise networks that will keep the cells as well interconnected within a system as possible.

In this way we define the future human city as consisting of cells of human communities and networks, operating in such a way as will guarantee to man the maximum of amenities under human conditions.

The key to the solution of the problem is the structure and function of the cell. Experience has shown that its dimensions should not be larger than 2,000 by 2,000 yards so that man can easily walk in it—ten minutes for the average maximum distance. Depending on the density which we accept, this cell can contain an average of 40,000 people and be built in such a way as will separate the movement of machines from that of man. Working on the basis of considerations related to man and his satisfaction, as already explained, we can define all characteristics of this cell for every special occasion.

It is in this cell that we can help the infant and the child to grow, and prepare it for life, in the same way in which the babies mature in the protection of the womb and later in their bed or room (Fig. 10).

To conceive and create this cell is not difficult if we consider the great experience transmitted to modern man by the cities of the past, whether in ruins or still alive. What we have learned from them confirms our experience from contemporary man completely: there is a natural human scale which has conditioned cities in the past, and which is still valid because man has remained basically the same.

When he moves beyond the cells, man does not need to move in the human scale, because he would not wish to walk 20 or 50 miles a day.

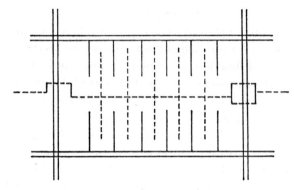

(a) ═══ speed 60-100 miles per hour (machine)
(b) ——— speed 10-20 miles per hour (machine)
(c) ----- speed 3 miles per hour (man)

FIG. 10. Human community, separating the paths of man and machine.

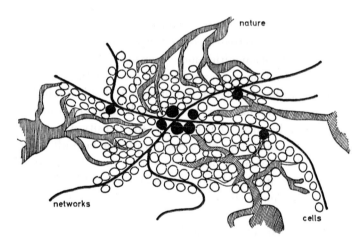

FIG. 11. Total settlement.

Beyond the cell we need much higher speeds and vehicles inside which there will be a human scale again. Travel in space, and the corresponding research, is going to help us understand to what extent this is possible and how. The very fact that inside the space capsule man's input and output of materials and information is controlled will help us to develop proper attitudes towards movements beyond the human cell of cities.

We can already foresee that modern technology can help us to build all networks of transportation and communications underground—the most important ones and those with high-speed traffic will be built deeper than the others, exactly as nature has done for the circulatory systems of the more developed organisms, such as the mammals (Fig. 11).

Moving in this direction, we can foresee that contaminated air will never be released into the open atmosphere, in the same way in which we do not throw the sewage into the streets any more. In the future, releasing the smoke of our fireplaces will seem just as unreasonable as letting the drain pipes empty into the streets.

In this way we can foresee that in the human city, the surface of the earth is going to be properly used, the landscapes will not be destroyed, and air and water will be as clean as before the unwise action of man started.

This is not easy and it is not going to happen tomorrow. If we can, however, care for the skin of our earth, which is our cosmos—the Anthropo-cosmos—as we do for the human body; if we will learn from medicine that our problems are not solved by surgery or curative methods alone, but only by the proper preventive methods and only where necessary by curative and surgical interventions; if we will love the system in which we live as we love ourselves, we can build the human city—and we shall.

DISCUSSION

Johnson-Marshall: Hitherto, as Dr. Doxiadis pointed out, cities have been small and there has been an idea of unlimited space being available for urban expansion, but we have at last realized that terrestrial space is strictly limited. The problem is one of balance of population in relation to the total space available, and we should not despair about this yet. We still have much to learn about the conditions limiting optimum settlement sizes, and this total ecological balance can only be achieved with the help of other types of scientist. Medical predictions and medical action may not be very effective in terms of population control, but the physical planners certainly need more help from the medical side before they can make any kind of planning predictions.

Certain needs in a civilized society will always exist but there are new urban conditions of which we are only beginning to be aware, and which Dr. Doxiadis brought out very clearly. We must grapple with the new ideas and new developments flowing from technology and go back to Dr. Doxiadis's point of family life—the family as the incubation stage of society. We must design our cities as groups of cells to enable this in-cubatory period to take place in a safe way. Many new and specialized work techniques have been developed, and some of these involve the total re-examination of the relationship between working and living. Here again we need to think in terms both of highly specialized work places and of a close relationship of spaces for working and living. The green regenerative spaces Dr. Doxiadis suggested were very significant. This should enable us to restore the "urban cores"—the real centre points of living—for basic sociocultural purposes which the 19th-century city almost destroyed. What the planners have to do today is to provide nearly everything for everybody, instead of for just a limited number, as in the past. We must start with the idea of reasonable fulfilment for every man and work from that in terms of availability of resources.

After this we come to the infrastructure, such as water supply and communications. This is really just a mechanical process of planning inter-communications and infrastructural networks so as to be really efficient for all purposes.

The regional concept, the concept of the city within a region and regional city complexes, is very important, and we can no longer have a contradiction between town and country; they must be complementary and this can only be thought of in broad regional terms.

Wright: Is Corbusier's Chandigarh the sort of city you are visualizing, Dr. Doxiadis?

Doxiadis: Chandigarh is the best example of an effort towards new city-building which we have, the most imaginative one, and in many respects in the right direction. As it was the first post-war attempt to build a new city it has many mistakes, but its value is very great. What Chandigarh does not represent at all is the fourth dimension, that of time. It is a static city, but we cannot have static cities any more—all our cities must be prepared for growth. Any study of any type of area or economy proves that all our major cities must be prepared for growth until the time comes when the population growth as a whole has levelled off. This time will come, as history and evolution show, but the question is where and when it will happen.

The experts accept that even if the United Nations passed a resolution today for compulsory birth control the minimum population of the earth would still reach 12,000 million simply because of the ongoing forces. But will the United Nations pass such a resolution in the year 1967? For all practical purposes the minimum population is somewhere between 20,000 and 50,000 million people, with an average of 30,000 million. However, when animals reach the maximum numbers at which food can be provided for them they level off much below that maximum, as studies of birds and deer have shown[4]. On the basis of this experience, if we assume that the earth can feed 30,000 million people, the population will be much beyond that estimate of 12,000 million and perhaps less than 30,000 million people. Therefore, I hope that Dr. Pincus and his colleagues will think in these terms and warn us to make the proper calculations for all our needs. As the builders of tomorrow we should not encourage the Utopian hope that we can plan for smaller or static cities when we have to expect a minimum of an additional 8,700 million people in our cities, whose population is now only 1,300 million people. The urban land which every person uses now is increasing, so it is probable that we shall need a minimum of 20 times the present area of cities in a century from now, even if the total population does not exceed the minimum figure of 12,000 million. These are facts established by the experts. We cannot avoid them. This is the trend and within this framework we have to start making adjustments and decisions. To avoid recognition of this is to be completely unrealistic.

REFERENCES

1. Huxley, A. (1962). In Preface, p. xxii (by Julian Huxley), to *Silent Spring*, by Rachel Carson. London: Hamish Hamilton.
2. Dubos, R. (1965). Technology and Man's Biological Nature. Paper presented at the *Symposium on the Technological Society*. Santa Barbara, California: Center for the Study of Democratic Institutions.
3. Hall, E. T. (1966). *The Hidden Dimension*. New York: Doubleday.
4. See ref. 3, p. 17.

II

POLITICAL, NATIONAL AND TRADITIONAL LIMITATIONS TO HEALTH CONTROL

K. EVANG

Health Services of Norway, The Royal Norwegian Ministry of Social Affairs, Oslo

PROMOTION of health, prevention and treatment of disease, rehabilitation, in short the *control of health*, nowhere takes place in a vacuum, but in a given political, national and traditional setting. To establish a general background for this paper we should remind ourselves that the unprecedented progress in health conditions during the last 100 years has taken place under the various political systems which we know today, with the national boundaries which existed during this period, and with traditions familiar to us all. Since neither man nor nature has changed fundamentally over thousands, indeed hundreds of thousands of years, there must therefore be something inherent in these political systems which—unlike the situation in all earlier systems—has promoted and stimulated the factors which lead to improved health. We live in the century of research, of science.

I have, however, been given the task here of trying to identify, not the many positive political, national and traditional factors, but some of the limiting ones.

Ecology is a key word in present-day health philosophy. Disease, infirmity, accidents, malformations, maladjustment, can only be understood and fought if one accepts the basic idea of the never-ending battle between man and the host of pathogenic agents in his environment. These unfriendly environmental factors are varied and manifold. New ones are being produced by nature and by ourselves all the time to add to or substitute for those which have already been recognized. Old ones with which mankind has lived unknowingly through the ages are still being isolated and identified.

This ecological approach was a logical step forward from the realization of the *multiple causation* of any disease, i.e. the interplay between the various environmental pathogenic factors. Clinical and experimental research could—and did—carry us a long distance, but only epidemiological research could handle the problem of the multiplicity of factors, try to quantitate them and arrange them in priority sequence for the health administrator to attack.

This is well and good, but how do the political, national and traditional factors which I have been asked to discuss fit into this broad ecological concept? No illustration ever shows the full truth, but we may come one step closer to its realization not only by distinguishing between man and his environment, but by accepting the splitting up of the environment into two basic elements: the active or causative agents themselves, and the structure through which they have to pass to reach the human being and which may be termed the milieu, in the widest sociological meaning of that term. There is nothing new in this simple concept. One of the German fore-runners of social medicine, Chajes, expressed it in these terms: "Between man and nature stands culture". ("Zwischen dem Menschen und der Natur steht die Kultur").

We are now in the process of coming to a keener realization of the two-way traffic by which man himself constantly produces new factors detrimental and dangerous to his health, both as far as the active agents are concerned and—even more—as parts of his milieu. This has been shown by the papers already given here on the major factors aggravating world health problems.

This picture only serves to introduce us to the importance of the type of society in which we live, which is everywhere the result of general political forces, of national factors and historic traditions, just as much as of geography, climate and natural resources. When some countries have mortality figures of between 15 and 20 deaths for infants up to one year of age, per 1,000 live births, while others still present figures of between 150 and 200, this must be mainly due, not to unchangeable biological components, not to climatic or other physical environmental factors, not to vectors which cannot today be controlled, but to the political, economic and social structure of the country concerned. Equally revealing is the comparison between countries, for example in regard to maternal mortality, mortality of children under ten, incidence and prevalence of certain preventable communicable diseases, etc. The average expectancy of life in certain parts of the world is still only half, or less, of that in the most advanced countries.

But one does not need to go to the poorer or the so-called "developing" countries to observe how factors of the type we are now discussing put limitations on health control. Technically it is possible to build an industrial plant which is relatively foolproof as far as accidents and industrial diseases are concerned. Politically, however, this is impossible. Technically it is feasible to produce a car which for all practical purposes is accident-proof as far as the occupants are concerned, of course including a built-in speed limit. Politically this is impossible. We have just heard about the pollution of water, air and food, the health hazards produced by bringing people together in cities, and malnutrition. And again we can solve these problems technically—in fact theoretically and scientifically most of them have been solved but politically we cannot solve them.

Analyses by the Food and Agriculture Organization of the relationship between growth of world population and world food production even seem to indicate that at least up till now we might easily have balanced the "population explosion" by a "food explosion" had it not been for limiting political, national and traditional factors, such as feudal and other motive-destroying systems of land ownership, lack of irrigation and proper fertilization, outmoded agricultural equipment and use of manpower under climatic and other conditions where machines should do the work. These and similar factors are rightly blamed. But we may go further and ask the question: why is it that countries which produce a large surplus of food in relation to an optimum consumption by their own population prefer to export that surplus—or at least part of it—instead of importing people to live in that country of plenty?

Migration has on many occasions in the history of man served to solve problems, as for example when the white man spread over the vast areas of North and South America, Oceania and elsewhere. Why has migration ceased to be a remedy, although we can easily define underpopulated as well as overpopulated areas of the world? Certainly it is not because we do not possess the means to move people from one place to the other. Most impressive "air bridges" have been established from time to time to move considerable numbers of people from one place to another, sometimes far away. But they did not always go to live there: on most occasions I am sorry to say they were sent to kill those who lived there already, and to spread fire, poison and misery, with disease following close on the trail.

We all know why migration on a larger scale is only an empty word: our world at present is deep-frozen in an unhealthy medium of national and political interests and traditions, made even more unappetizing by the generous addition of racial and religious prejudices. We simply do not yet dare to live at close range with other peoples on this globe.

We are not willing either, for much the same reasons, to share with others what we have got or produce. When in 1943 the great statesman Franklin Delano Roosevelt called the Hot Springs Conference of the United Nations to discuss post-war problems, he was in fact urged to do so by his vice-president, Mr. Henry Wallace, and by close friends of Mr. Wallace, including some of those who had been active in the Health Section in the League of Nations. The president received the delegates in the White House at Washington after the conference and his speech to us included approximately the following words:

"After the war the greatest problem will be the gap between the poor and the rich in the world. If we are not able to bridge this gap, we will not avoid a new war. We must therefore establish a system which makes it possible for the poor Chinese labourer to enjoy the surplus which we produce, for example of wheat. This is necessary so that the Chinese people can build their own productive machinery. However, the Chinese labourer cannot pay the price per bushel which the American farmer on the prairie asks for, and we cannot reduce the price which the American farmer will have. We cannot reduce his standard of living—on the contrary. Therefore we must establish an international credit system in such a way that food from surplus countries can be used by the hungry populations in the poor countries without these countries thereby becoming politically dependent upon those who present the gifts."

As we know, the Director-General of FAO at that time, Sir John Boyd Orr, tried to give life to this idea by suggesting to the second conference of FAO (Copenhagen, 1946) the establishment of a World Food Board. The terms of reference were to:

(1) Stabilize prices by buffer stocks schemes;

(2) Hold a world food reserve against famine;

(3) Finance surplus disposal programmes to needy people;

(4) Co-operate with a credit-issuing agency (to be created);

(5) Co-ordinate bodies dealing with individual commodities.

The conference—which I attended as a member of the Norwegian delegation—accepted the idea "in principle". However, when politicians use the term "accept in principle" it means, as we know, that they do not accept the principle. The old story repeats itself—when God does not want a thing to happen, he appoints a committee! A "Preparatory Committee" with Lord Bruce as chairman went to work and the mountain gave birth to a mouse. The more essential parts of the body of this mouse were then put on ice at the next conference of FAO.

At its tenth anniversary (1955) FAO produced a book entitled *So Bold an Aim. Ten years of International Co-operation Toward Freedom from Want*[1] which contains (pp. 80, 83), the following laconic description of what happened at this cross-road of world health:

"This was manifestly asking too much of governments. They would have to subscribe extremely large sums of money at a time when they needed every penny to restore or maintain their own solvency. In addition, they would be expected to part with sovereignty over a number of matters which they regarded as vital to the management of their own economies and their policies of full employment; and all this in favour of a scheme the practical operation of which had not been adumbrated in any way."
"Thus ended Sir John's grand design. As a practical proposal it was a non-starter. As a platform for ventilating the heartfelt ideas of many governments, mainly the smaller and poorer ones, it was invaluable. And the issues it raised and faced still come up year after year at one meeting or another and will so continue until in prosperity or crisis the groping nations find some acceptable solutions."

Economists can tell us that while poor, so-called developing countries no doubt develop, the richer countries which are supposedly in the process of assisting them in bridging the gulf, develop even more quickly, so that the distance is growing. Whether we name the influences which bring this about political or economic is mainly a matter of taste. What the health of the peoples of the world might look like if these national and political forces could be controlled and directed for positive purposes defies imagination.

What might be called a "world conscience" is no doubt growing, most clearly and strongly in the younger generations, but so far international co-operation is working in an iron cage, able to observe everything outside, but unable to get out and really grapple at close range with the enemies. One of the tragic side-effects of this is to my mind the alienation of youth, disgusted and frustrated by the discrepancy between the never-ending lip service and the modest results.

This alienation (in German *Entfremdung*) or lack of involvement of young people, which from the mental health point of view is rightly a matter of great concern in many of the rich countries, has many more aspects to it than this. But in the final outcome the chaotic and depressing political situation in the world, the brutality, the cynicism, the killing and the lies, have an indirect effect on the health of many of the younger generation. The well-known quotation from one of Ludvig Holberg's plays "Everyone says that Jeppe drinks, but no one says why Jeppe drinks" may equally well be applied to the tragic and dangerous spread of marijuana, LSD and other hallucinogenic agents amongst young people.

But you do not want me, I am sure, only to give general illustrations of the basic influence of national and political factors on the health of people.

If one observes these matters at closer range, meaning by country, one will quickly realize that the way in which a given country serves its people in the field of health can only be understood in the light of the political, economic, social and administrative structure of the country concerned. Therefore I think no two countries with identical organizations of health services, in the widest meaning of that term, will be found, just as no two countries exist with identical political, social and administrative structures. As a consequence one can also easily identify three main types of health services in the world today, just as one can identify three main types of political and economic systems:

(1) The "Western European" type developed in its original form in central, continental Europe, but gradually characterized by the "welfare state idea" in the Nordic countries and United Kingdom.

(2) The "American" type to be found in its most characteristic form in the United States of America, and partly in other countries ideologically close to the USA. Here the health services are guided by the ideas of free enterprise and free competition. As much as possible is left to the initiative of the individual, as little as possible being accepted as a responsibility of society.

(3) The "Soviet Russian" type which was introduced through the Russian Revolution in 1917 and spread from the USSR first to other eastern European countries, later also to China and certain countries in Asia and Africa. The dominating health philosophy under this system is that health and disease cannot be regarded as private affairs. Society must take the full responsibility for organizing health services, from planning and co-ordination to execution.

Each of these political systems has, in other words, developed its special patterns for health control, and there are most interesting dissimilarities from system to system, for example in the priority given to the various basic functions or components of the health services:

(a) Promotion of health;
(b) Primary prevention;
(c) Curative medicine;
(d) Secondary prevention and follow-up;
(e) Rehabilitation and tertiary prevention;
(f) Care of the "weak" (non-rehabilitative);
(g) Medical research;
(h) Medical education, including postgraduate training.

Political factors also of course finally decide—within the individual country—the degree to which the various social classes will be reflected in their morbidity and mortality data, differences in economy, education, etc.

In the poor, newly emerged developing countries, no single pattern has as yet been developed. Since assistance to developing countries in the field of health is being offered by advanced countries representing all three main systems and variations thereof, developing countries find themselves in a most confusing situation. One could not say that their attempts to choose from each system the best parts and drop the less valuable have been convincingly successful.

What may be achieved under favourable political conditions even during periods of great economic difficulties has been convincingly demonstrated in our time, for example by the USSR after the Russian Revolution in 1917 and by China after the Chinese Revolution in 1949. In both cases a country which would in today's terminology be termed underdeveloped succeeded over a short period in improving the health status of its population to an unbelievable degree. One of the keys to this staggering success is, I think, to be found in the priority given to primary prevention: another lies in the identification of human health problems with those of other mammals and certain other animals, and generally in a sound ecological approach.

Do not misunderstand me: in the last 10–15 years many—in fact, most—developing countries have made remarkable progress in improving health conditions, but they demonstrate at the same time very clearly the limitations put by political and national factors. Politicians are like other people in the sense that one of their fundamental motivating fears is fear of death, fear of the end which will come to us all. We are faced here perhaps with one of the main psychological reasons for the ambivalent attitude of politicians towards health matters. They hate disease and death and like to forget about them.

One interesting historic example is that health was "forgotten" when the Covenant of the League of Nations was drafted after the first World War. Only at the last moment was world health brought in, producing the Health Section of the League of Nations, one of the forerunners of the present FAO, as well as of WHO. Although international participation in the League of Nations was limited*, the Health Section of the League developed into one of the most successful and non-controversial parts of the organization, making itself indispensable through its statutory functions.

Who would have thought, therefore, that health would again be "forgotten" when the Charter of the United Nations was drafted at the end of the Second World War? However, this was exactly what happened, and the

---

* The USA was never a member, Germany withdrew in 1933, after seven years' membership, Japan withdrew in the same year, Italy in 1937, and the USSR was expelled in 1939, after five years' membership.

matter of world health again had to be introduced more or less *ad hoc* at the United Nations conference at San Francisco in the spring of 1945*. I have described the attitude of the politician towards health matters as ambivalent; yet when forced into a corner by health problems he cannot escape, the politician may act with unusual speed and generosity. Thomas Parran, Surgeon General of the United States Public Health Service at that time, made use of this psychological law in his bold move to incorporate medical research on a large scale in the United States Public Health Service. To use American phraseology, Parran ''sold'' to Congress the idea of doing something about four selected groups of diseases: heart and circulatory disease, cancer, rheumatism and diabetes. These diseases happen to be those most prevalent amongst congressmen and those most heartily feared by them.

From the point of view of the health of the peoples of the world at large, I think we would agree that other health problems should have had priority over most of those chosen. Whether a highly specialized interest of this type should be named healthy or morbid is of course a matter of taste, but it resulted in the National Institutes of Health in Bethesda, an institution of unprecedented character, which has been invaluable in the promotion of medical research not only in the United States itself but in many other countries of the world.

There are other occasions also on which politicians may act quickly and decisively in matters of health, namely when an accident occurs, as for example the thalidomide tragedy, or when—for this or other reasons—public pressure is brought to bear on a specific point. Under the guidance of existing mass media, the public will now perhaps react more quickly and concretely than before. Unfortunately in most cases it is the new ''wonder drug'', or wonder methods such as intermittent renal dialysis or the latest advances in brain and heart surgery, which most frequently attract attention. But there are also many encouraging examples of well-informed public opinion exerting increasing pressure upon politicians in important and fundamental health matters, thereby bringing about reforms and improvement. In my part of the world we have over the last 10–15 years observed quite a number of most interesting examples of these tactics: a ''pressure group'' is formed by citizens who for some reason or other have taken special interest in parts of the health services. With the various means at the disposal of such pressure groups things may gradually move more satisfactorily.

* Initiative was taken by the advisers in health matters to three national delegations: the Brazilian (Dr. De Paula Souza), the Chinese (Dr. Szeming Sze) and the Norwegian (myself).

Under circumstances where the political balance in a country is at stake and where individual parties therefore have to think of something special to attract votes for the next election, this may sometimes lead to political "overbidding" in the field of health. Legislation is promulgated and promises are made for which there exist no services—neither institutions nor personnel. The health authorities will not infrequently have to take the criticism as scapegoats for the politician, weakening the position of the health authorities generally.

Add to this behaviouristic pattern of politicians their ever-existing tendency to save money, to ask for minimum standards or "permissible levels" instead of optimum standards in the field of health, and you may understand why I have always been a strong advocate of bringing in a medically trained person as the responsible overall administrator and co-ordinator of health services, in direct contact with the political people who make the decisions[2].

When the constitution of the World Health Organization was drafted in Paris in the spring of 1946 by the so-called Technical Preparatory Committee appointed by the Social and Economic Council of the UN the sixteen members of the committee, from as many countries, acted in their personal capacity as technical experts in the field of health and not as representatives of their governments. During the drafting process an interesting attempt was made to substitute international democracy for international anarchy in the field of health. Some members of the group suggested an article in the constitution which would give the World Health Assembly (the yearly conference of all member states) the status of a World Health Parliament. The World Health Assembly would have had the power to pass, by simple majority, health regulations which would have been binding upon all member states, regardless of whether they had voted in favour or not. This is, as we know, normal procedure for legislation passed by the relevant body within a country or state. Was it too ambitious to think that this simple democratic principle could now also be introduced into the friendly and constructive relationship between nations with a common interest in world health? It was: even in this group the attempt failed. A formula was found which preserved the sovereignty of the individual member state, regardless of whether or not this was in the interest of the world at large. What was no doubt technically and scientifically highly desirable in the interest of controlling world health, and also administratively possible, had again proved to be politically impossible.

But the battle was not completely in vain. A small piece was saved which in fact puts the World Health Organization in a somewhat more fortunate position than all the other specialized agencies of the UN. I refer to Articles 21 and 22, under which the World Health Assembly may adopt "health regulations". Unlike other specialized agencies, including ILO, where resolutions and recommendations have to be ratified through relevant constitutional processes by the individual member state before coming into force, a health regulation adopted by a world health assembly "...shall come into force for all members after due notice has been given of their adoption by the Health Assembly except for such members as may notify the Director-General of rejection or reservations within the period stated in the notice." (Article 22.) The two health regulations passed so far (on Quarantine and on International Statistical Classification of Diseases, Injuries and Causes of Death) have proved to be highly acceptable.

A relevant question therefore is, why do we not proceed? We have the opportunity under article 21 also to adopt regulations concerning "standards with respect to the safety, purity and potency of biological, pharmaceutical and similar products moving in international commerce; advertising and labelling of biological, pharmaceutical and similar products moving in international commerce."

In spite of increasing efforts in recent years, relatively little has been achieved, and again I do not think that we can find the limiting factors in the scientific, technical or administrative fields, although of course some of these problems are formidable. Why do we not widen article 21 to include more fields which might now be fruitfully covered by health regulations? Why not, through a widened article 21, pass health regulations on non-dangerous levels for air pollution, radioactive fall-out, noise and vibration, food additives, insecticides and pesticides, standards for immunization of children under various epidemiological conditions in the world, and the labelling and declaration of content of poisonous substances used in the household?

The World Health Organization came into being just at the time (1948) when the political honeymoon which the United Nations had enjoyed for a short period after the Second World War had definitely come to an end, and the "cold war" had started. It was of course a most unfortunate political climate for a newcomer which was supposed to act non-politically in the field of international health, but which was built and run by member governments. The withdrawal for a short period into "inactive membership" of the group of eastern European countries was a blow to the organization, from which, however, it recovered. The lack of success in bringing the People's Republic of China in as a member, was—and still is—

much worse*. It means that a whole wall is missing in the building. The Arab-Israel conflict also created some trouble. As if this was not enough, influential political forces of a more general character made themselves felt through the UN itself, threatening the independence and technical integrity of WHO and other specialized agencies. The very principle established at San Francisco in 1945, namely to give scientists, technicians and administrators a chance, in the specialized agencies and independently of political considerations, to build international co-operation on a broad scale, was in the process of being betrayed.

The most dangerous attack came through the proposal in the UN for a ''consolidated budget''. In principle this meant that all the member states of the UN would have had to pay only one contribution, namely directly to the United Nations. Like the individual ministries in a national government, the various specialized agencies would have to produce their separate programmes. A clear-cut political body, namely the UN itself, would then have discussed, accepted or rejected these programmes, decided priorities and finally allotted to each specialized agency one part of the total consolidated budget.

If I am not wrongly informed, high credit goes to the Directors-General of the most important specialized agencies at that time—Morse, Huxley, Boyd Orr and Chisholm—for stopping this frontal attack to get political control over the specialized agencies.

A weaker and more indirect attempt was made later when the UN programme of technical assistance was introduced, but this also worked out in a satisfactory way on the whole. Again great credit for political wisdom goes to the non-political heads of these organizations, including Dr. Candau, who is present at this symposium. I think the well informed will agree that when Dr. Candau's plan for the establishment of a World Health Research body was torpedoed, it was national prestige, combined with political ambition, which was the driving force in shelving the idea—of course supported by the wish to save money.

An example of the way in which national prestige may hamper efficient international health activities is found in the principle of ''equitable geographic distribution'' in WHO. Article 24 of the constitution, dealing with the establishment of the Executive Board of the Organization, states that ''The Health Assembly, taking into account an equitable geographic distribution, shall elect the Members entitled to designate a person to serve on

* China is one of the founding members of WHO and the countries which have recognized the People's Republic of China take the official attitude that that country is the rightful possessor of the seat now occupied by Taiwan.

the Board.'' Since the Executive Board of WHO is an instrument of the World Health Assembly, ''equitable geographic distribution'' in this context has rightly been interpreted to mean that the selection of member states entitled to designate a person to serve on the Board should reflect as closely as possible the number of member states in the respective geographic areas into which the world has been split, that is, the ''regions'' of the World Health Organization. Less helpful but still understandable is the close adherence to the same principle in regard to employment of staff in the secretariat. It is understandable because member countries of the organization would not like to see this secretariat dominated by a small group of states, the nationals of which, for example, had one of the working languages of the organization as their mother tongue. On the other hand, it means in practice that if a top psychiatrist is needed to fill an important position and the person obviously best qualified for that particular job is an American, the Director-General would be prevented from appointing him because the ''quota'' of American staff members in the secretariat has already been filled.

The principle becomes completely meaningless when it is stretched also to include the selection of experts for field projects undertaken by the Organization in collaboration with the government of a member state. One may have to go a long way down the ranking list based on qualifications until a person is found who happens to be a citizen of a country whose quota has not been filled.

The higher the degree of specialization, the more destructive this principle becomes. But it is being pressed all the time, even in regard to the selection of scientists and other highly specialized experts for advisory panels, expert committees, etc. We have even experienced the baroque situation that a country on the one hand has criticized the Director-General for not applying the principle of equitable geographic distribution strictly enough and on the other hand has complained that WHO has taken away one of the very few individuals representing that particular specialty in the country concerned. As will be understood, the small and poor developing countries will here find themselves in an exposed position.

The fact that two standards of health services can exist in one and the same country, based on racial, religious or other types of discrimination, is obviously incompatible with the improvement and control of health. The countries of Africa, supported by many other developing countries, have to my mind therefore carried their main point when they argue that such health discrimination is also incompatible with the ideas underlying the World Health Organization. The situation is intolerable. However, I think it is highly questionable whether the situation is improved if one hurts the World Health Organization by violating the principle of universality of membership of that organization.

Generally speaking, formation of political blocs of countries operating as such within WHO are not conducive to international health work, regardless of whether such a bloc is composed of developing African countries or of highly developed western countries. A number of the richest countries in the world have set a bad example by forming in Geneva a permanent committee which discusses the problems of international health at a nontechnical and political level before the same problems reach the proper bodies of WHO.

One should not of course speak of political limitations to health control in an informal group like the one at this symposium without pointing out that at present international co-operation in the field of health, as well as the improvement of health conditions in the countries concerned, is hampered or made impossible by the old and too well-known destructive political instruments: racial discrimination and war. Apartheid in the Union of South Africa, the white supremacy rule in Rhodesia, and—worst of all—the war in Vietnam, are the most drastic examples at present. Others could be added.

If we turn to what may be termed *traditional limitations* to health control a very wide field presents itself for comment.

Traditions in public administration, in the relationship between lay and medically trained administrators, and between public and private (voluntary) bodies working in the field of health in fact decide to a surprisingly high degree how health problems are tackled in individual countries, as well as the list of priorities.

Traditions play an important role in deciding whether special groups of people should enjoy health services at a higher or lower level than others, for example war veterans, the elderly, indigent, mentally retarded, physically or otherwise handicapped, etc.

Traditions rather than medical considerations contribute towards the fact that a person suffering from self-induced, acute intoxication is regarded in some cases 100 per cent as a patient, in other cases 100 per cent as a criminal, in others again as a mixture of both, and this is dependent not on his condition but on the toxic agent: barbiturates, marijuana, morphine or alcohol. This also varies confusingly from one part of the world to the other, being highly dependent upon ethical, legal and other social traditions. Much the same holds true for the ever-increasing groups of maladjusted children, adolescents and others.

Traditions rather than rational thinking also contribute highly to the varied patterns found in regard to the splitting of responsibility in health matters between various groups of health personnel: medical doctors, dentists, clinical psychologists, medical social workers, nurses, teachers, vocational therapists, physiotherapists, health inspectors, etc. Even between members of the same ''profession'' the distribution of roles may be a matter of controversy.

While family planning and sex education, medically speaking, are accepted everywhere as indispensable prophylactic health measures which should be generally available, traditions of various types—especially religious—still prevent effective and rational programmes from being carried out in practice everywhere.

Pre-scientific schools of curative medicine, carried on by tradition, still play a more or less important role in most countries, depriving the health services of personnel and exploiting the public ideologically as well as economically.

When the ''marriage between sociology and public health'', long overdue, in the future becomes more of a reality, these and many other tradition-borne limitations to health control may be analysed and eventually removed. At present we seem to live in a period in which the non-rational forces are on the offensive.

Let me finally touch briefly upon some problems of an even more delicate and controversial nature, that is on what may be named the iatrogenic traditional factors limiting the improvements of health control. By this I mean the traditional factors found within the medical profession itself, and which at the present stage of development prevent, hamper or distort the optimum development of health services.

To avoid misunderstanding, let it not be forgotten that the medical profession on the whole has been a driving, dynamic force in the development of effective health control measures. My task here, however, is not to enumerate the many positive aspects, but to point to some negative ones.

By tradition medical doctors belong to the conservative forces in society, as do most other social groups with higher education, secured economy, monopolistic status and other prerogatives. This is apt to produce a number of unfortunate attitudes during a period—for example, the last 30–40 years —when the explosive development of medical science and technology called for radical changes in the tools by which scientific insight should be spelled out in health services for individuals, special groups of individuals, and whole populations. This holds true for medical institutions as well as for the activities of the individual doctor.

The term "hospital" in general has become more or less meaningless. One has to specify which of the many types of hospitals one is talking about: what type of patient does the institution care for—bed patients and/or out-patients? Does it aim only to cure or to prevent and rehabilitate as well? What degree of specialization does it have? And so on. The medical profession has no doubt been instrumental in developing these new types of institutions, but all too frequently vested economic interests and traditional attitudes are hindering progress.

All over the world the general practitioner, the traditional family doctor, is disappearing. This branch of medical activity is recruiting very badly in most countries of the world and the reasons given are everywhere practically identical: loss of "status" in relation to specialists and medical institutions, heavy work load, irregular working hours, bureaucratization of society with too much paper work, professional isolation and therefore reduced possibility for postgraduate training, and on the whole professional frustration. The many attempts to remedy this situation seem so far to have given very modest results, to my mind because the medical profession itself is still hypnotized by the old traditional conception of the general practitioner as the "backbone of the health services", and through fear of losing traditional sources of income.

The adequate handling of patients—in the widest sense of this term—based on today's insight has reduced to practically zero the situations which should be handled by one isolated M.D.: the patient with his four "dimensions" (somatic, mental, social, and in interrelation with therapeutic forces) can only be understood and properly handled by a team. Nevertheless, medical doctors are very reluctant indeed to adapt themselves to this situation. They are not willing to play their new role as members, sometimes as leaders, of the team. Fear of changing the traditional role of the doctor seems to lie at the bottom of this attitude.

The costs of health services in most countries are increasing at a higher rate than the rise in national income. Under these circumstances the rational and effective use of the many types of medical and paramedical personnel and of medical institutions is becoming an urgent matter. The medical profession has demonstrated relatively little interest in these and other administrative, or should we rather say functional, aspects of the health services.

By leaving these tasks to others, by resisting in many countries the introduction of prepaid medical care and broader health programmes, by refusing to consider seriously a new role in the medical team, and also by using their "seller's market" to create inflation in the costs of health services, the medical profession is to some extent putting brakes on the organic growth of measures for health control. The medical profession has reached a cross-road where a choice has to be made: should the medical doctor be regarded in the traditional way as a "free lance" or as an integrated part of the total social structure? New terms such as "medical sociology" or "sociological public health" point to the direction in which we have to move, whether we like it or not. It would be a tragedy if the medical profession, bound by traditional pride and fears, should forfeit its natural, fundamental role in this dynamic process, which will under any circumstances continue rapidly to change the health status and health problems of the world population.

SUMMARY

Over the last 30–40 years and especially after World War II health problems have become important political issues, nationally and internationally. It is now the openly declared policy of governments of all descriptions to create living standards and health services which would produce optimum conditions for the attainment of " . . . complete physical, mental and social wellbeing and not merely the absence of disease or infirmity."*

Internationally the countries of the world have also subscribed to the idea that "The health of all peoples is fundamental to the attainment of peace and security and is dependent upon the fullest co-operation of individuals and States."*

These are not empty words. All nationalities, assisted by mass media, are keenly aware of the potentialities of present-day medical science and technology, and are pressing hard everywhere for the fulfilment of what the politicians promise.

Economically as well as scientifically and administratively the situation seems most favourable for major steps, nationally and internationally, towards the improvement of health status. Although many encouraging achievements may be demonstrated, the health situation in many parts of the world is still deplorable. Even in highly developed countries there exists a wide gulf between the health services which might be established, based on present-day scientific insight, and the services which the public is in fact enjoying.

An attempt is made briefly to identify some of the political, national and traditional limitations to health control at present.

* Constitution of the World Health Organization, preamble.

DISCUSSION

le Riche: In North America there is also a development towards a welfare state. In Canada, for instance, the health services have provided prepaid hospital care since 1959 and soon there will be completely prepaid physicians' services. Whether the welfare state is always the best thing, I don't know.

Kaprio: One of the problems of the developing countries, as Dr. Evang mentioned, is the difficulty of choosing which system to follow. Some former colonial countries have systems even more tradition-bound than anywhere else, because of their links with the former metropolitan countries. They stick to the system because it is the only one they know from the colonial period, and they have very great difficulty in starting to change and modernize the system.

Then there is the question of the flexibility of a system. England created a very admirable national health service, but it was divided into three branches and it is now so firmly fixed that nobody seems to be able to move on to the next step. There are similar difficulties in the USSR, where there is also an excellent comprehensive system for the purposes for which it was originally created.

Lambo: The selection of a national health framework is also tied up with economic and political issues. In some developing countries the psychological reaction after independence has been so powerful that these countries have chosen the complete opposite of whatever existed previously. Some measure of flexibility is needed so that a young country can experiment and evolve patterns or institutions which have some affinity with the projected social structure and culture of the country. The tradition which has been mentioned is one which is artificial and is bound up with political and economic considerations.

Florey: Are you optimistic that people will take to more flexible methods?

Lambo: A great deal is being done in some countries, certainly in mine. Again, one cannot separate this from economic freedom, which many young and developing countries do not yet have. The greater the freedom, the easier it is to experiment.

Dogramaci: Dr. Evang said that when members of the medical profession form a union for the protection of their own prestige this is against the common good and welfare of the community. There is a great deal of truth in this, but it is not emphasized as much as it should be.

Turkey receives quite a bit of financial aid from the U.S. Agency for International Development and uses this for the improvement of the

212

health services. For the past five years we have had a socialized system; almost one-third of the provinces are now included in this scheme. This is an example of a developing country receiving aid from a developed country but not using their methods.

Evang: The question, what system is the best—the capitalist, the totalitarian or the welfare state?—is meaningless, because each system is just thinkable in its own context. You cannot overnight revolutionize one single part of a structure. Canada has been moving for some time in the health service field towards what is regarded as a welfare state approach in Europe. The United States is taking the first legal steps in establishing a prepaid medical programme.

It is interesting to note that the welfare state idea is being attacked both by the East and by the West. Our Russian friends would say that this is deceiving the population—it just tries to satisfy and pacify them without giving them real control, and our American friends would say that the welfare state in introducing "socialized" medicine takes away people's initiative by supporting them from the cradle to the grave. Historically, both these systems were derived from the original European system. They both came into being in opposition to what existed at that time in western Europe.

The difficulty in criticizing certain attitudes of doctors is of course that generally speaking the medical profession has been and still is a driving and dynamic force in the development of health services. Who developed all these health services if they didn't? They therefore have a very strong platform. Just now in many countries a battle is being fought between the medically-trained administrators and the administrators without technical knowledge. The politicians are much in favour of this, because they frequently do not like to have technically-trained administrators close to them; they want to have somebody in between to interpret what the experts are saying. I am a very strong believer in the medical profession also taking the administrative tasks upon itself.

Querido: You referred to the proportion of the national income used for the health services. There is still a big gap between what can be done and what is done even in the highly-developed countries. I suspect that economists will say that health services could never have much more than 5 or 6 per cent in countries with a high national income. Do you think it is feasible in a national budget to go up to, say, 8 per cent?

Evang: There are two sides to this. First we have the question of what percentage of the national income should or might be used for medical and social services, and this will vary from country to country—in some countries it has now reached 10-12 per cent if you include all the social services. This money is not being poured down the drain. Seventy or 80 per cent of this goes in wages, a large proportion of which will be paid back again in taxes, so to a certain extent it is a self-financing system and it is not non-productive as the politicians and economists often seem to think. However, during certain periods of scientific growth I think the services we are able to render increase at an abnormally rapid speed. We are in such a period now, so that if the percentage of the national income which the medical services use doesn't rise more rapidly than the increase in the national income itself, the gulf between what we could do and what we are doing will become deeper and deeper.

Querido: As soon as a competitive industry loses its markets because its products are too costly, it investigates to see whether it can operate on a cheaper basis. It seems to me that before we try to go up to 6·5 per cent we should first see whether the system is run efficiently, and I am sure it is not carried on efficiently in many countries in the West. A general practitioner in the Netherlands probably spends much of the day on activities which could easily be done by cheaper labour.

Evang: I agree. This is one of the most difficult and important problems in the world today—to utilize the various types of medical personnel, including doctors, more rationally than is being done at present.

Kaprio: WHO has recently analysed the costs of health services[3, 4]. In several countries the expenditure on health services has already gone higher than this figure of 5 or 6 per cent of the national income. As health expenditure grows the economists get more interested and the pressure to make internal economies in the health services grows; at the same time the health administrators want to keep their right to increase expenditure because they are the ones who can see the benefits to society of doing so. That is why it is so important that at the head of health administrations there should be technically and professionally trained people, so that these services are not restricted by questions of cost. England for a long time had restrictions on new hospital building—though this may have been right because it was a question of priorities between education and hospitals. The struggle between the politicians, the economists and the medical administrators must be continual.

Pequignot: The growth in national income in France is about 5 to 6 per cent per annum and the growth in the cost of medical care is about 8 per cent. It is remarkable that the income tax increase in France for the same period was also 8 per cent. Perhaps both phenomena reflect the rise in the standard of living.

Katsunuma: The question of whether or not the health services are economically productive has been much discussed. Shell[5] is working on the possibility of introducing change in technological development as a working variable of the production function in addition to labour and capital, and a formula for transformation was suggested. On the same sort of thinking, health data can be the variable for the production function. I am extremely interested in this matter and we have been trying the same line of work in Japan. Mushkin[6] suggested that the rise observed in the United States during the period 1900–1960 depended on a health improvement of about 13 per cent, while Schultz[7] pointed out that the money invested in education resulted in a contribution of about 33 per cent to the gross national income. So I think it is worth while trying to improve health education in the developing countries.

Florey: How would you define health in this connexion?

Katsunuma: We use the WHO recommendations, in other words, the death rate, life expectancy and proportional mortality.

Evang: It is a fact now that health services have a higher priority than certain other commodities, with the result that the "demand" for health services is different from the "need", and one of the problems in health services today is to say where to draw the line. I think John Maynard Keynes was the first economist to explode the original theory of "the full glass": that is that the first task of an economy was to produce all the "necessary" commodities—food, clothing, housing and so on—and only when there was an overflow could a country have luxuries like health services. Keynes, however, said this was nonsense—the most important factor in production is labour and if a country doesn't take care of its labour force it cannot produce. The situation has changed radically. In the old days there was always a surplus of people who were used as slaves, soldiers and unskilled labour. Now there is no place for unskilled labour either in peace or war—they are of no use in our days. We have now to invest large amounts in the form of educational and health services to make people useful.

Lindop: You were concerned about the slow rate of disappearance of non-scientific methods, Dr. Evang. I understand that the Chinese medical services recently found they had to maintain their traditional medical practices as well as introducing scientific medicine, just from the man-power point of view. How much should one try to remove some of the traditional medical practices in developing countries before one has actually instituted scientific methods?

Evang: The Indian attitude and the Chinese attitude differ fundamentally in this respect. India had two traditional systems, the Ayurvedic, which is Hindu, and the Unani, which is Moslem. The Unani system was politically not important but figures obtained in 1951 showed that there were so many Ayurvedic doctors that they represented a political force that could not be ignored. The result was a dual system of western medicine and Ayurvedic medicine, with special Ayurvedic universities.

In China they also accepted both traditional and "western" medicine but they amalgamated them: for example, when an appendicitis case was brought into the surgical department of a hospital in Shanghai which I visited in 1960, according to the Chinese maxim that "The patient must have all chances" he would be seen by both the western surgeon and the traditional Chinese physician; he would have blood counts and so on and if the situation developed in a drastic way he would be operated on. The Chinese seem to feel that if they bring these two systems together they will merge.

Doxiadis: If an ancient Greek had been present at this discussion he would have protested about one thing that you mentioned, Dr. Evang: Unani means "Greek"; it is derived from the word "Ionian". In Alexandrine times Greek medicine entered the East and was later adopted by the Arabs and others and called Unani, or Ionian Greek. Its teachings go back to Asclepios and are related to the teachings of Aristotle and Plato, as I had the occasion to find on many occasions in Asia.

Banks: My understanding is that the Indians have endeavoured to bring Ayurvedic and western medicine together. When this happens there is a tendency to upgrade traditional systems to western medicine. The Unani system of medicine still exists, and the practitioners of both systems also use modern methods.

Florey: What we have really been discussing here is the allotting of priorities. This is what politicians do, but I am not sure that any country has yet devised a system by which it is done satisfactorily: what we usually do is to form another committee to place over all the existing committees. Perhaps we can hope that the comments of our group here will help to guide the politicians who are deciding the priorities.

REFERENCES

1. Food and Agriculture Organization. (1955). *So Bold an Aim. Ten Years of International Co-operation toward Freedom from Want.* Rome: FAO.
2. Evang, K. (1966). The Position of the Medically Trained Person in the Administration of Health Services. *American Journal of Public Health,* **56,** 1722–1733.
3. Abel-Smith, B. (1963). *Paying for Health Services: a study of the costs and sources of finance in six countries.* Geneva: WHO, Public Health Papers, No. 17.

4. Abel-Smith, B. (1967). *International Study of Health Expenditure and its Relevance for Health Planning*. Geneva: WHO, in press.
5. Shell, K. (1966). Toward a theory of investive activity and capital accumulation. *American Economic Review*.
6. Mushkin, S. J. (1962). Health as an investment. *Journal of Political Economy*, **70**, suppl. no. 5 (part 2), 129–157.
7. Schultz, T. W. (1963). *The Economic Value of Education*. New York: Columbia University Press.

12

SIZE AND DISTRIBUTION OF PRESENT WORLD RESOURCES OF DOCTORS, SPECIALISTS, NURSES, MIDWIVES, MEDICAL TECHNICIANS, SANITARIANS AND OTHER HEALTH STAFF

LEO A. KAPRIO

Regional Office for Europe, World Health Organization, Copenhagen

A T the United Nations Conference on Application of Science and Technology for the Benefit of Less Developed Areas, in Geneva in 1963, international concern and interest was expressed in the education and training of human resources. It was stated there that[1]: "The most important investment any country can make, whatever its stage of development, is its human resources, that is, in the education and training of its population under institutions which create incentives and which make it possible for the individual to realize his aspirations." We at this symposium all agree on the importance of the proper use of some portion of the pool of human resources for the care of the sick, prevention of disease, and maintenance of the health of the population as a whole. Indeed, unless the health of a country is well managed, the effectiveness of a nation's human resources may be dissipated or squandered.

Several earlier papers here gave examples of the vast potentialities of the application of present medical knowledge and of the new challenges in research work that await us and promise new solutions. But what are the real possibilities arising from this new knowledge? How many doctors, nurses, midwives and other skilled workers are available to carry through the programmes which could improve the health of people in many parts of the world? My task is to try to give you at least a reasonable answer.

Most of you probably expect me to give long lists of numbers and produce a series of tables to describe the information available on the health manpower of the world. That, at least, was my own first reaction when I saw the title suggested for my paper. But then I realized that I almost had to avoid numbers. Instead, I thought it would be useful to go deeper into the dynamism of health manpower and the question of utilization of health staff both by the health administration and by the general public. This may lead me away from hard facts to some speculations. These will still be worthwhile if they help us all to see more clearly the problems facing world health leaders today.

As national or international medical leaders or policy makers we may have a rather simple approach to the problems of medical manpower. Whatever new challenges we have—whether the elimination of smallpox from a rural province of a developing country, or keeping out of hospitals the 70- to 80-year-olds in a highly urbanized community—we tend to ask for more staff of all kinds, and this has been typical of the development of organized medical services, either for preventive or for hospital work.

Two different factors of the health manpower situation are sometimes confused with the manpower needs. Every community has a deep-felt need for medical care. This also applies to the "ritual" services expected from the entire medical and paramedical personnel. This includes all situations where medical personnel are needed, starting from birth and ending with death—aspects concerned with prolonging life, treating even hopeless cases, providing security in cases of anxiety, and being available day and night. These are all factors closely related to a social-cultural setting rather than needs that can really be met. However, in many communities we have to consider the manpower needs in relation to this type of total setting.

In a traditional community, a great part of this need is met by healers, witch doctors, etc., but even in a modern society some magical aspects are expected from the medical personnel. As people who deal with public health, we often look at the manpower situation from a much more "specific" point of view. We look for the way to prevent or control all diseases on a community scale when we know that we have the tools or the methods to do so. We feel that we should demand manpower to meet such needs. The needs, however, are not necessarily always those felt by the population concerned.

DEFINITION AND CLASSIFICATION OF HEALTH MANPOWER

The usually accepted definition of "manpower" applies to persons who participate in some way or other in the productive efforts of the community. Medical or health manpower would therefore include all those persons who are participating directly in the health and medical services and activities of the community.

Every nation has indigenous health practitioners working productively

LEO A. KAPRIO

in the health field; most of these may be officially recognized but there are others who are not part of the official health system. In some countries the bulk of the health work may indeed be carried out by indigenous and illegal health practitioners. However, the quantity and quality of indigenous health workers must be ignored here, and only officially recognized categories of health personnel can be reviewed.

Although each country has a varied range of health personnel, attempts have been made to establish—for purposes of international comparison—special classifications. The International Labour Organization (ILO) recommends for census purposes a list called the *ILO Classification of Occupations*[2]. WHO has assisted ILO to define their classifications more sharply, and it is hoped that the next census of the world in 1970 will provide more exact information than is available today.

In a questionnaire sent to all national health administrations, WHO requested them to indicate, as on the 31st December 1962, the total number of medical and paramedical personnel practising or working in the country, either in the government services (full-time or part-time) or exclusively privately or serving non-governmental bodies like religious missions or industrial concerns. The various professions enumerated in the questionnaire[3] were as follows:

(1) Physicians (graduates of a medical school)
(2) Medical assistants (for countries and territories where this heading is applicable)
(3) Dentists (graduates of a dental school)
(4) Midwives (excluding nurses with midwifery qualifications):
    4.1 Fully qualified
    4.2 Assistants with certificate
    4.3 Others (to be specified)
(5) Nurses (excluding nurses with midwifery qualifications):
    5.1 Fully qualified
    5.2 Assistants with certificate
    5.3 Others (to be specified)
(6) Nurses with midwifery qualifications (for countries and territories where this heading is applicable)
(7) Pharmacists (graduates of a pharmacy school)
(8) Assistant pharmacists (for countries and territories where this heading is applicable)
(9) Veterinarians (graduates of a veterinary school)
(10) Sanitary engineers
(11) Sanitary inspectors and sanitarians

(12) Physiotherapists (excluding physicians specialized in physio-
therapy)
(13) Laboratory technicians
(14) X-ray technicians
(15) Other scientific and technical paramedical personnel (to be
specified)
(16) Other health auxiliaries (to be specified)

A rather sharp distinction is made by WHO between professional
health personnel who have received education and training beyond secondary school level and auxiliary health personnel who have less than full professional qualifications and require supervision by fully trained high-level
health personnel. The term "paramedical health worker" has been used to
cover all professions allied to medicine which together make up the health
team.

Definitions in an abstract sense can, of course, readily be made, but in a
given country the health manpower education and training programmes
may be in such a state of change and revision that comparisons of various
categories of health personnel within the country, or from one country to
another, are virtually meaningless. In short, today's physician may be the
equivalent of the Russian "feldsher" tomorrow.

REVIEW OF HEALTH MANPOWER STATISTICS

A host of information is available on health manpower in many countries
of the world. The information WHO has is usually only a summary, based
on the reports of governments or member states. As we are all aware, some
countries have very good and exact registers of all legalized health professions, but too many countries do not know their total health manpower
situation exactly. During the last few years interest in the dynamic aspects
of health manpower has grown and new approaches have been developed.
One example comes from the United Kingdom, where the "brain drain"
has promoted studies of the flow of physicians in and out of the country and,
at the same time, deeper analysis of the reasons for these movements. Such
studies and research on health manpower problems are increasing. They
often reveal amazing gaps in our knowledge of situations we thought we
knew well. Methods are also being developed to determine manpower
trends in countries which have no proper statistics or registers.

(1) *The world picture of health manpower*

The only comprehensive source of information on all groups of recognized health workers is the *World Health Statistics Annual*, volume 3 for

1962, with the title "Health Personnel and Hospital Establishment".[3] The information given is mainly from 1962 and 1963 and it was published in 1966. I have already referred to the classifications used in collecting information for this document. The replies from governments were analysed and checked by the WHO secretariat and are listed in the document country by country. This WHO information has already been utilized and more deeply analysed in some other publications, including *Manpower for the World's Health*[4]. The Third World Health Conference on Medical Education in New Delhi also utilized in its publications material from this report, as well as from the *World Directory of Medical Schools* published by WHO in 1963.

Table I gives, continent by continent, the totals of the various groups of medical and paramedical personnel as reported in the WHO *Statistics Annual*[3]. This is not of course a true picture but only a summary of whatever information the various governments have been able to submit. Several countries have given only the figures for government health personnel, and it would not be advisable to rely too much on the totals in Table I for any real comparative purposes. One should go back to the original document for information given country by country and look for the reservations, omissions and footnotes there. However, for the purposes of this symposium I have dared to show the total picture because this is the only answer I can give to the question put in the title of my paper. Some conclusions may even be drawn from these figures. If one compares the various continents with their total populations in mind, one soon realizes that in some parts of the world even minimal health services for the total populations are dreams and not realistic thinking.

The less developed the country, the smaller—usually—is the number of doctors per population unit. And the smaller the number of doctors, the smaller the number of other health personnel. For example, the United Kingdom has one doctor to about two fully-trained nurses, but in India, which has few doctors per population unit, there are two doctors to one trained nurse. However, there are interesting variations even between countries which seem to be on the same technological level. Some of them are clearly based on different traditions and patterns of health services, but they also demonstrate that some service can be given in different ways and sometimes through a more economic or effective solution. We are all aware that in the United States there are practically no midwives and that delivery is performed by the doctors, but countries like the Netherlands or Finland have relatively large numbers of midwives who are responsible for most normal deliveries either in homes or in hospitals.

Table1

MEDICAL AND PARAMEDICAL PERSONNEL[3]

	Africa			America			Europe	Asia			Oceania	USSR
	UAR	South Africa	Rest of Africa	USA	Canada	Rest of America		India	Japan	Rest of Asia		
Physicians	10,929	8,968	12,871	272,502	21,000	117,931	525,882	77,780	102,906	91,386	19,416	443,300
Medical assistants	—	—	3,307	—	...	874	24,490	...	—	1,378	302	364,100
Dentists	1,042	1,337	1,044	105,549	6,103	44,613	132,866	1,426	33,182	19,456	5,305	20,200
Pharmacists	3,278	3,211	3,224	117,400	8,322	36,777	162,869	58,172	62,645	34,925	11,947	20,872
Veterinarians	1,008	474	727	21,600	1,524	6,501	61,674	6,500	17,463	4,627	1,759	...
Sanitary engineers and other sanitation and health personnel	589	50	3,917	26,200	1,410	2,825	13,411	...	17,620	16,013	1,921	28,500
Midwives	1,778	16,714	13,818	—	—	13,706	109,403	46,232	30,000	42,000	416*	231,600
Nurses with midwifery qualifications	—	—	2,091	...	—	4,467	4,451	...	15,955	14,673	1,153*	—
Nurses	768	25,351	28,622	550,000	50,730	70,647	752,049	39,350	122,834	86,790	4,477*	684,100
Assistant midwives	3,841	—	7,311	—	—	2,935	5,944	...	—	4,375	188*	...
Assistant nurses	3,335	9,939	25,656	225,000 }	62,553	24,365	140,240	...	82,253	20,057	1,696*	...
Midwifery and nursing auxiliaries	9,998	4,445	12,901	413,900 }		49,466	176,846	...	106,331	9,370	7,154*	...

—: None.
...: No data.
* No figures for Australia.

223

There are also differences even between developing countries in approximately the same stage of development. A few, like the Sudan, have trained a large number of auxiliaries, but others, with approximately the same type of resources available, have done nothing. Many other interesting examples could be given, and numerous articles and books have been published since 1960 on health manpower. However, this is not the place to go into these details.

There is only one factor to which I should like to draw attention, and even that is a well-known fact:

(2) *The geographical distribution of manpower inside countries*

WHO has recently requested member states to provide information on the geographical distribution of staff by administrative units inside the country, as well as giving total numbers in the country. The information available, both from the national studies as well as from WHO, indicates that in practically any country the big metropolitan areas have the highest number of doctors, and often also the highest number of other health staff, again by population unit. There are a few interesting exceptions. A recent study from western Europe[5] shows that in the highly industrialized metropolitan centres nurses are not so easily available as in more provincial cities of the same country. This study opens up interesting questions regarding the availability of female manpower for health services in highly industrialized countries.

In developing countries, the capital city has practically all the health personnel which exist in the country.

In addition to the geographical distribution, one should also pay attention to the utilization of health staff and health facilities by the population. Utilization studies show that even if health staff is available, the insured or well-to-do population groups and middle and higher social classes utilize the health services much more than, for example, the lower income group or rural population or old-age groups. This, in a way, means that the well-to-do, well-educated city dweller has a much higher ratio of health personnel to serve him and his family than the rural, remote, less literate, underprivileged population groups. If this is related to the prevalence of infectious diseases, especially, and the programmes and plans to eradicate or control these diseases, we realize how the manpower question enters into the picture.

STUDIES AND RESEARCH ON HEALTH MANPOWER

The numbers available now should be used as a base for national or international manpower policy discussions. As the figures are sometimes too incomplete for planning purposes, manpower studies and research are necessary.

(1) *Need for research*

It has been suggested that we, as health leaders and health policy makers, should go deeper into the health manpower situation and support more research in this field. It has been said that to be able to establish a proper and workable manpower policy we should know the ecology and dynamics of health manpower much better; this applies to both the developing and the developed countries. The research into manpower for health services could, to quote Hiestand[6], concentrate on six major subjects:

(1) The availability of basic data on health manpower;
(2) Shortages and future demands for workers in particular fields;
(3) The inflow of workers into particular fields, including the development and training of personnel, the incentives, disincentives and opportunities to enter various fields, etc.;
(4) Losses from the health fields through retirement, leaving the labour force, transfer to other occupations, etc.;
(5) Current manpower utilization patterns and their changes over time;
(6) The qualitative dimensions of manpower in the health services.

Hiestand claims that even in the USA, which already has a long series of statistics on health manpower published by the Federal Government, very little analytical work has been done.

However, to provide a concrete example of a study in developing countries which already have large-scale problems, I shall give a summary of the findings of a Johns Hopkins team which worked for the Turkish Government on a manpower study.

(2) *Ecology and dynamics of medical manpower in Turkey*

For the past three years the Ministry of Health and the School of Public Health in Ankara, Turkey, have participated in an intensive health manpower study, assisted by the Johns Hopkins School of Hygiene and Public Health with funds from the US Agency for International Development[7]. Turkey nationalized its medical and health services in 1961 and it has been preparing a long-range plan for health services, beginning in the eastern part of Turkey and spreading over a 15-year period through the whole population of 30 million. Therefore, a careful and valid health manpower study was deemed vital if the human resources were to be invested in a pattern which made sense socially and economically.

LEO A. KAPRIO

Turkey is by no means an "underdeveloped" country and indeed sophisticated western health services have been developed and provided in parts of the country for over a century. Table II provides a comparison of Turkey's health manpower and economic development with several selected countries to point up the similarities and differences.

Table II

HEALTH MANPOWER AND ECONOMIC RESOURCES IN TURKEY
COMPARED WITH SOME OTHER COUNTRIES

Country	GNP per head (US dollars)	Level of human resource development*	Physicians and dentists per population of 10,000
Turkey	220	II	3·5
USA	2,577	IV	18·0
Nigeria	78	I	0·2
Colombia	263	II	5·0
Chile	379	III	7·5

* Level I: Underdeveloped.
Level II: Partially developed.
Level III: Semi-advanced.
Level IV: Advanced.

Note that there is a general correlation of gross national product (GNP) per head, level of human resource development, and ratio of high-level medical manpower, namely physicians and dentists per 10,000 population.

The Health Manpower Study in Turkey has provided us with a detailed and dynamic picture of the medical manpower that goes far beyond assumptions which might be made from the official statistics for health manpower. The methodology used for this study will not be reviewed here; it suffices to say that modern statistical principles of sampling and a dedication to detailed collection of all valid information were followed throughout the investigation.

A few of the findings of this study are reviewed here to depict the ecology of health manpower which must be understood if health manpower resources are to be efficiently and effectively developed, organized and utilized for any action.

(3) *Official statistics on health manpower in Turkey versus research survey data*

Two major census studies were completed in detail, one for physicians and another for nurses and midwives (Table III).

These findings show gross errors of from 3·6 to 23 per cent in the more easily counted categories of professional health workers. Such errors could result in grave mistakes in health and medical planning. Of course,

226

head counts per 10,000 population for the country's high-level professionals alone do not reveal the necessary health manpower dynamics which can provide useful planning guidelines for the country. Table IV reveals the startling figure of 2,248 for Turkish physicians (18 per cent) under age 65 who were not practising medicine in Turkey in 1964. Thus, in the face of an already short supply of doctors, 18 per cent were abroad either permanently or for varying periods of time, measured in years rather than months.

Table III

HEALTH MANPOWER IN TURKEY

Professional category	Official WHO statistics (1964)	Research survey data (1964)	Difference
Physicians	9,664	10,027	+363 (3·6%)
Nurses	2,383	1,852	−531 (22%)
Midwives	1,356	1,048	−308 (23%)

Table IV

TURKISH PHYSICIANS GRADUATING 1923–1963

Number of graduates from Turkish medical schools	12,687
Number of graduates from foreign medical schools	188
Total	12,875
Estimated number of deaths	600
Estimated to be abroad	2,248
Available supply of doctors in Turkey 1964	10,027

MALDISTRIBUTION OF PHYSICIANS

Probably no country in the world can escape some problem of maldistribution of its professional health personnel. However, only a careful assessment of how many health personnel are actually rendering what kind of services in a given community can document the extent of this maldistribution pattern.

For the whole of Turkey there was found to be 1 physician per 3,063 inhabitants. However, such a global figure disguises the serious imbalances which are found from one region to another, and even within provinces or within sectors of large cities. In Turkey the European region had the most favourable ratio of 1 doctor per 761 inhabitants; the least favourable ratio was in the Black Sea Coast region, where it was 1 : 8,841. This is a difference of more than tenfold!

However, even regional figures and provincial figure averages are mis-leading. It was found, for example, that 64·5 per cent of physicians were actually practising in three major metropolitan areas, Istanbul, Ankara and Izmir. In rural villages and towns, where 68 per cent of inhabitants are located, only 13 per cent of physicians are practising.

Even the geographical distribution is not the total story, because 75 per cent of doctors are specialists, with only 25 per cent in general practice. Therefore only a small portion of first-line physician care is available to the population generally, and of course the disparity between urban and rural populations is exaggerated even further.

Maldistribution within the specialties of medicine produces even greater inequities. For example, only 1 per cent of specialists in Turkey are qualified in the fields of public health and preventive medicine—fields of professional competence that the Ministry of Health urgently requires for managing comprehensive health service programmes and policies. Even more significant was the finding that only 1 per cent of specialties were concerned with basic science in medicine, and these are also urgently needed for medical school faculties.

CONDITIONS RELATED TO MEDICAL MANPOWER PROBLEMS

(a) *Education:*

A number of factors lead to the ultimate loss of physicians abroad and to serious maldistribution within the country. Several studies were carried out and the conclusions of a few can be cited to emphasize the major elements in this situation:

(1) Medical education is cure-oriented with little emphasis on preventive and community medicine;

(2) Post-MD education is almost exclusively available in clinical disciplines, thus fostering specialization;

(3) Wastage of medical student material contributes to medical manpower shortage. In a 10-year review of 7,006 students registered in three Turkish medical schools only 3,912 eventually graduated (55·7 per cent);

(4) Problems in general and particularly in secondary school education.

(b) *Imbalances in health personnel patterns:*

There are on the average six doctors for each nurse in Turkey—a ratio which should be completely reversed. This means that most patient care must be given by low-level nursing auxiliaries and that physicians must

228

spend more of their time in direct or indirect (by supervision) patient care. Indeed, in Turkey as a whole there is only one nurse per 18,070 inhabitants, or 5·5 nurses per 100,000 population. Regional rates vary and range from 1 per 5,264 in European Turkey to 1 per 94,071 in Eastern Asiatic Turkey. The imbalance between nurses and doctors is even further exaggerated when the urban-rural differences are examined (Table V).

Table V

URBAN-RURAL DISTRIBUTION OF DOCTORS AND NURSES IN TURKEY

Urban-Rural	Distribution of nurses (%)	Distribution of doctors (%)	Population (%)
Rural villages and towns	9·6	13·4	68·1
Cities	24·5	25·2	26·8
Metropolitan areas	63·9	61·4	5·1

Thus, even more than doctors, nurses tend to cluster in the metropolitan areas of Turkey.

Time does not permit additional analysis of health personnel imbalances, but the critical doctor-nurse ratio is so distorted that it is obvious that health services cannot be efficiently and effectively organized and deployed under these circumstances.

(c) *Work conditions for high-level health personnel:*

Generally the salaries and job responsibilities for doctors and nurses in Turkey are uniformly bad. Indeed, doctors who have gone abroad cite economic factors, job opportunities and advancement as major reasons for leaving Turkey.

Long hours, uncertain responsibilities, inadequate salaries, poor living conditions in hospitals, lack of professional recognition, and inflexibility of work schedules for part-time and married nurses are only a few of the myriad reasons producing problems for nurses. Many of the most competent and most highly educated nurses in Turkey in fact leave for better conditions abroad! There are many social and cultural factors relating to the role of women in Turkish society which also significantly affect the situation.

IMPLICATIONS FOR HEALTH MANPOWER DEVELOPMENT AND POLICY

First, public health administrators must not plan future national health programmes without recognizing the complex elements which affect health manpower development, organization and use. Crude figures of

229

doctors per 10,000 population must be carefully scrutinized and reviewed within a country to discern distribution patterns and final patterns of effective use.

The imbalances of health personnel that were so strikingly shown in Turkey must be carefully evaluated and appropriate corrective steps developed. Obviously a piece-meal correction cannot be successful, but a comprehensive and long-range replanning of the medical manpower system must be implemented. Legal, political, social, economic and cultural factors are so interrelated in any manpower problem that national policy formulations must take cognizance of all the relevant components that affect development, organization, and deployment of medical manpower.

Perhaps the major defect in medical manpower statistics is in the assemblage of the data into individual categories, i.e. doctor, nurse, midwife, etc. A new system of collecting data on the health team *in toto* may need to be developed. Perhaps a ratio of doctor:nurse:midwife and auxiliaries should be given an index value that might indicate "underdevelopment" in the health manpower system.

The example of Turkey also emphasizes the defects in the educational process for a given health manpower role. If what is needed in Turkey is more physicians competent to work in health teams in rural communities, how does medical education really meet the needs and demands of society? Is Turkey, in point of fact, training "universal doctors" capable of supplying curative medicine for an affluent society? Is there a need to train "culture-bound physicians" geared to the medical-social problems of Turkey, rather than the ultra-sophisticated urban hospital-bound variety? Perhaps the two "types" of physicians are not mutually exclusive. Indeed, if an imaginative, creative, and strategic national policy were developed for the conditions and ecology of health services for Turkey, perhaps in the foreseeable future manpower development and organization would be in harmony with the nation's needs. National health policies can at least begin with those steps which ensure proper registration of medical manpower so that this high-level professional resource can be properly "invested" in the nation's future.

I have given you the example of Turkey; however, for many countries—for example in Africa—the situation is even more difficult. There is the question of establishment, within a reasonable future, of what I would call medical or health independence. In developed countries such as the UK, USSR or Sweden, we are already taking it for granted that the major unit for the health service is a region of one or two million people, served at the centre by a medical school, by all other teaching institutions for health personnel and by a system of continuous education. At the community level the front-line services consist of either general practitioners or real health centres with supporting staff, or polyclinics or group practice, or whatever the country's health pattern may provide.

In Africa most of the new countries should, of course, be like the regions of more developed countries, but they have a long way to go. On the central level they have to establish medical schools, nursing schools, and schools for sanitarians and auxiliaries. There should be, of course, an effective Ministry of Health, a central laboratory and a network of hospitals. Most of the African countries will need infrastructure—which we call the basic health service—but, of course, in the beginning, this can be only minimal and concentrated in a few major problem areas.

To analyse the manpower needs, one has to establish a realistic model for a health service that fits in with the resources and economic development of a country at that moment, and this, of course, will differ from country to country.

CONCLUSION

Finally, I would mention that on an international level we must realize that we have to try to support the various countries so that they can obtain their medical independence. If they cannot do this from their own resources we have to try to find ways and means of assisting them, either through international organizations or bilaterally by friendly countries. If the international community insists on speeding up the present rate of development of health services to achieve world-wide eradication of one or several diseases, there will be a tremendous need for international assistance, not just funds, to establish more teaching institutions—but that is the subject of the next paper.

DISCUSSION

Dogramaci: Turkey is not a developed country. It is certainly developing, but rather slowly.

Today in Turkey we have more women doctors than fully-qualified nurses. In the past hardly enough applicants came forward for the available places in schools of nursing. When nursing was included in university training its prestige immediately rose. In one school of nursing we planned to take 100 students in three classes of 30–35 each and we received 600 applications for the 100 places. Lowering of standards, at least in our case, was not an attraction, while with added prestige candidates became more abundant.

It is true that about 75 per cent of our doctors are specialists and that more than half of the remaining 25 per cent are in the process of specialization. In a country like the United States this shows how advanced medicine is, but in our case it is a handicap. We discovered that our graduates did not think that they were eligible or capable enough to go and practise, and they thought that another three to five years specializing in one branch of medicine would give them security. Our training system was based on the European medical education system, with very large classes and very little clinical or practical work. Now we are trying to change the entire system. We established two new medical schools, one of them trying to evolve beside an already existing medical school in the same university (Ankara), but starting from scratch with an entirely new philosophy; the other one was established two years later at Erzurum, again with an entirely different philosophy and resembling the second medical school in Ankara University. We tried to eliminate what we considered to be deadwood and to take the greatest advantage of curriculum time. Our efforts have aroused a lot of interest, so much so that members of the Royal Commission on Medical Education in England came and studied our system; this was very flattering and at least it helped us when we needed further financial help. We try to train doctors for the rural areas without lowering the standards. We have discovered that it is the insecurity of working unsupported in a rural area rather than the hardships of life there that has made it difficult to find doctors to go the villages.

Our experience in the two new medical schools has influenced the other medical schools and they are also trying to change their curricula. Medical schools have complete autonomy in administration, teaching, and to some extent in financial affairs, within the universities, and the changes have to come from within.

Wright: The ratio of doctors to nurses which both Dr. Kaprio and Professor Dogramaci referred to is of great interest. It would be useful also to know the total populations of the areas to which the figures in Dr. Kaprio's table apply.

How much can auxiliary personnel be used in medical work? In veterinary work they are used, for instance, for giving inoculations. In Italy, once a doctor has prescribed a series of injections, it is often the portiere's wife who administers them! The use of auxiliary personnel does seem a possibility, certainly in underdeveloped countries, simply because much of the medical attention in these countries is now preventive rather than curative, due to the very lack of doctors, the difficulties of communications, and so on. Can any provision be made for such personnel in regard to family

planning? Clearly the number of doctors and midwives is utterly inadequate to face the enormous problems presented if family planning is to be
introduced on a large scale.

Fanconi: The problem of physicians and medical personnel is also a very
big problem in the well-developed countries. When I entered the
Children's Hospital in Zürich many years ago there were only five doctors
and two volunteers. At that time we had no specialists in the hospital, but
we had the same number of beds and even more outpatients than we have
today. Now there are 25 specialists in this one hospital, and 70 doctors.
During the 1930's the cost per patient was 7 Swiss francs, while in 1960 it
was 74 Swiss francs, more than 10 times as much. Twenty-five years ago we
had a third of the personnel who are in the hospital today, yet personnel
costs today are 22 times as much.

This over-specialization is happening all over the world, even in Turkey,
as we have just heard, and it is necessary because of the enormous pro-
gresses in somatic medicine. In the United States in 1900 there were 170
general practitioners per 100,000 inhabitants, in 1962 only 33. Specialization in the United States has gone up from 30 per cent in 1930 to 82 per
cent in 1960. The consequence is that we have fewer and fewer general
practitioners and the general practitioners have much more to do with
patients who are not really ill but have psychological problems. In
Switzerland in 1938 for every 100 insured patients there were only seven
consultations, while in 1962 the figure was 105.

We cannot discuss here the definition of health. Furthermore the
general practitioner is now often overwhelmed with red tape and bureaucracy. Therefore it is more and more difficult in Switzerland, and also in
England, to find general practitioners for the rural areas. The shortage of
nurses is also a very big problem. It is important to stress the problems in
the developed countries and not to refer only to the undeveloped
countries.

Candau: Really we are in a strange world—we are talking about things
which are completely different. A little over a year ago I attended the
White House Conference on Health in Washington. There I got the greatest
surprise of my life and it really broke my heart when people started telling
me how bad the situation was in New York—so bad that I couldn't sleep for
worrying about it! When I look at the rest of the world I don't know what
we are talking about. I know the situation is difficult in Switzerland, but if
we wish to do something we have to realize that the situation is completely different in the countries where the need is greatest. If not, we are
going to leave this conference making an appeal *for* the brain drain,

because the only solution to the problems of the developed countries, like the United States, is by brain drainage: instead of having one office in London to recruit personnel, the U.S. should open three or four more in different cities in Europe.

The problem of population will not be solved unless we can develop sufficient manpower. Auxiliary personnel can do a job but they cannot do it without proper supervision. One country, after starting a programme of birth control with auxiliary personnel and using the intrauterine device, wanted to prepare a request to an international organization for drugs to treat the complications resulting from the use of the intrauterine device. If a request of this kind has to be considered, certainly the birth control programme cannot be a success. In one country the number of withdrawals of the intrauterine device is greater than the number of insertions. Unless we have enough personnel we cannot do anything, however important the problems are.

We have to decide for what purposes we need the doctors before we decide on a curriculum for our medical schools. At present both preventive and tropical medicine should be part of the basic curriculum in many countries. The medical profession in the developing countries must recognize that the training of their nationals must differ from the training given to nationals of, for example, England, France and Belgium, which they still try to copy. The colonial heritage is not altogether to blame. Certain doctors in the developing countries are fighting to maintain a system and standards which are completely unrealistic.

Beer: A revolution is going on both in the appreciation of auxiliary medical personnel and in the techniques and limitations of their use. Dr. Candau, Dr. Kaprio and their associates in WHO are very actively involved, as we also are in the Red Cross and other organizations, in seeing what can be done in this field.

In health education the professionals could help us to define what the auxiliaries could do. A very important aspect is to get the public health-minded, and in this respect a lot could be done. The time-honoured methods of training the public in first aid, mother and child welfare and home nursing need to be completely revised and adapted to the new realities. In some countries in Latin America, in Nigeria, and in other parts of the world, new and revolutionary programmes of health education are being organized by WHO and the national health educators, in co-operation with the Red Cross. But even in this field programmes have to be adapted for each country; that is why we have no standard solutions to offer but can only ensure that we start anew on a fresh basis. The Red Cross has made some very promising beginnings. Old British and French manuals are still used for first-aid training in Africa; we are now trying to rewrite them and our British and French friends have been the first to help with this. New courses on health in the home and mother and child welfare are being prepared for Africa and South East Asia; we are putting the emphasis on elementary hygiene, encouraging people to make proper latrines and kill off the flies.

We get an almost frightening feeling in some countries that the people we have trained are already being given too much to do, because of the lack of doctors. Where there is only one doctor to 40,000 or 80,000 people the first aiders are called on to do things which they definitely should not do, but there is no one else to do them.

Conflicts have occurred between the volunteers and the professionals in the paramedical and welfare fields. We are now trying to break down the causes of conflict. We want the professionals to tell us what to do and help in training and defining the fields of volunteer activity. We must also get away from the class differences which in Latin America and other places have existed between the people doing voluntary welfare work and the professionals. It is very important that WHO and the medical profession should interest themselves in helping the volunteer organizations to recruit and train their personnel.

In some European and other countries we have to break down resistance from some professional circles. Nurses, for example, tend to say that in a hospital the nurses should do everything, but many welfare and technical jobs in a hospital could be done by non-nursing staff after proper training.

Some medical associations, like the International Organization against Tuberculosis, have stated that they cannot, in the new countries, organize local branches—there are not enough interested persons available to staff a number of "specialized" local committees. They would therefore welcome it if *one* health organization, like the Red Cross, expanded its local organization and took care of the follow-up of campaigns against different illnesses, and helped to organize vaccination programmes and health education.

Lambo: The long-term investment needed for health and educational programmes is almost out of the normal economic range of many developing countries. What is needed may be a modest beginning but flexible experimentation in medical education. The type of training is very important, especially in terms of the national objectives, but the most important thing is probably the quality and relevance of medical education to local needs. A certain amount of specialization is needed, but the types

235

and priority should be decided after careful consideration. Patterns of care which may evolve are also very important and this may reflect the political and administrative structure of a society. Another type of parameter which one may use is the available infrastructure.

Seventy per cent of the population of many young countries live in the rural areas and are without the usual infrastructure needed to build upon. Any health programme needs a certain amount of basic infrastructure before it can really be successful. Probably more important in this particular area of experimentation in medical education is the role and status of the doctor in a particular society. One feels that training of the doctor who is going to practise in Washington, D.C., or San Francisco or Bombay should be different from that of the doctor who is going to practise in Ibadan. Many English-speaking or French-speaking countries in West Africa still cling to their colonial traditions, for fear of not being recognized internationally and because they are economically tied to their colonial past.

I would very much like to see national research on manpower but I would also like to see as a matter of urgency research into the effectiveness of different types of medical training and all types of services. This may be very difficult from the point of view of methods but it would yield more relevant information than just research into manpower.

Pincus: From our experience so far, of fertility control measures and the type of personnel needed, it appears that roughly one-third of the time of a physician plus the full time of a nurse (or social worker) would take care of 1,200 patients in a clinic. This is not a very enormous demand and I think it can be fulfilled.

Furthermore, in many cases paramedical personnel or nurse's assistants can be quite effective in birth-control programmes, particularly once a project has been launched.

The need for physicians to do things like withdraw intrauterine devices is the real problem. I fully agree with Dr. Candau about the need for simpler methods. As newer methods evolve many of the problems associated with intrauterine devices or the present-day oral contraceptives will tend to disappear. Nonetheless, medical personnel and auxiliaries will always be essential for birth-control work. Paramedical personnel alone are not enough.

In terms of the availability of personnel for health programmes there is one overall consideration which ought to be discussed, i.e. we talk very glibly of the brain drain and the movement of medical and trained personnel to where the money is—the Sutton law! I think we have to start a movement in the other direction. It seems to me that training for foreign service in the medical and health fields is not an inconceivable thing, even in the developed countries. I have personally had so many appeals from people who wanted to go into this work but who had no special training that I feel that if this were set up as a regular professional training service for work in overseas countries, not only in the field of birth control but in any aspect of public health, we might see a new trend in the developed countries.

Kaprio: I did not have an opportunity to go into what type of administrative pattern and service one can envisage for auxiliaries in a given country, i.e. what the national leaders planning the service would like to have and what they can afford to have and where they can get the manpower. For instance, in many countries the political system is such that you cannot control the doctors, but you can control the auxiliaries. In India, for example, a system has been set up for training malaria workers, medical health workers, and the female workers who are the auxiliary nurses; they try to cover the country with about one worker to 5,000 individuals and there is a chance of this working out. These people deal only with malaria, smallpox, some first aid, some health education and some aspects of family planning, and they can be supervised to do only these things. The big difficulty in India is the supervisory system, but there is a possibility of building up a limited service that could have an impact.

The USSR did something similar in a certain phase of its development and Dr. Evang referred to what was happening in China. Whatever emotional feelings we may have about such schemes, with discipline and a supervised though limited staff one can do a lot. Many countries which have only a few staff will have to find some such means of controlling their health services.

I think the solution to the tremendous demand for medical care in the developed countries is to organize new forms of administration through which all medical workers, including general practitioners, will become part of a team. The individual doctor should be part of a regional system which would co-ordinate all aspects of administration, continuous education and finance. Scarce highly qualified people must not be wasted on trivial tasks.

There is also the socio-cultural aspect: what is expected from a health service and what can really be effective? We continually struggle with this problem in many countries. The future pattern, both immediate and long-term, of health services in any country must always be kept in mind—without that we cannot rationally discuss manpower.

REFERENCES

1. Lubin, I. (1963). In *Science, Technology and Development* (United States papers prepared for the United Nations Conference on the Application of Science and Technology for the benefit of the less developed areas), Vol. XI, pp. ix–xii. Washington, D.C.: U.S. Govt. Printing Office.
2. International Labour Office (1958). *International Standard Classification of Occupations*, vol. III. Geneva: ILO.
3. World Health Organization (1966). *World Health Statistics Annual*, 1962; Vol. III: Health personnel and hospital establishments. Geneva: WHO.
4. Hyde, H. van Z. (ed.) (1966). Manpower for the world's health. *Journal of Medical Education*, 41, no. 9 (part 2).
5. Donald, B. L. (1966). *Manpower for Hospitals: a Study of Problems in some West European Countries*. London: Institute of Hospital Administrators.
6. Hiestand, D. L. (1966). Research into manpower for health services. *Milbank Memorial Fund Quarterly*, 44, 146–181.
7. Taylor, C., Dirican, R., and Deuschle, K. *Health Manpower Planning—Turkey*. (To be published in the International Health Monograph Series, Johns Hopkins Press.)

238

13

EDUCATION AND TRAINING FACILITIES, PRESENT AND POTENTIAL; AND RESEARCH

H. Pequignot and A. L. Banks
*Department of Medical Pathology, Faculty of Medicine,
University of Paris; and Department of Human Ecology,
University of Cambridge*

No health service can survive unless it has competent medical and ancillary staff. The relationship between the level of health and personnel resources is certainly not a simple one, but at any one time the benefit the population receives from medicine is in direct proportion to the efforts made to train personnel and to undertake scientific research. The chief problem for a health organization or institution is how to make the best use of its costly and valuable staff, for the nature of medical work is such that once they are appointed, they must be trusted to carry out their work in their own way. And just as present-day communities benefit from past efforts, so their future health can be forecast on the basis of what they are doing to train tomorrow's professional men and to encourage research.

For the public, and sometimes for the health and welfare authorities, the above truisms are unfortunately often obscured by certain frequently held illusions, which we shall now analyse.

(a) One fallacy stems from the enrichment of certain communities without effort on their part. When Jenner discovered vaccination against smallpox, Roentgen the X-rays, and Pasteur the bases of asepsis, the entire world profited without having made any contribution. One can always hope that a similar miracle will be repeated many times. But has there been a miracle? Although such discoveries were immediately made known to all mankind, they were only utilized by communities which had reached the same level of scientific development as those where the discoveries had been made. Others wait even today to benefit. There are still unvaccinated populations and even more without adequate X-ray equipment. Similarly, even in the largest hospitals the problem of asepsis has not yet been resolved.

Moreover it is less and less likely that such a miracle could be repeated gratuitously. Today most important discoveries involve the products or apparatus of large industrial organizations, which usually sell their discoveries rather than give them away.

(b) A second illusion arises from the fact that there is no simple relationship between the existence of an effective staff and the realization of the need for medical care. Thus, in France after the Napoleonic wars all the surgeons of the Emperor's armies had to retire on half pay to the provinces and the rural areas, and thus an elementary system of medical care was diffused which consisted merely of their presence. In a developed country, the very fact that a new technique is introduced or a new service created may itself lead to consciousness of the need for that service, just as the addition of a small crystal to a supersaturated but normal-looking solution results in mass crystallization. The rapid rate of increase in the use of medical care services and of the health budget reflects a similar situation of supersaturation, but even in the most prosperous and developed countries the population as a whole does not benefit from all that modern medical science can offer. In this direction it has been shown that lack of apparatus and drugs is the limiting factor that is easiest to overcome, the lack of money raises more difficult problems, while the lack of qualified personnel is at present insurmountable.

(c) Another illusion, increasingly recognized as such, is that increasing mechanization and automation and greater productivity will compensate for lack of staff. However the development of such techniques in medicine has resulted in an even faster increase in the number of specially qualified people required.

(d) It could perhaps be argued, without being paradoxical, that the strongest limiting factor affecting the availability of medical services is the lack of capable teachers. It is not necessary to emphasize the special medical aspects of this lack of teaching staff. Essentially, in all classes and branches of the teaching profession, the office of teacher is being devalued. This term, devalued, is used by teachers at all levels to imply that their social and financial status has been lowered and that they are dissatisfied with their reduced prestige in the professional hierarchy.

Much emphasis has been placed on this reduced prestige and it must be taken seriously since it contributes to the drying up of the supply of teachers. But the devaluation of the teaching profession in the minds of the teachers themselves is even more serious. The general tendency is to give priority to research and to regard teaching as a less interesting and subordinate task, unworthy of highly qualified people. The master tends to think of it as a necessary evil, as a tax which he pays to the community in order to obtain from it facilities for research and the ability to select, from a mass of students, a few well-chosen disciples.

Specialization in research progressively worsens the position of teaching as a duty. The full-time research worker is better able to obtain grants, facilities and buildings than the part-time worker, who is being reduced to the status of an amateur in the eyes of those who hold the purse strings. It is not at all certain that the isolation of the research worker from the teacher is not detrimental to the former, but it is clear that this segregation may have catastrophic results on the recruitment of teachers with faith in their task.

(e) In many countries professional and financial considerations have led to pressure being exerted to limit the numbers of the medical profession. Such pressure has been the more powerful because several opposing interests have been converging in the same direction: some members of the medical profession hoped that their numbers would be increased as little as possible so that their living standards might be maintained; some health and welfare authorities hoped to economize by having fewer staff to pay and therefore they encouraged the aims of the doctors. This attitude may of course result in serious difficulties in staff recruitment by some authorities, including health administrations, and may greatly hinder aid to developing countries. But, even more important, a monopoly profession which is not able to respond to the needs of the public is very badly placed to get its legitimate demands accepted, and the minor economies made by the health and welfare authorites are not on the same scale as the increase in the cost of medical care.

These preliminary considerations over, three questions will be discussed:

(1) How to recruit the professional men we need.

(2) How to ensure that they meet the needs of the public.

(3) On what bases the necessary research can be financed.

It is easier to increase the list of difficulties than to solve some of them.

RECRUITMENT

(a) First, students must be volunteers. Experience has shown that of those who join the medical profession unwillingly (through family pressures, for instance) a high proportion later leave it—in France, for example, a good third of medical qualifications are not used in professional practice[1].

The question therefore arises of the appeal of medicine to the young. Many people, in many countries, think that the position, already difficult for medicine, is even more serious for nursing. The doctor's image in society (in literature, newspapers and on films) and the image that the profession has of itself play a part in determining the attractiveness of medicine. In this connexion it is very disquieting that in some countries such as Switzerland, Italy, Belgium, Austria and even France, professional discontent has led to strike action.

(b) The most important point is undoubtedly the bottleneck of university training and this requires special consideration.

Medicine has become more scientific during the last hundred years, and it is now based on mathematics, physics, chemistry and mathematically orientated biology. The mathematico-physical standards for entry to medical studies and throughout the course have been raised, although insufficient efforts have been made to enable students who are only moderately good at mathematics and physics to acquire sufficient knowledge of these subjects.

It is by no means certain that these higher standards are fully justified, but in any event they ignore two fundamental considerations. The first is that students who excel in the exact sciences are increasingly drawn to the numerous openings in those sciences. Thus some of the best brains are attracted away from medicine. Further, secondary education in some countries tends less and less to direct towards science those students who show no early promise in this field. Medicine thus receives fewer of the intermediate class of well-educated but not scientifically gifted students who used to go into medicine.

The second and much more important point is that it is not usual for students interested in mathematical and physical sciences also to have a taste for human contacts, with the ability to create and sustain them and an inclination towards psychological enquiry and the understanding of other people. Yet such qualities are increasingly necessary in many branches of medicine, while the mathematical knowledge now insisted upon is not used. Too much stress on mathematics may exclude excellent practitioners not only from specialties like psychiatry or paediatrics, but above all from general practice.

(c) In a Utopia it might be possible to direct students towards medicine by vocational guidance methods, according to requirements, but no country has yet been able to forecast correctly its needs in doctors and professional staff. The errors of the professional organizations have been surpassed in this respect only by those of the health administrations. This does not give confidence for the future, and the distrust for compulsory direction remains. Further, it seems unreasonable to suggest that there should be a preliminary selection or direction of those entering particular branches of medicine or science. No one who is now a physician of any kind could have foreseen the particular course he took in his professional life, his interest in it, or the difficulties he encountered during his early studies. In short, there are too many facets of medicine for the future student to obtain a standard picture of the doctor that he might become: he cannot draw on his own experience, even as a patient, to visualize what medicine means.

A wide basis of recruitment is therefore required, and courses of study should be designed to impart a minimum of mathematical knowledge to students interested in people, and a knowledge of human requirements to those more inclined towards mathematical and abstract problems. Ideally, methods of entry should include promotion from the paramedical professions. In many countries this method of recruitment appears to be essential, since many of the medical students come at present from the same social class and their experience is purely academic. All these methods of entry should of course converge to one common course of study, so that the seeds of later divergence are not sown at the beginning. The basic medical sciences can retain their contact with medicine only if they are fertilized by elements from the clinical side, and the latter must be prepared to absorb some of those who initially believed themselves to be destined for a purely scientific career.

MEETING THE NEEDS OF THE PUBLIC

When medical training was by apprenticeship, the student learnt by contact with practical problems. There was what Leibnitz would have called a pre-established harmony between precept and morbidity. When teaching hospitals began to select patients according to the interest of the heads of the various departments in their special problems, the gap between teaching and the needs of the public widened. This becomes especially obvious when graduates of such hospitals go to a developing country, but it is apparent everywhere and there is a danger that the situation may become worse.

There was general agreement at the second World Conference on Medical Education in 1959[2] regarding the dangers of specialization, but no-one then questioned whether this might be the result of current methods of teaching. Is the lack of general practitioners not simply because we seek less and less to train them? It would be possible, without exaggeration, to

243

describe as follows the medical student's progress. First, an attempt is made to turn him into a research biologist and then he is dazzled with the enchanting possibilities of clinical specialization. This is tantamount to directing towards general practice those who have failed in the other two directions. It then becomes apparent that those who have drifted into general practice are not necessarily those who might have been interested and found satisfaction in it. This negative selection is all the more likely to produce bitterness when these doctors find that they have unfavourable working conditions. In all countries the general practitioner has the hardest daily routine, the biggest responsibilities and the lowest social standing in the profession.

The present position is therefore the result of known conditions, but where is the remedy to be found? A reassessment of general practice on the professional level would require such radical changes both at the professional and administrative levels and in the popular image that it is hardly feasible. Academic measures offer more promise. A return to clinical studies in contact with the patients, not with specially selected but ordinary patients—possibly from the less selective hospitals and out-patient departments—should be the point of departure for all medical studies and not merely an applied course at the end of them. Elementary nursing duties, raised little by little to the level of simple medical tasks for the benefit of these ordinary patients, should begin on entry to the basic science studies and should come before specialized clinical training.

During this preliminary training the students would be in close contact with the psychological and psycho-sociological problems of their patients, and those interested in the nature and variety of these could be directed positively towards general practice. They would then continue their studies knowing what they required from the basic sciences and clinical specialization, and would thus benefit more from them. For the other students, destined for specialization or scientific studies, this experience would engender a wholesome respect for general practice and a better understanding of its problems, and it would undoubtedly improve the relationship between the various categories of doctors, which now deteriorates because they are so remote from each other. Encouraged by these better teaching methods, the moral and material standing of the general practitioner would improve and the unity essential to good medicine would be re-established.

The seriousness of this problem must be stressed. If internationally coordinated measures are not taken the present trend, of which everyone complains but to which each contributes, will result in a separate category of "feldsher" (as in the USSR). Such a solution is already being recommended to the developing nations and it may soon be found that the developed countries are moving towards the organization of the former, and not the reverse. Countries which have retained their existing medical structure (and this is already the case in the big capital cities, with their chronic illnesses, ageing of the population, and increased life expectation) may find themselves with patients with less and less specialized illnesses being served only by doctors practising in increasingly narrow specialties.

RESEARCH

One of the central and most recent problems of medical research is finance. The research which created modern medicine from the 16th century to the dawn of the 20th was the result of unconscious and implicit financing. Essentially it was founded on the affluence in which rich patients enabled a relatively small number of doctors, often already well endowed, to live. These doctors were thus able to limit their private practice and spend part of their time in intellectual pursuits, at the same time caring for patients who could not afford to pay. Thus the rich paid for research without being aware of it or even expressly wishing to do so. Under such a system research was undertaken voluntarily and with complete intellectual freedom.

Local communities (lay or religious) provided the material for research, again unknowingly, by means of hospitals for the poor where these doctors could care for them. Their use as teaching hospitals was not improper, for the apprentice doctors or surgeons also followed their masters when they attended private patients. Research was distinguishable from the primary task of healing only by the psychological attitude of the investigator.

In the last hundred years powerful and self-contained research institutes have developed throughout the world. Medical research took on a new lease of life from the concomitant development of physics and chemistry, and later from biology, which has become independent of medicine only in the last few decades. Today the emphasis is on fundamental biological research, the clinical applications of which may be immediate or far in the future. These comments do not imply any criticism of this kind of research, but the fact that it is the centre of attention is not without its drawbacks. This fundamental research is the only type of biological research which receives the same order of financial support as physical and chemical research, but the considerable though insufficient efforts made on its behalf are made at the expense of traditional methods of research because the role of the latter appears to be regarded, subconsciously, as having ended.

Although undervalued by many theoreticians, clinical research remains indispensable for it plays the double role of providing the clinical experience which comes before research and for the application of research. The method is extraordinarily simple and its social importance is so great as to merit serious consideration. It rests on the observation and treatment, in the best possible conditions for clinical and biological supervision, of the maximum number of patients followed up for as long as possible.

Two examples will illustrate this type of research. The first is the study of the Hiroshima and Nagasaki populations, though this is highly specialized. A more recent example is the discovery of the part played by thalidomide in the aetiology of limb malformation in newborn babies. It is interesting to note that the work of the chemists who developed the thalidomide molecule and of the pharmacologists and clinicians who discovered its tranquillizing properties would be popularly accepted as research, whereas the work that showed its harmfulness might not, although the latter has had the impact of a fundamental discovery because it has changed world opinion on malformations.

This kind of research at the patient's bedside will never be out of date. Advances in medicine, whatever their origin—even purely physical, as for instance Roentgen's discovery of X-rays, which has been part of medical routine for a long time—can only be effective through actual diagnosis and treatment. The results of a diagnostic technique, of a new drug or of a surgical procedure must, after all, be assessed in a number of individuals. Whatever the quality of preliminary laboratory experiments on tissue culture or animals—when they are possible, which is not always the case— the application of the results to man requires rigorous and systematic verification. Clinical research will only be dispensed with when all progress in therapeutics, diagnosis and treatment has stopped—that is, it is to be hoped, never!

The use of modern therapeutic measures imposes an increasingly rigorous discipline on clinicians and the day may come when no therapeutic agent will be administered to a patient without the diagnosis, the dosage and all side-effects being recorded, together with a post-mortem examination in case of death (whether expected or not) and the comparison of its results with the diagnosis and treatment. Only a prospective and systematic study of this kind will enable untoward results to be ascertained. The practitioner, even if working alone, cannot be excluded from this system of surveillance, especially since certain medicaments given to ambulatory patients are almost exclusively prescribed by him (e.g. thalidomide or phenacetin). It goes without saying that what we said about drugs applies *a fortiori* to all therapeutic measures.

This example takes us into the field of medico-social research, or what the English-speaking countries now call epidemiology. Some biological phenomena are not capable of resolution by individual observation. For example, only by carefully planned study by age groups of the clinical and post-mortem appearances of congenital cardiopathies or any other congenital malformation that can endanger life is it possible to ascertain their precise significance. It was necessary to wait for adequate statistics compiled by the life insurance companies to learn the importance of obesity and to modify our views on normal weights. Only by rigorous retrospective and prospective investigations can the effects of smoking or the daily consumption of wine not involving drunkenness be assessed, and so on.

The solution of the medico-social problems of modern communities depends on the study of the long-term effects of changes in the way of life, food and environment. The epidemiological work carried out at Hiroshima to discover the remote results of the atomic bomb should be applied with the same strictness to the effects of air pollution or of the daily use of progestational drugs.

The time taken (several years) to relate phocomelia and thalidomide caused surprise. In fact the incidence of malformations had gone up from 3 per 100,000 to 5 per 1,000 births. It is difficult to see how, in present circumstances, it would be possible to detect the cause of an increase of from 2 to 4 per cent in the incidence of a common anomaly, of a two or threefold increase in an individual's chances of developing asthma or migraine, or a 50-fold or even a 100-fold, increase in the number of carriers of a rare enzyme defect such as analbuminaemia.

To sum up, while fundamental research can be financed in the same way as, for example, space or atomic research, clinical research requires to be sponsored quite differently and in line with the traditional manner described above. It is suggested that whenever a payment is made for a medical service or to the doctor something should be included for research. The client, whether a national health service financed by the State, a social insurance organization, or a private insurance company, should agree to pay for research—just as people throughout the world, when they take a train or a plane, or buy a car, a suit of clothes or a household detergent, pay each time for the development and research which have made the service or the article possible, whether it is provided by public or private enterprise. To say that clinical research is similar to applied and developmental research implies that it needs special methods of organization and financing, but not that it is of inferior quality to fundamental research. It is not only in medicine that so-called fundamental research may end in the development of a "gadget", and applied research in an intellectual revolution.

All doctors, whatever their type of practice, would be able to take part in this type of research, provided that they had the spirit of enquiry and the wish to do so, and this may be one way of restoring the status of the general practitioner.

SUMMARY

Just as societies benefit today from past investments, so the future of their health services depends on the efforts made now to prepare future physicians and to undertake research.

In this paper various difficulties are examined which are not specific to the health sector, including those of education in general, and three subjects have been chosen for special consideration in this field:

Is the selection of future members of the medical profession satisfactory, with particular reference to teaching?

Do the medical men whom we now train answer the requirements of the population? On this point, the problems involved in the training of general practitioners have been stressed.

Is the financing of true clinical research neglected in the current organization of research?

DISCUSSION

Wolman: In the developing countries many of the opportunities for disease correction lie in non-medical application, yet the training problems and opportunities for non-medical personnel in these countries have not been mentioned in your paper.

Pequignot: It is very difficult to do anything in the field of health for the paramedical workers when there is no collaboration with medically qualified personnel. This type of personnel must therefore be available before the use of non-medical workers can be considered. In the developing countries it is not possible to provide only preventive medicine without curative medicine.

Garcia: Modern medicine needs the team approach and the effective use of leadership, but how much are we teaching medical students about the different skills that can contribute to medical work? How much are we

248

teaching them about working as a team, or acting as leader of a team in conditions that may not be ideal? How much enthusiasm are we infusing in them for working in a team practice instead of private practice? How much do we tell them about the cultural background or limitations of the community where they are going to work? These things should be introduced in some way during the early part of the curriculum in the medical schools.

To decrease unnecessary demands from the public takes time, but it can be done. In Chile we have been trying to educate the public not to abuse the existing facilities. We also try to educate the medical people to establish a better relationship with the patient and his family so that they co-operate better. We use nurses, pharmacists and health educators to resolve any doubts the patients have about the treatment and follow-up.

Too many of the doctors are in the big cities, of course, but it is not easy to redistribute them, because there may be legal problems which prevent this, and such measures might work against the security of the medical personnel. But something can be done.

Pequignot: I think it is not a good thing to separate the university and the community. It is difficult to explain to students their work in the community if they are isolated in the university; it is difficult to send students out to treat all the classes of a nation when all the students come from the same class of the population. Medical students must come from all classes of society and be more representative of the population as a whole.

Regarding the abuse of the health services, I have made a study[3] of this in France and I think it is very exaggerated. Perhaps the demands are not good demands, but the needs are very real.

le Riche: In the past I have helped to force the medical profession into asking for more training in mathematics. If we are selecting cold introverts, mathematicians and physicists, and pushing them into medicine, this is a wrong development, but I do not know what to do about it. All universities have these requirements now; it is a trend which is probably unfortunate, but if people cannot add up figures, they won't be able to plan the research work you want, Professor Pequignot. The dichotomy between the cold arithmeticians and the warmer-hearted extroverts may be inevitable.

Evang: The type of students recruited means a great deal. The remedy was suggested that ordinary patients should be used more for training possible future general practitioners. In Norway we have some experience with this method; unfortunately there is no sign that it makes any difference to the recruitment of general practitioners.

When the prepaid medical programmes under which most practitioners work in the developed parts of the world were established 40–50 years ago, people were of course thinking only of curative medicine, and that is the only thing which the doctor is paid for. To my mind the way to make general practice attractive again is to widen the scope of activity of the general practitioner, to include preventive medicine and rehabilitation and to pay him for this as well. This can only be done by creating a new type of general practitioner and introducing him into a public health service in which he plays a role which gives him some status. I can see no opposition between the clinical and epidemiological approach. It is the epidemiological handling of the clinical observations which we sometimes miss.

Dogramaci: In the selection of students the developing countries tend to copy the pattern in Paris, for example—a large intake in the first year, with many later dropping out. This is a great waste of manpower. Many of the students take up medicine for family reasons, as Professor Pequignot says, but others enter because they think it is a good profession to be in. They rarely know whether they are really fitted for the profession. A system of premedical education, within the universities but outside the medical schools, where students could study physics, biology, chemistry and the social sciences and where, if they decided not to continue in medicine, they could go on with some other scientific career, might solve this problem. A student could go on to study social science and still take advantage of the knowledge he had already acquired in natural sciences. Some of these students might become biochemists or microbiologists or physiologists, without necessarily spending many additional years in becoming physicians.

The point about facilities for research, especially in epidemiology, being available for general practitioners is a good one. But I am afraid the clinical specialists would probably snatch the opportunity to do these studies. To make general practice more attractive, would it be feasible to make a specialization of it? Students could be given a grounding in the 50 most common diseases encountered in general practice. In England the general practitioner refers the patient to a consultant or specialist, so that no element of specialization comes into general practice. All the developed countries should look at this question in order to try to solve the problem of recruiting adequately trained general practitioners.

At least in Turkey the possibilities of fundamental research have acted as a bait to bring back from abroad some of our qualified personnel.

Candau: What Professor Dogramaci said about the recruitment of students is extremely important. Extra training for students before they enter medical school is a good idea. The standards of secondary education are becoming lower in certain areas of the world and the only way is to bring the available students up to the level needed for medical training. In certain medical schools in Africa 65 per cent of the students are eliminated in the first year: this is not only a waste of manpower—it also does tremendous harm to the students themselves to fail.

Burkitt: In the selection of future doctors I think we have underestimated the question of motivation, of character and of vocation. Choosing doctors purely on academic standards may lose the most valuable people to our service. Many otherwise excellent doctors have been lost to medicine because they have been discharged for drunkenness or some other failing, whereas others (not nearly so clever) are highly respected because of the men they are. It is very hard to assess this aspect in selecting students, but I do feel that the attempt should be made.

Pequignot: It is not the same thing to give students a lecture on psychology or on social science as to get them to understand life in the community. Contact with all kinds of people, of all ages and from all types of cultural background, is necessary.

Banks: I strongly support what Professor Pequignot said about the training of general practitioners, but it is important to know first what we mean by a general practitioner. The term can mean different things in different countries. I much prefer a term Professor Pequignot himself uses—the omnipractitioner. What is needed in developing countries is a doctor able and willing to work among his own people as the leader of a team of paramedical workers and auxiliaries suitable for the area concerned. The training of such doctors and teams is of fundamental importance to the developing countries.

Candau: A teaching institution has to take part in research but it should be first and foremost a teaching institution. In many areas, for example in Africa, we find that the teaching staff are giving 75–80 per cent of their time to research and not paying enough attention to teaching. They regard teaching as an extra, and the number of students is sometimes unduly limited for this reason.

Lambo: That is the fault of the entire system of promotion. To become a professor one has to spend almost the whole time in research. When we look at medical education, we should look at the total picture, including the promotional system within the medical hierarchy.

Pincus: Many people go into research, yet the research worker is the poorest paid in the profession and he works the longest hours. So what are the attractions of research? One answer is that it satisfies intellectual needs which are not met in teaching or clinical practice. The solution is not to downgrade research and try to get doctors out of research into teaching, but to raise the values of teaching and the values of clinical work.

Querido: Professor Pequignot has dealt with very important problems affecting curricula and student selection in western countries. What criteria should be applied in the developing countries if they are to fulfil their own needs? As Professor Wolman said, these criteria might be non-medical. Is it possible to define what is needed in these countries according to the level of national income per person? That is, a developing country should perhaps spend 5–10 dollars of the first 100 dollars of its national income per head per year for health services and on the education of the necessary medical personnel. The people to be trained within this budget should perhaps be sanitary engineers and not medical specialists, though these may be trained in a neighbouring country which has a medical school. When a country can afford to spend, say, 30 dollars per person for health services and the training of personnel, there should perhaps be one medical school for every 10 million people so that leaders can be trained to take over the next step of development. A country which has 50 million people and a national income of, say, 200 dollars per head should perhaps (following this line of thought) provide one medical school in addition to training sanitary engineers. If we knew more about what was needed along these schematic lines of thought, we would be better able to assist these countries in the right way.

Kaprio: Only very recently WHO was asked by several governments to analyse their actual resources for developing health services in a more systematic way. The establishment of a medical school is such a big investment that most of the smaller African countries have tremendous difficulty in establishing one on their own. Some countries have difficulty even in keeping up the standards established in the previous colonial administration period and there is a tremendous need for outside assistance. The question of when one should establish a medical school depends very much on the help available from outside, the emphasis on sanitation and nursing education, and whether the personnel in these fields can be trained in the country concerned. It is only since the dust of independence has settled down that we have been able to see what the actual situation is in many countries and to start discussion with the national leaders. It will take time before an effective system can be established. WHO hopes to be able to provide leadership here.

One of the big problems is that we have not been able to convince the bankers that investment in human resources in a medical school is worth while as against investment in, say, a motor plant. The United Nations Special Funds have provided money for setting up an engineering school and a veterinary school but not yet for a medical school. This is partly the fault of the doctors themselves because there is such an emphasis on the individual right of doctors to practise whatever and wherever they like. There is no understanding that the medical profession forms part of the overall services of the community and has an impact on the economic and social development of the country. This image of the doctor prevents us from getting outside investment for medical schools.

Banks: Dr. Candau some years ago pointed out that certain areas of the world, especially in Asia and South America, already had a university structure on which to build, but that in parts of Africa there were neither medical schools nor universities.

It should be possible to share the resources for teaching the basic sciences between several countries in such circumstances, with students returning to their own countries for clinical training.

A danger which has not been touched on so far is the problem of dilution of staff. Where medical schools and universities are built up too rapidly, people who are not good enough to be promoted in the old-established universities may reappear on the senior staff in newly-created schools and universities. That is dilution carried to the point of ridicule but it is particularly dangerous in medicine.

It seems to me that research must also be suitable for the needs of the country. It is useless to encourage a man to embark on an M.D. thesis on a rare or non-existent condition when the real problem in his community, for example, is a high mortality in children under the age of five. One feels great sympathy for these young men who have got to publish in order to advance their careers: for them it may be a question not of "'publish and be damned'", but of "'publish *or* be damned'"!

REFERENCES

1. Lethielleux, P. (ed.) (1966). Démographie médicale. *Cahiers Laënnec*, No. 3, September.
2. Clegg, H. (ed.) (1961). *Medicine: a Lifelong Study*. Proceedings of the second world conference on medical education, Chicago, 1959. New York: World Medical Association.
3. Pequignot, H., Rosch, G., and Voranger, J. (1957). Remarques sur le coût du petit risque. *Revue d'hygiène et de médecine sociale*, **5**, 450.

14

OUTLINES OF A WORLD HEALTH SERVICE, AS A STEP TOWARDS MAN'S WELL-BEING AND TOWARDS A WORLD SOCIETY

G. E. W. Wolstenholme

Ciba Foundation, London

So far in this meeting we have been largely concerned with needs and difficulties—needs which are near the heart of all human problems; difficulties that are compounded by the self-centred forms of society in which we choose or are obliged to live. It is now high time to speak of achievements and opportunities.

In our modern world good news is no news. Unfashionable Christmas carols may sing of "tidings of comfort and joy" but journalists are expected to write only of friction and disaster. How often does any national newspaper in any country headline the constructive work of the United Nations' special agencies? The Children's Fund, the Commission for Refugees, the Bank for Reconstruction and Development, the Civil Aviation, Maritime, Food and Agriculture, and Educational, Scientific and Cultural Organizations, the International Monetary Fund, and other UN agencies make a great positive contribution to the world. I do not ignore the human failures and deficiencies of some of the international civil servants who work for them, but these agencies provide a scaffolding which perhaps alone in this world gives the outline and promise of the building of a new and more cooperative international society. Of all these agencies none contributes more to current improvements in our daily lives and gives more hope of a better future for all mankind than the World Health Organization (WHO).

Is there general recognition of the work of WHO? No; it is too easy to sneer at its mother the General Assembly—in itself so much better than nationalistic anarchy—and ignore the enterprise of the adult and legitimate offspring. When preparing this symposium I have felt humiliated to uncover the total ignorance of many people, in positions of responsibility, about the work of WHO. One eminent Londoner asked if I ran WHO from my office here in Portland Place!

People who do have a little learning about the UN and its ramifications might suppose that the earlier emphasis in this symposium on a stressful, diseased, crowded, ill-educated and unco-operative world implies criticism of or a lack of faith in the work of WHO. Let me therefore try to give some impression of its achievements, although I am vividly aware of my own inadequacy and the fact that as I present this paper I am surrounded by the masters—including Dr. Candau, the distinguished and humane Director-General of WHO. At least if I do this the Londoner mentioned earlier may get a glimpse from the written record of what is being done in his name.

The World Health Organization is an agency of the United Nations, created in 1946 and ratified by member States in 1948. Membership, open to all States, at present numbers 127, but regrettably it does not include the country with much the largest population and the longest history of civilization. Its aim is the "complete physical, mental and social well-being" of all men, women and children on the surface of our globe.

Its annual budget is US $50 million, roughly doubled by grants shared with related agencies and from private gifts; the whole is almost doubled again to about $170 million when expenditure by governments in association with WHO is included. The budget therefore approaches $200 million a year for projects initiated or assisted by WHO for the whole world. This is to be compared with the National Health Service annual budget in Britain of $3,750 million, much the same sum as we British spend on tobacco or on alcohol in one year.

The headquarters of WHO is in Geneva and it has regional offices in Africa, the Americas, South East Asia, Europe, the Eastern Mediterranean and the Western Pacific. Expert consultants in 44 panels include over 12,000 scientists, educationists and health administrators. The permanent staff numbers about 3,500 doctors, nurses, engineers, administrators and interpreters.

WHO is a world intelligence agency for communicable diseases, on which all quarantine measures are based. It sponsors international reference laboratories for diseases which scorn national frontiers. It is the ultimate authority on the health standards of food, on vaccines, drugs, systems of disease classification and diagnostic procedures, and it runs the counter-spy system against the traffic in illicit and dangerous drugs of addiction. As the recorder of rare reactions to drugs, it may forestall another thalidomide-like tragedy. It awards some 2,500 fellowships a year for postgraduate training in medicine, nursing and environmental health. It organizes each year about 40 short instruction courses and around 80 technical conferences.

It contributes at any one time, in manpower and in money, to 1,000 health projects in 150 countries.

WHO is an organization which between 1948 and 1963 treated, for example, 43 million people in 45 countries for the syphilis-like disease of yaws, and set 190,000 trained workers to the task of essentially eliminating malaria, to which half the world's peoples were exposed—and almost one-third of the world's population has by now been given protection from malaria, though 360 million remain at risk. It is WHO which lends hundreds of experts and teaches thousands of health workers to attack a host of disorders and diseases: for example, smallpox (a campaign to vaccinate 220 million in one year has just begun, to continue over ten years); tuberculosis (still some two to three million preventable deaths each year); leprosy (about 15 million people in 50 or 60 countries blighted by its mutilation); maternal and infant mortality (a tenfold difference between the most fortunate and the unhappiest countries); cancer, heart disease, rheumatism (the big killers and cripplers with widely varying incidence in different areas): water, soil and air pollution (in the world as a whole it is said that one in four hospital patients is ill because of infected water); blindness (10 to 12 millions sightless); deafness (millions still uncounted); infestations by parasites (many hundreds of millions of people chronically weakened and defeated by three or four such diseases together); mental illness; senility; accidents; malnutrition; and animal diseases.

The last details in this hasty, impressionistic sketch of WHO refer to its work on the co-ordination and stimulation of medical research, such as that on human genetics, heart diseases, cancer, dental health, bacterial resistance to insecticides—wherever a comparison from different areas may be revealing, or where a condition, a reaction to a drug for instance, may be too rare to excite attention in any one country.

It is an impressive record—yet this is only preliminary work in bringing to most people in the world a modest chance to enjoy the health which until recently has been the blessing of a privileged few. And already we have such an increased expectancy of life and so many more children survive that the problem of population growth makes almost every other problem trivial.

Impressive—but WHO can only act on request from governments. Its expert advisers operate only within national limits. And because of lack of money or skilled manpower not all requests can be met. Where it is able to help, WHO does its best to encourage the mobilization and creation of the local infrastructure which will maintain, or at least not wholly throw away, the value of WHO's efforts in disease control.

What more should be done—in self-interest, even if not in a spirit of humanity? What more *could* be done? We are accustomed to a world of major inequalities: for example, in the ability to grow food, in provision of clothing and shelter, in survival, in sanitation, and not least in medical care. Some of the most fully developed countries have one doctor for 750 people or less, whereas in Africa the situation averages out at least a hundred times worse at one doctor to 75,000. In Britain nurses exist at the level of one to 500; in India at one to over 10,000. In Ethiopia, for instance, the few doctors and nurses naturally congregate in Addis Ababa and Asmara, leaving a tiny handful to care for some 20 million people. Even the fortunate countries such as the USA and Britain beg or borrow doctors from other parts of the world to maintain their present levels of medical service. And recruitment in quality, and proportionately in quantity, falls because many of the existing doctors feel wasted and frustrated.

It has been estimated that the world could do with 750 new medical schools, with perhaps 75,000 teachers, but whether they come or not manpower in medicine and health work is certain to become more precious, and to require greater and more intelligent economy in use, throughout the next 30 years. The answer seems to me to lie, first in an infinitely wider measure of medical and medical auxiliary collaboration; secondly, in international co-operation; thirdly, in a high mobility of services whereby they are applied where the need, and only so long as the need, is greatest; and fourthly, in the creation of local services which can consolidate the advances made.

This implies some extension of the present great work of WHO. But for me there is an even more important consideration. No one country can solve, or indeed should attempt to solve on its own, this problem of medical care. If there is any such thing as a "health of mankind" it must be seen in its world context. If ever there was a problem ready made for international co-operation, this is it. Health should be the model, the pilot plant for a world society, a community of man. With this in mind and with a somewhat desperate diffidence I wish to make the following suggestions for a World Health Service (WHS).

First of all, we need an assessment of what would be required in the way of medical teams, or combinations of teams, to provide the basic essentials of medical therapy, of disease prevention, and of health education throughout the world. This assessment must be broken down briefly in terms of men, materials and money.

The men, and women, will be doctors from all specialties, including general practice, every variety of medical auxiliary, with abundant openings as well for orderlies, clerks, drivers, and so forth.

The materials will be those found necessary for medical work in any emergency such as a major natural disaster or in the unnatural horror of war.

The money to pay the staff, to buy the materials, to move both staff and materials to and from the places where they are needed, to provide the essentials of administration and interpretation, and to set up and maintain schools for training and technical services, on a scale which would make a minimum but a telling response to the outstanding needs of mankind would, I believe, be of the order of US $100 million a year. This figure may be compared with the $100 million which according to President Johnson is the cost to the USA alone of less than two days of "unofficial war" in Vietnam.

But, for some odd reason, survival in war and survival in disease are entirely different things, by at least a hundredfold, and it will be looked upon as quite a task to find $100 million a year. One appropriate solution would be to require each State to count, on one day in the year, the number of medical doctors within its frontiers, excluding any in a World Health Service or employed by WHO, and then to make a contribution to the WHS equivalent to US $100 for each doctor. A suitable census day would be that of the patron saint of physicians, St. Luke's Day (18th October) each year, payment to be completed by 31st December of the same year. A WHS would also perhaps commend itself to younger people as a worthy cause for which to collect voluntary subscriptions.

A WHS should be an expansion of WHO; certainly there should be no duplication of technical or information services. At the very least, they should be closely integrated, the WHS as a Division of WHO or with its own headquarters no further away than, say, Lausanne, and with an Executive Board on which WHO would be strongly represented, together with the Red Cross and similar organizations and relevant UN agencies such as UNICEF, FAO and the International Telecommunication Union.

The recruitment of all members of the WHS would be expected to establish standards for the world as a whole. To be selected would be an affair of pride, and to have served in the WHS a recommendation for one's future career!

The special training for work in particular environmental conditions and the preliminary building up of the various teams found to be required would be the task of educational establishments set up at headquarters and, I suggest, also in connexion with the present Regional Centres of WHO in Copenhagen, Brazzaville, Alexandria, New Delhi, Manila and Washington.

Pilot work by the teams, to gain experience of field conditions and of working together, could be carried out wherever there occurs a catastrophe such as a major epidemic, earthquake, hurricane or flood.

The teams I have in mind would regularly have a nucleus of nurses, engineers, clerks and drivers. The medical staffing would be varied according to need, from perhaps an eye surgeon with his operating theatre nurse and his anaesthetist, to combinations able to staff a small general hospital.

Apart from all medical specialties, the Service would employ and give initial and continuing training to nurses, midwives, sanitary engineers, dentists, opticians, radiographers, pharmacists, laboratory technicians, social and psychiatric workers and general duty orderlies.

The drain on valuable manpower from the richer countries might be regarded as robbing Peter to pay Paul. There are times and places, however, when even the richest State would be pleased to call on the aid of WHS. The loss of medical manpower would at least force out into the open a review by each country of its medical staffing and educational facilities, not only in self-interest but also in the full consciousness of the needs of those less fortunate.

When they review their own health services, the more prosperous countries are faced with a choice either of rapidly producing large numbers of doctors with inferior training, or of concentrating every effort to select the best students available, to educate and to continue to educate them to the limits of medical and social science, and then to free them from all duties which can and should be carried out by auxiliaries with a shorter and simpler training. A World Health Service would encourage this second choice, giving international opportunities for both doctors and auxiliaries to work to their utmost ability and so gain a satisfaction far beyond financial rewards. Stronger recruitment and higher standards in all countries would follow.

Recruitment to the WHS would be for varying periods, not excluding service as short as six months, perhaps repeated. This might be on secondment from a national health service, but one would want recruits to come forward from a great variety of backgrounds. The benefit of such experience, working with one's peers in a professionally élite service, regardless of nationality or other difference, would not be wasted on return home.

In time, every State would contribute men and women to WHS. During their service, they would have supranational citizenship so far as movement was concerned. A State in the early stages might refuse entry, until confidence in WHS is achieved, but at times, in the interests of world health, a body such as the General Assembly, or one formed by it for the purpose,

259

might require entry on pain of withdrawal of other UN assistance. Perhaps this is the point at which a World Health Parliament might be expected to support and facilitate WHO and WHS both legislatively and financially.

Members of a WHS could be expected to take pride in their own country's contribution to its work, whilst sharing in loyalty to the Service, and at the same time learning to understand and engage heart and soul in tackling the problems of the areas in which they are called upon to serve.

The pay of all members should be at agreed international rates; nevertheless, some form of national taxation could reasonably be levied to sustain a continuing sense of responsibility in their own national affairs.

Whilst all qualified staff should receive appropriate pay, there might be some who would choose to return all or part of it to the general funds of the Service. In any case, there would be room for voluntary part-skilled or unskilled service on a remarkable international scale. Algeria, Iran and Yugoslavia have all been reported to accept some form of health work in place of military service. A period of six months training at a school at WHS headquarters or a regional centre, followed by 18 months in the field, with a chance to develop some form of technical proficiency, would provide a demanding outlet for the idealism and energies of youth in every part of the world.

I use the phrase "in the field". In some parts of the world this would be literally true, but my own meaning includes the staffing of a network of health centres and hospitals, previously existing or not, until indigenous medical and health workers can be found and trained to accept responsibility. We are all agreed that a minimal permanent health service is necessary for that most pressing of all problems, birth control, if for nothing else; and a great deal could be done by sanitarians alone.

It might be suggested that a reasonably prosperous country should refund the cost of any aid received from WHS; even the poorest might make a return contribution in food and transport to WHS teams within its territory. There would be many instances, however, in which the ability to make a payment, or its extent, would be debatable. It appears to me, therefore, that WHS should meet from its central funds the whole cost of its work wherever it may go. Countries which benefit would not be discouraged from expressing their appreciation as generously as they wished, by providing additional men and women, equipment or money to the WHS as a whole.

A vital part of the World Health Service would be the free flow, or feedback, of information about the effectiveness of its activities throughout the world, in co-ordination with WHO in all its ramifications. The existence of such a society of trained scientific observers covering every habitat of mankind would be of immense value in research—for example in such things as geographical pathology, in epidemiology, in the detection of relationships in disease, and in the definition of reservoirs of infection, to name but a few. One would hope that the most sophisticated mechanized systems of information storage, analysis, retrieval and dissemination would be employed. Could one also hope that in this work bureaucracy would always be more concerned with the task to be done rather than with the records of what has already been done?

With up-to-date information, flexibility of constitution and movement would be of the first importance, teams or combinations of teams being moved and modified wherever the need was greatest.

Language barriers need not be severe, provided that one or two members of a team are capable of establishing essential contacts with the people to be given aid. Real need is a very efficient interpreter.

These notions for a World Health Service may be received with immediate complaints about infringement of sovereignty, spying, charity beginning at home, levelling down, a threat of a World State and so forth.

Maybe it would be open to abuse, but can we close our eyes, ears and hearts to the opportunity a WHS presents? Our record as human beings in this century so far makes it, for all its high standards of living in some areas, the darkest age of man. Two most fearful wars, killings on a scale exceeding all previous slaughter, exposure to radiation of all living creatures and plants, devastation of our natural environment, negligent waste of soil, isolation of a quarter of the human race, callous disregard of deaths and injuries on the roads, indifference to the implications of the population growth—it is a long indictment. The forces of sickness, injury and infirmity face us with a worthy and a shaming challenge. WHO has made a great beginning; in the closing years of this century could we gain the saving grace of taking a further vital step towards a healthy fraternity of nations? In so doing we might awaken a wider consciousness of the community of man.

DISCUSSION

Pequignot: We have discussed political problems, but we are not governments, we are scientists. Perhaps a scientist's first duty is to help man to decide what is of greatest importance to mankind—to go to the moon or to feed the millions of hungry people? We scientists are perhaps the only men who can ensure that mankind asks itself these questions. A world health service might have the same significance and force a decision in the medical field as to which diseases require the most urgent attention—leukaemia, or malaria, or schistosomiasis?

de Haas: To me an international health service seems somewhat Utopian, but it would be a very important achievement if these ideas could be fulfilled. In earlier discussions I realized that we talked mainly from our own point of view, and not from that of the so-called developing countries. Concerning medical manpower, for instance, it is a fact that developing countries give more technical assistance to industrial countries than we give to them. More doctors from technically underdeveloped countries are working in industrialized countries than the reverse, which is supposed to be the case—not to speak of the financial advantages industrialized countries slip into their own hands in handing out so-called technical assistance. If technical assistance could actually go in the right direction, from industrialized to developing countries, we would be doing a great service.

Would an international health service stress the preventive or the curative side of medicine? In all western countries curative medicine still seems as dominant as it was in the 19th century.

Developing countries need intellectual and economic independence even more than so-called political independence. Would a world health service increase or decrease this intellectual independence?

Wolstenholme: It seems to me it is inevitable that in seriously under-developed areas we would impose our point of view until many more of our people have intimate experience of other parts of the world. After such experience they should adapt their aid to the needs of the local society. I am certainly not oblivious of the fact that this idea appears to come only from our end, but the formation of a world health service which is truly independent would establish a non-national organization in which people from all nations could eventually meet to contribute. This might very soon provide an opportunity for educated people in any country, no matter how underdeveloped, to begin to measure up to and work side by side with members of the service at all its different levels. This intellectual challenge could be very profitable.

Regarding curative and preventive medicine, I am convinced that our own increasing shortage of medical manpower can only be met by changing the emphasis within our national health service. We must ourselves produce teams of doctors to work in collaboration with hospital and community health services at all levels, and inevitably, therefore, a much greater part of the work of even our big teaching hospitals will be in connexion with community services and much more concerned with preventive medicine.

Lambo: I compliment Dr. Wolstenholme on his insight and sensitivity to world needs, his fertile ideas and his imagination. It is from similar nebulous and imaginative ideas in the past that concrete actions have come. In the organization of such a body as WHS, a parallel might possibly be drawn with the organization of the Boy Scouts, which was a local body which became an international body. WHS could similarly eventually end up as a world body, after a first phase as a local organization.

Do you envisage specialization of labour between the WHO and the WHS, Dr. Wolstenholme? This, again, might be part of the first phase until WHS is more highly developed and able to cover a wider area of activity.

Wolstenholme: It would be a misfortune to base a world health service on combinations of different kinds of national health service, although I think it would be highly desirable for members of a national health service such as our own to spend part of their careers in this international work. But the recruitment must also come from every other possible source of medical manpower and *not* be restricted to those who are already members of a national health service.

The question about specialization in connexion with WHO is difficult to answer in any detail because I am not properly informed about the internal workings of WHO.

Dogramaci: Such a service is needed but I feel the creation and establishment of an altogether new system would not be an easy matter. An alternative would perhaps be to establish within WHO a special system called something like "The International Health Workers Service Fund", where all the advantages of being within an already well-established organization would still exist, but any danger of duplication would be avoided. Even if WHO were widely represented in a new service, the actual domains of authority might not be clear, whereas an extension within WHO where international health workers could be pooled, organized, and channelled, and for which new sources of funds could be raised, might be simpler.

Wolstenholme: I suggested that a WHS might be a division of WHO, but in any case a WHS and the WHO must be extremely closely integrated and share technical and information services. If representatives of WHO itself thought such an extension was a good idea and in no way crippling to their own efforts, I would certainly think it most desirable that it should be a part of the WHO.

le Riche: As to the financing it seems perfectly possible that Canada alone could pay \$100 million dollars for the service because they have something like $300 million already budgeted for external aid for 1966–1967. The sum of money is not great to people who are really interested, and I think people could be interested. It is not really Utopian—it is something that could be tried. It would obviously have to start on a relatively small scale, so it would not come into conflict with the work of WHO, and WHO activities will inevitably have to expand as the world grows more into one world. The financial side should not be difficult, but manpower will probably be a greater problem.

Evang: What Dr. Wolstenholme has outlined to us today is nothing less and nothing more than a further logical development of what was started between the two wars and since carried on. The first stage in the history of WHO was of an administrative and compiling organization, carrying out only the few statutory functions of the Health Section of the League of Nations. In 1949, at the Second World Health Assembly, we passed the first barrier and started to be an operating agency in the field. At that time the question raised by Dr. Wolstenholme as to whether it should also be a supply agency for material supplies, medical schools, drugs, and all that sort of thing was discussed, and this idea was defeated. As a result, UNICEF had to be started to undertake that part of the emergency supply business which the conscience of the world could not leave undone, namely, for the children. A merger now of UNICEF and WHO would be the first logical step towards the world health service.

When Truman in 1949 in his presidential address introduced for the first time what later became the Technical Assistance Programme of the United Nations, capital investment was among his points, but the politicians castrated this idea of capital investment from the beginning, so that UN technical assistance was deprived from the outset of one wall of support. After some years the developing countries were all filled to the brim with technical know-how, and were shown how they could save lives and so on, whereupon many of them replied, "We know now, we are perhaps not less intelligent than you, but now we need assistance to do all this". On several occasions the United Nations has tried to establish an organization for capital investment, and now there is the International Development Administration which has to extend to something called "preinvestment".

Lindop: Naturally I welcome everything Dr. Wolstenholme has said, but since we are not politicians, it is extremely difficult for a group of scientists or medical people to present such a scheme to governments, who put up all sorts of criticisms of what might go wrong or what might be the effects. In the interim period before we can actually get the scheme presented to governments perhaps we ourselves, from this body even, could start a feasibility study by selecting one area in the medical field which could be tackled on such an international basis. This would show that such a scheme can be carried out and accepted, and that the feedback mechanisms in terms of education and development of centres in developing countries, and the feedback to our own country's requirements would be demonstrated. Then in two or three years we would be able to answer some of the criticisms politicians are likely to put up against such a scheme. I feel very strongly about this since Lord Boyd Orr's proposals for a world food organization obviously failed because no scientific data from a feasibility experiment were available with which to answer the objections of the politicians.

Wolstenholme: This is a most admirable idea, if it could be realized.

Querido: This scheme seems Utopian because it is only a drop in the ocean, but this is no reason for not carrying it out. It could be the one thing which in turn sets in motion other things. What appeals greatly to me is that if the scheme succeeded a large number of people would acquire knowledge of all the situations needing attention, simply because this is a temporary service—unlike WHO where most people are lifetime officials, and consultants only come in sometimes for a short period. When I was a student I wanted to go to what one called at that time a colonial country, to spend a few years there, but instead I went into research and a university career. Later in my university career I went to these countries and became acquainted with their situation, which made me personally engaged in it. I have seen this happen to many of my friends. Something I have always regretted about decolonization is that so many people have thereby been deprived of an opportunity for maturation and experience which they do not get in their own nicely organized countries. If the scheme proposed by Dr. Wolstenholme could be realized it would benefit not only the developing countries, but also those who participate in it. And these persons will also form a kind of pressure group in their own countries which would press for more assistance to the developing countries.

What Dr. Wolstenholme said about a reassessment in our own countries also appealed to me very much, as I am sure that we can be much more efficient with what we already have, once we are forced to face our own problems.

Lastly, I wholeheartedly support the ideas of Professor le Riche; 10 per cent of any technical aid programmes might well be used for health care as this will ensure a more logical development of the country.

Candau: I need a little time to think about what Dr. Wolstenholme said, as this was a surprise to me. The source of money is very important, because it is very idealistic to think countries would be willing to give 10 per cent of their technical assistance money for health. I do not believe we would meet with much success if we tried to get this $100 million from governments. My first reaction to the suggestion is that this service would fill a gap, utilizing money from sources independent of governments and at the same time making use of the goodwill which exists and which cannot always find an outlet. It would be a kind of international peace corps without the political implications of the peace corps.

Beer: Two types of ideas are presented on occasions like this: those which can be realized immediately and those which might seem almost hopelessly difficult to execute on a short-term basis. But the second type are very often necessary ones. They force us to think, and perhaps even irritate us when we imagine all the difficulties involved. Dr. Wolstenholme's proposal for a World Health Service definitely belongs to the second category. It is easy to say how difficult it would be to realize it now. But the needs are there—we have heard that from several speakers. So something has to be done, and a public discussion on the ways and means must start, and that is why we should be grateful to our host that he has forced us to take position, and to continue the debate! And I would even add that this scheme might be broadened by a parallel mobilization of trained volunteers to assist the professionals.

Wolstenholme: I put forward these ideas with more than one object in mind—not only the relief of suffering but the consequent necessity to review our own privileged positions in the wider context of world needs, and also as an exercise and example in international co-operation.

GROUP DISCUSSION

Candau: It is extremely difficult to summarize or make an assessment of the present ills of mankind, and more difficult still to find a therapy. I do not think we can produce a world therapy. That would mean disregarding the patient and just considering the disease, because for all cases of a specific disease one would give the same medicine without taking into consideration the individual patient. Very great differences exist between one region and another and even within the same region or country. At this symposium people from undeveloped countries, like myself and Professor Lambo, know how difficult it is in our countries to apply a uniform therapy. I come from a country which includes some highly developed areas and also the Amazon region, one of the most backward areas in the world. This is one extremely important point which has emerged from our discussion.

Analyses of the world health situation will make it much easier to understand the difficulties. Yesterday when we started analysing the problem of malnutrition we began to see where the core of the matter lies. This applies also to problems of population, communicable diseases and so forth, and one of the most important things we have mentioned here is population and its associated problems of malnutrition and undernutrition. In the present year of 1967 when I consider all the pressures of eradication of disease, of malnutrition, undernourishment, population and many others, I cannot see any bigger problem than the lack of manpower. There are rich countries unable to develop their own services and economy for lack of manpower. Professor le Riche mentioned Libya: the problem of Libya is manpower. They cannot produce food because they have to produce petrol; they have more money for hospitals, for health services, for schools, than they have manpower to build and staff them.

In the medical field this is the general problem all over the world. We talked about family planning and came to the conclusion that one doctor could deal with 3,600 individuals, but a country like Pakistan has only one doctor for every 8,000 people, so practically all the doctors in Pakistan would be needed for family planning to the exclusion of all other medical activities—and Pakistan is a country with more doctors than many African countries.

It seems we have a blockage and this blockage is tradition. We are trying to do things in the way we did before, forgetting that medicine is an

267

evolutionary science. No country can expect to start off training doctors in universities like Oxford or Harvard, for example. We did not start like this. We started in a much more modest way. My country has been in the business only about 150 years and we now have 32 medical schools, the standards of which differ from one part of the country to the other, but they provide the doctors the country needs. The 110 Latin American schools have no equivalence with any schools in the USA or anywhere else, with the exception of the Haiti Medical School which has equivalence with schools in France. The Africans have become independent too recently to be able to deal with their problems alone and we need imagination to help them. When I visited Dr. Dogramaci in Turkey I saw the great effort he is making to find a solution. I do not know whether he is right or wrong but it is good to have new ideas and to use imagination. My impression is that we are not going to have students of the level we are talking about, and to solve our problems we shall have to use the raw material which exists, the students who are available. The USSR takes students with whatever knowledge they already have, completes their secondary education and then starts them on their medical training. This is the secret of the success of Lumumba University in Moscow, where to my surprise I found 62 students from Latin America!

To obtain teaching staff, the nationals of a country must be trained for this purpose. The Libyans said they could not have a medical school because of the difficulty of finding staff. I told them that to have a medical school in 1972 they must send their people now to be trained to take the responsibility of becoming faculty members. In one French-speaking country the Dean of the University told me the associate professors were too young to become established professors. I suggested they go to France for three or four years to complete their training for "agrégation" and the answer was: "It is not possible, they are too young. They are only 35 years old." A young country must use young people. Foreign professors may go to a country for two or three years to help, but the nationals must be prepared to take over their own responsibilities.

The most important problem in the world is manpower, because no other problems can be solved unless we have adequate manpower. From the political point of view manpower is the only thing which causes no trouble and the only thing that is permanent in a country is brains. All the rest—money, the construction of hospitals, a cobalt bomb in a country which does not know what to do with it, big trucks equipped with dentist's and X-ray equipment for Latin American countries which would be better off with 100 jeeps for the same price to carry out smallpox eradication—all these are temporary. The thing of real value and of political importance is what a foreign student gains from the institution in which he studies abroad. The often lifelong contacts he establishes there with the teaching staff are of abiding value and can lead to a much more permanent kind of international understanding and co-operation.

We are all anxious about nutritional problems, family planning, communicable diseases and the other big problems of health but if we could find a way to improve the manpower situation of the developing countries, they will then find their own solutions with only a little guidance from us.

Payne: We have been considering solutions to manpower problems in developing countries in a rather traditional way, adapting old methods to new situations—and by and large we have come to recognize that there are no easy or early solutions. We need a new approach.

The thing we have not done is to consider how advances in modern technology can help us. Our main difficulties are:

(1) Lack of doctors and other health personnel, but especially doctors because of the time and cost of their training.

(2) Maldistribution of the few doctors available.

(3) Lack of communications with rural areas.

There is quite a simple way in which these problems can be *partially* overcome, and the coverage achieved by a physician increased—for some functions at least—by a factor of approximately ten.

Small transceiver transistor radio links would enable a physician to keep in constant touch with paramedical personnel in an area of about 1,800 square miles. If these personnel are given elementary training to which is added the ability to describe symptoms, these could be transmitted to the physician who in a high proportion of cases—perhaps nearly 90 per cent—could arrive at the most probable diagnosis and order the treatment from the standard kit with which the personnel are supplied. This approach has been used extensively in Alaska where one Eskimo woman from each village is brought in for training and on her return to the village is linked with a medical centre by radio. It has worked very well. Of course in Alaska it is backed up by a plane or helicopter service to bring serious cases to hospital. We cannot expect this in developing countries yet but we should keep it in mind for the future.

But even the simplest scheme as outlined would extend some medical coverage to areas where now there is none—and at very low cost compared to the cost of training a physician.

Pincus: I sympathize with Dr. Candau about manpower but in the United States within the past three years approximately eight million women have come to use oral contraceptives, whereas three years before that the number was only 50,000. The medical personnel that achieved this must have already been in the country. Does this mean that the United States medical service has been drastically bogged down because doctors have supplied oral contraceptives instead of devoting their time to normal practice? I think not. Maybe the training for some of these jobs is not quite so difficult as we think. In Puerto Rico and Haiti we had one physician for 3,600 women but perhaps we could develop a situation where this ratio would be much higher.

I think the rate of training can be accelerated, especially in contraception, which is inexpensive and does not require very sophisticated understanding. Over the past five years we have perhaps trained a little over a hundred people in the programme supported by the Ford Foundation. These people then go back to their own countries and the repercussions are extremely wide. They in turn train other people. I do not think we can ignore the possibility of increasing the training very largely at a budgetary cost which may not be extraordinary. For certain specialized services Dr. Candau is absolutely right—I cannot see us training someone in three months to be an expert in radiography or any of the medical disciplines but in some fields where we consider the problem is sufficiently important maybe we can.

Lindop: In any discussion on the shortage of manpower, I think we must re-examine the status of women, because from our discussions during the last three days it is clear that women are the ones responsible for contraception, they are the ones responsible for water transport in the rural areas, and they are the key figures in health education and nutrition. Also, there is at present a fantastic wastage because of the social attitude towards working women, which is even worse in highly-developed countries than elsewhere. Women cannot do an adequate job of work because the social system is not yet adjusted to the fact that they should be doing it and that women are at least half the existing potential manpower. Certainly in Britain, and also in any consideration of potential manpower in the developing countries, the status of women, particularly trained women, really must be re-examined.

Wolman: I accept Dr. Candau's emphasis on manpower as our main problem, but I would like to point out there can be danger in over-emphasizing the restraints caused by lack of manpower. Experience has shown how the problem itself often forces the generation of manpower, though not in the orthodox curriculum preparation sense. In our discussions on medical, engineering or nursing manpower, we have been bound to the concept of time and curriculum which, as Professor Payne pointed out, may lead us into a blind alley. Perhaps manpower of a different nature and equipped with a different methodology, which modern technology can and does provide, could be generated more rapidly. It might not meet the accustomed specifications, which I suspect we are not going to meet for a very long time, but we should not be bound too heavily by this manpower restraint, which exists in every country in the world. In every problem in the United States we are confronted with a manpower crisis. At one time admissions to medical schools were superabundant in our country, but then the climate changed, as Professor Pequignot pointed out, and the bright young people moved into other categories for a number of socioeconomic reasons: better pay, better opportunities, more jobs, more glamour and the like. I am inclined to believe exactly the same thing will occur provided we ourselves are not so psychologically restrained that we just go home from this conference and say: "Well, it's too bad we don't have professional and subprofessional people, so let's quit."

I am sure, of course, that Dr. Candau is not surrendering, but we have to escape from the way in which the more sophisticated and the more affluent societies are generated. Professor Payne suggested two routes: firstly by aiming at the best technological accompaniment of service, and secondly by starting from scratch. As already pointed out, we had to start from scratch in England, in the United States, in Germany, in Holland and indeed everywhere else, but we forget this. We had to manage without full complements until resources warranted the generation of greater numbers of professionals. Another resource, as has just been pointed out, is the women, who in these countries may be untutored, but are nevertheless bright. We must not get too pessimistic about the lack of manpower.

Lambo: We should not disregard local cultural and social attitudes towards the utilization of women. Certainly this particular suggestion could be examined and full utilization made of womanpower, but there are difficulties in this respect in other countries and I feel the scientific tendency to make use of all manpower should not violate the sacred attitudes of certain societies.

As well as local talents and material, we should also use local institutions as much as possible. In some English-speaking countries in West Africa we have lost within the last ten years one in ten of our highly-trained people to North American countries. Perhaps this is because they are so supertrained they are miserable working in Nigeria or Sierra Leone and so they want to stay in North America. This must be taken into consideration in planning the training of manpower in developing countries.

Wright: Although agreeing with Dr. Candau that manpower is the key problem, I was a little disappointed he did not refer to training of manpower in the context of local needs. Great differences in techniques exist between different areas—in the tropical and subtropical as against the temperate areas. Perhaps the same sort of differences should be considered in the training of doctors—are we at the moment simply adopting the western curriculum and hoping that these doctors will be able to cope with local tropical and subtropical problems? Or are we looking at the local problems, as we should, to devise a curriculum on that basis? I mention doctors, but this applies throughout the medical services, as in all other services. Manpower should be adapted to the local needs of the country.

Beer: I agree about Dr. Candau's points on manpower, but some things could be adjusted to offset the fact that greater economic development leads to a severe brain drain in the medical field. The developed countries offer better jobs and research opportunities. Bilateral "aid" programmes with scholarships for medical students and postgraduates in America and Western Europe are sometimes a sign of hypocrisy because one knows that many of the best students will probably remain in the developed countries. In French West Africa, for prestige and other family reasons, many people want to get scholarships to French universities instead of studying at the faculties of Dakar or Ibadan, with a better chance of remaining in Africa when they have completed their training.

Much progress in Africa and Asia is held up because of the exclusive use of "outside" languages also for paramedical training. This is not necessary. In Bulgaria, instead of Turkish-speaking girls being made to learn Bulgarian and go to Sofia for training, doctors and teachers run three-month basic courses for "rural nurses" in Turkish in their own districts and these girls then remain in their villages. So it would be better when training auxiliaries to find ways to train people locally in their own languages.

Evang: We cannot end without mentioning one highly complicating factor in the general impact of world health services. Regardless of whether we are bothered with problems at home, the major problems are in the developing countries. Sir Norman Wright referred to the vicious circle and the Utopian philosophy that an attack on the weakest links—poverty and lack of food production—should improve the situation. We now know that unfortunately one cannot succeed this way but that a simultaneous *multiphasic* attack must be launched on health, on education, on production, on family planning. This is extremely complicated, as anyone who is familiar with the developing countries will realize.

Querido: Shortage of manpower is the problem but this need not prevent a world health service of the kind Dr. Wolstenholme suggested. Obviously people will have to be trained and if a world health service could train people locally according to schemes planned by technically well-informed people with a curriculum based on local needs, this would be an enormous contribution. Those of us who have taught in a developing country know that the curriculum does not always fit the local needs adequately.

As regards the money for this, there are bilateral arrangements for technical aid and teaching might be considered as technical aid. I see no contradiction.

Candau: I do not object to this service at all but I was trying to define the field! The financing of such a scheme is extremely important in the sense that I think the money will not come from governments, because I have had long experience of special funds and of voluntary funds and the voluntary contributions from governments have been practically nil. The money could be found from other sources which already exist in Britain, Switzerland, France, and the United States, for example, and a fund could be organized through voluntary contributions to ensure a long-term scheme. I have little faith in bilateral programmes because it is extremely difficult to find out what is being done under a bilateral programme—no government will tell us. We do not know what Canada is doing, what the United States is doing, what the USSR is doing, and sometimes they do not even know themselves! I am not against this scheme at all and I hope I did not give you the wrong impression. I think this service will be able to achieve a great deal over and above what WHO can do and that the only real problem is that of finance.

Wolstenholme: In Britain many people have been very dissatisfied for some years because we could not find out from government, from universities, or from philanthropic institutions just what is already being done by this country in the medical world as a whole. During the last year the Royal Society of Medicine has set up a committee under my chairmanship and with the support of the Royal Colleges of Physicians, Surgeons and Obstetricians the Ministry of Overseas Development, and the British Council, and we are now trying hard to set up a register of international relationships between this country and all other parts of the world in regard to exchanges of medical manpower, examiners, teaching material and so on, in either direction. I do not know whether we can achieve this but once the register is reasonably complete, we may see where there is undue emphasis or an extravagance of aid, and where there is none at all.

CONCLUDING REMARKS

Professor A. L. Banks

The subtitle of the Ciba Foundation states that it exists for the promotion of international co-operation in medical and chemical research, and I venture to think that we have had as good an example of international co-operation throughout the last three days as during any of the preceding 99 symposia.

The first thing which impressed me during our discussions was the importance of comparative medical studies, and the close relationship between pathology of disease in man and in animals. I hope something further will develop from this.

Out of the valuable discussion on malnutrition the need clearly emerged for a developing country to measure its progress against the conditions formerly existing in that country, rather than by comparison with conditions in a European country.

Another highlight was the discussion on "the inhuman city". We are deeply indebted to Dr. Doxiadis and Professor Johnson-Marshall for venturing into an alien environment to confront us with what is even for them new territory. I was reminded of Leonardo da Vinci as I watched Dr. Doxiadis with his drawings and diagrams. I think the "mushroom" cities of the developing countries constitute the greatest single health problem, for they are the danger spots—physical, mental and moral. Of course, the Doxiadises of the world cannot demolish all these cities and build new ones, but their concept of the city as a living place and a place in which to live properly is a fine one.

Our discussions on medical education and manpower are so fresh in our minds that I need say no more.

Finally, we come to Dr. Wolstenholme's proposal for a World Health Service as a step towards man's well-being and towards a world society. We here are all professionals, and it is not part of a professional's stock-in-trade to be either optimistic or pessimistic, but I think we can go away reassured that our discussions have clarified some of the problems relating to the Health of Mankind, and hopeful that we may see the concept of a World Health Service become a reality.

Members of the Symposium

Publications include: *Food Shipment from Australia in Wartime*; *Challenge to Education*; *Scientist in Russia*; *Technology and the Academics*; *Community of Universities*; *African Universities and Western Tradition*; and papers on aspects of experimental botany and on education.

A. L. BANKS

Professor of Human Ecology, University of Cambridge, since 1949.
English—Middlesex Hospital Medical School, University of London, and Lincoln's Inn. Divisional Medical Officer, Public Health Department, London County Council (duties included special public health enquiries and slum clearance), 1934–37; Ministry of Health, 1937–49. Formerly Principal Medical Officer, Ministry of Health. Member: General Medical Council; General Dental Council; WHO Expert Advisory Panel on Organization of Medical Care; Building Research Advisory Committee; Registrar-General's Advisory Committee on Medical Nomenclature and Statistics; Medical Geography Committee, Royal Geographical Society, etc. Barrister-at-Law (Lincoln's Inn); Fellow of the Royal College of Physicians; Fellow of Gonville and Caius College, Cambridge, since 1951; Fellow of Royal Society of Medicine.
Publications include: *Social Aspects of Disease*, 1953; (ed.) *Development of Tropical and Subtropical Countries*, 1954; (with J. A. Hislop) *Health and Hygiene*, 1957, and *Art of Administration*, 1961; private and official papers on medical and related subjects.

H. BEER

Secretary General of the League of Red Cross Societies, since 1960.
Swedish—Graduated in History and Political Science, Stockholm University; organized relief within and outside Sweden to university students from war-ravaged countries; Executive officer, Swedish Governmental Relief and Rehabilitation Commission, 1944; joined Swedish Red Cross as Consultant, at the request of the late Count Folke Bernadotte; Secretary General, 1947–60; served as Secretary General, 17th International Conference of the Red Cross in Stockholm, 1948. In Swedish Red Cross, organized relief for disaster victims, refugees, etc., and planned Field Hospital in Korea, 1950; visited Korea and helped plan Scandinavian Medical Centre there. Interested in Adult Education and Training; and a Founder of Stockholm's People's University. As Secretary General of the League since 1960, has carried out 160 missions to 65 countries, inspected League operations in many disaster areas, contributed towards strengthening Red Cross medicosocial activities in the world, represented the League at numerous international conferences, and reinforced League collaboration with UN and other international bodies, especially WHO. Set up and supervised League's Red Cross Development Programme with Five Year Plans for assistance to Societies in newly independent countries and in developing areas.
Publications include: brochures and articles on various subjects, especially on Red Cross activities and on the international refugee question.

W. I. B. BEVERIDGE

Professor of Animal Pathology, University of Cambridge, since 1947.
Australian—Research bacteriologist, McMaster Animal Health Laboratory, Sydney, 1930–37; Commonwealth Fund Service Fellowship, Rockefeller Institute, Princeton and Bureau of Animal Industry, Washington, 1938–39; Research Officer in Virology, Walter and Eliza Hall Institute for Medical Research, Melbourne, 1941–46; Visiting Worker, Pasteur Institute, Paris, 1946–67; Visiting Professor, Ohio State University,

1953; President, Permanent Committee of the World Veterinary Association, since 1957; Consultant in Comparative Medicine, World Health Organization, 1964–66.
Publications include: (with Sir Macfarlane Burnet) *Cultivation of Viruses and Rickettsiae in the Chick Embryo* (Medical Research Council's Special Report No. 256), 1946; *The Art of Scientific Investigation*, 1950; and articles on infectious diseases of man and domestic animals, especially virus diseases.

D. BURKITT

External Scientific Staff, Medical Research Council, London, since 1966.
Irish—Qualified Trinity College, Dublin, 1935; Army Surgeon, 1941–46; M.D. Dublin, 1946; Service in Uganda, 1946–66; Final appointment: Senior Consultant Surgeon, Ministry of Health, Uganda, and Teacher in Clinical Surgery, Makerere University College Medical School. Fellow of the Royal College of Surgeons of Edinburgh; Foundation Fellow of the East African Association of Surgeons; Honorary Member of the Sudan Association of Surgeons and South African Association of Surgeons; Corresponding Member of the American Association for Cancer Research.
Publications include: numerous papers in scientific journals on the African lymphoma.

M. G. CANDAU

Director-General, World Health Organization, Geneva, since 1953.
Brazilian—Graduated in Medicine, School of Medicine, State of Rio de Janeiro; and received special training in public health at University of Brazil and Johns Hopkins University, Baltimore. In charge of various health services in State of Rio de Janeiro, 1934–43, and was appointed Assistant Director of State's Department of Health. Participated in eradication campaign, undertaken by Brazilian Government in co-operation with Rockefeller Foundation, against the mosquito *A. gambiae*. Director of Division, Assistant Superintendent, and later Superintendent, Serviço Especial de Saude Publica, 1943–50. Assistant Professor of Hygiene, School of Medicine, State of Rio de Janeiro, since 1938. Director, Division of Organization of Health Service, WHO, Geneva, 1950; Assistant Director-General of Advisory Services, 1951; Assistant Director, Pan-American Sanitary Bureau, Washington, 1952. Honorary Fellow (Foreign): Argentine Medical Association. Honorary Fellow: American College of Dentists; American Public Health Association; National Academy of Medicine, Peru; Peruvian Public Health Association; Royal Academy of Medicine in Ireland; Royal Society of Medicine, London; Royal Society for the Promotion of Health, Great Britain. Fellow of the Royal College of Physicians, London. Honorary Member: American Hospital Association; American Venereal Disease Association; Bolivian Public Health Society; Canadian Public Health Association; Geneva Medical Society; National Academy of Medicine, Brazil; Panamanian Public Health Association. Member: Brazilian Society of Hygiene; Society of Medicine and Surgery, State of Rio de Janeiro; Royal Society of Tropical Medicine and Hygiene, Great Britain. Doctor *honoris causa*: University of Brazil, 1963; University of Sao Paulo, Brazil, 1965. Honorary Doctor of Laws: University of Michigan, 1961; Johns Hopkins University, Baltimore, 1962; University of Edinburgh, 1963; Queen's University, Belfast, 1965; and Seoul University, Korea, 1965. Honorary Doctor of Medicine: University of Geneva, 1963. Honorary Doctor of Science: Bates College, Maine, USA, 1963. Awarded Bronfman Prize for Public Health Achievement by American Public Health Association, 1961; Eduardo Liceago Medal and Diploma by President of Republic of Mexico, 1963; Mary Kingsley Medal, Liverpool School of

Tropical Medicine, 1966; and 1st Award of Royal Society of Health's Gold Medal, 1966. Publications include: scientific papers covering a wide range of subjects, including malaria, parasitology, public health administration, biostatics, rural hygiene, etc.

LORD COHEN OF BIRKENHEAD
Emeritus Professor of Medicine, University of Liverpool; and Senior Physician, Royal Infirmary, Liverpool, since 1934.
English—Visiting Professor of Medicine, New York State University, 1958; and McGill University, Montreal, 1959. President: Royal Society of Health, since 1958; General Medical Council, since 1961; Royal Society of Medicine, since 1964; (Life), Institute of Health Education; National Bureau for Co-operation in Child Care, since 1965; UK Foundation of WHO, since 1966. Chairman: Central Health Services Council, 1957–63; Standing Medical Advisory Committee, Ministry of Health, 1948–63. Member: Expert Advisory Panel on Professional Education, WHO; Moynihan Lecturer, Royal College of Surgeons, 1948; Bradshaw (1939) and Croonian Lecturer, Royal College of Physicians, 1963, etc. Fellow of the Royal Colleges of Physicians of London, Edinburgh, Glasgow and Ireland. Hon. Freeman of Birkenhead; Associate Knight of St. John of Jerusalem. Created Baron, 1956.
Publications include: (Editor-in-Chief) *British Encyclopaedia of Medical Practice*; *New Pathways in Medicine*, 1935; *Nature, Method and Purpose of Diagnosis*, 1943; *Sherrington: Physiologist, Philosopher and Poet*, 1958; *The Evolution of Modern Medicine*, 1958; and contributions to many books, and medical and scientific journals.

J. H. DE HAAS
Head, Department of Health Development, Netherlands Institute for Preventive Medicine, Leiden; and Professor of World Health, Leiden University.
Dutch—Lecturer and Professor in Paediatrics, University of Indonesia, Djakarta, 1934–48; Internment in Japanese camps in Java during World War II; Chief, Child Health Section, Netherlands Public Health Service, 1950–60; Netherlands Institute for Preventive Medicine, since 1953. Visited many industrialized and developing countries as WHO consultant and lecturer, and on other missions.
Publications include: works on child development, morbidity and mortality and nutrition in tropical and western countries; epidemiology of tuberculosis and accidents; child health and school health services; changing mortality patterns and cardiovascular diseases.

I. DOGRAMACI
President, Hacettepe Science Center and Hacettepe Medical Center, Ankara, since 1965; Professor of Paediatrics, Ankara University, and Head of Department, since 1954; and Director of the Institute of Child Health, Ankara University, since 1958. President, Board of Trustees, Middle East Technical University, Ankara, since 1966.
Turkish—Graduate of Istanbul University Faculty of Medicine; Postgraduate training in paediatrics, 1939–46: Ankara Numune Hospital; Boston Children's Hospital; and St. Louis Children's Hospital. Lecturer in child health, Ankara University, 1947–48; Associate Professor of Paediatrics, Ankara University, 1949–54; Dean of Hacettepe Faculty of Medicine and Health Sciences, Ankara University, 1963; President of Ankara University, 1963–65. Represented Turkey on UNICEF Executive Board, since 1960. Hon. Fellow, American Academy of Pediatrics; Hon. Member, British Paediatric

278

Association; Corresponding Member, American Pediatric Society. Hon. Doctor of Laws, University of Nebraska.

Publications include: *Annenin Kitabi* (Mother's Handbook in Child Care) 5 editions; *Premature Baby Care*; Porphyria in Childhood (chapter in *Advances in Pediatrics*); and numerous papers on paediatrics and medical education. Editor, *Turkish Journal of Paediatrics* (Ankara); Consulting editor, *Clinical Pediatrics* (Philadelphia).

C. A. DOXIADIS

President of Doxiadis Associates—Consultants on Development and Ekistics, since 1953; and Chairman, Board of Directors, Athens Technological Institute, since 1958.

Greek—Graduated as Architect-Engineer from Technical University, Athens, 1935; graduate work at Berlin-Charlottenburg University, and received the degree of Dr. Ing. Chief Town Planning Officer, Greater Athens Area, 1937–38; Head, Department of Regional and Town Planning, Ministry of Public Works, Greece, 1939–44; Lecturer and Acting Professor of Town Planning, Technical University of Athens, 1939–43; Visiting Lecturer: Universities of Chicago, Michigan, Yale, Princeton, Harvard, Massachusetts Institute of Technology, etc. Minister and Permanent Secretary of Housing Reconstruction, 1945–48; Minister-Co-ordinator of Greek Recovery Programme, 1948–51. Member, Greek Delegation, San Francisco Peace Conference, 1945; Greek Representative to France, England and USA on problems of post-war reconstruction, 1945; Head, Greek Delegation at: International Conference on Housing, Planning and Reconstruction, 1947; and Greco-Italian War Reparation Conference, 1949–50. Greek Representative on Housing, Building and Planning Committee of the Economic and Social Council of the United Nations, New York, 1963 and 1964; Chairman, Session on Urban Problems, UN Conference on Application of Science and Technology for the Benefit of Less Developed Areas, Geneva, 1963. Consultant to: UN International Bank for Reconstruction and Development; Agency for International Development; Redevelopment Land Agency of Washington, DC, Ford Foundation, and Governments of: Brazil (Rio de Janeiro), Ethiopia, Ghana, Greece, India, Iraq, Jordan, Lebanon, Libya, Pakistan, Spain, the Sudan, Syria, and USA. Honorary Corresponding Member, Town Planning Institute of Great Britain, 1947; Honorary Corresponding Fellow of the Royal Incorporation of Architects in Scotland, Glasgow, 1964. Awarded: Sir Patrick Abercrombie Prize of the International Union of Architects, 1963; The "Cali de Oro" Award of the Society of Mexican Architects, 1963; Award of Excellence, Industrial Designers Society of America, 1965; Aspen Award for the Humanities, 1966. Greek Military Cross; The Royal Order of the Phoenix (Greece); the Order of Cedar (Lebanon); and the Order of the British Empire.

Publications include: *Ekistic Policies for the Reconstruction of the Country with a Two-Year Programme*, 1947; *Our Capital and its Future*, 1960; *Architecture in Transition*, 1963; *Urban Renewal and the Future of the American City*, 1966; *Between Dystopia and Utopia*, 1966; *An Introduction to the Science of Human Settlements*, 1967; *Building our Cosmos*, 1967; *Entopia*, 1967; Forthcoming: Ecumenopolis, Toward a Universal Settlement, 1968.

K. EVANG

Director-General, The Health Services of Norway, The Royal Norwegian Ministry of Social Affairs, Oslo, since 1939.

Norwegian—Studied medicine at the University of Oslo; served on staff of Oslo Municipal Hospital, and did postgraduate work in England, France and Germany. Entered

Government service, 1937, and during World War II accompanied the Norwegian Government into exile, serving in London, Washington and Stockholm organizing the Norwegian overseas public health services, the provision of medical supplies to the Norwegian resistance, and assisting in the planning of health and social services for post-war Norway. Closely associated with WHO from the beginning and headed the Norwegian delegation at every World Health Assembly; President of the Second World Health Assembly, and Chairman, Executive Board at its 36th and 37th Sessions; Member, WHO Panel on Public Health Administration; has also served on a host of expert groups and international conferences. Awarded the Léon Bernard Medal and Prize "for his unremitting service and outstanding achievements in the field of public health and social medicine".

Publications include: *Health Service, Society, and Medicine*, London, 1960; *Health Services of Norway: The Norwegian Joint Committee on International Social Policy*, Oslo, 1960; *Medical Care and Family Security (Norway)*, New York, 1963; and various publications in medical journals, etc., related to health administration and social medicine.

G. FANCONI

Professor of Paediatrics, Faculty of Medicine, University of Zürich (Retired).

Swiss—Graduate of Bern University; Assistant: Pathological-Anatomical Institute, University of Zürich, 1918; Physiological Institute, University of Bern, 1919; and University Children's Clinic, Zürich, 1920–26; Head Physician, Children's Clinic, Zürich, and Lecturer in Paediatrics, 1926–29; Director, Children's Hospital, Zürich, and Professor of Paediatrics, Faculty of Medicine, University of Zürich, 1929–62. Dean, Medical Faculty, University of Zürich, 1946–47. General Secretary, International Paediatrics Association, 1950–66; President, International Cystic Fibrosis Association, 1964; President, Swiss Association for Nutrition, 1966. Hon. Doctor, Universities of Turin, Geneva, Paris, Uppsala, La Havana, Guadalajara (Mexico), and Rio de Janeiro; Hon. Professor, Universities of Guatemala and Santiago (Chile).

Publications include: various articles in medical books and journals; Founder and editor of *Helvetica Paediatrica Acta*, since 1945.

LORD FLOREY

Provost of the Queen's College, Oxford, since 1962; and Chancellor of the Australian National University, since 1965.

Australian—Educated Adelaide University and Magdalen College, Oxford. Rhodes Scholarship for S. Australia, 1921; John Lucas Walker Student, Cambridge, 1924; Rockefeller Travelling Fellow in America, 1925; Huddersfield Lecturer in Special Pathology, Cambridge, 1927; Joseph Hunter Professor of Pathology, University of Sheffield, 1931–35; Nuffield Visiting Professor to Australia and New Zealand, 1944; Professor of Pathology, Oxford University, 1935–62. Awards include: Lister Medal, Royal College of Surgeons of England, 1945; Gold Medal, Royal Society of Arts, 1946; Royal Society of Medicine Gold Medal, 1947; USA Medal of Merit, 1948; Royal Medal, Royal Society, 1951; Copley Medal, Royal Society, 1957; Lomonossov Medal, USSR Academy of Sciences, 1965. Foreign Member, American Philosophical Society, 1963; Foreign Associate, National Academy of Sciences, USA, 1963; Foreign Hon. Member, American Academy of Arts and Sciences, 1964. Fellow of Lincoln College, Oxford; Honorary Fellow, Gonville and Caius College, Cambridge; and Magdalen College, Oxford. Fellow of the Royal Society, 1941; President of the Royal Society, 1960–65.

Trustee of the Ciba Foundation, since 1964. Awarded Nobel Prize for Medicine, 1945; created Knight, 1944; Commander, Legion of Honour, 1946; Order of Merit, 1965; and created Life Peer, 1965.
Publications include: contributions to scientific journals on physiological and pathological subjects: *Antibiotics* (with co-workers), 1949; (edited and contributed to) *General Pathology* (3rd edn) 1962.

VICTORIA GARCIA
Professor of Health Education, School of Public Health, University of Chile, Santiago, since 1957; and Assistant Professor in Public Health Administration, since 1955.
Chilean—Graduate of University of Chile, Santiago, 1935; First Assistant, Chair of Internal Medicine, San Vicente de Paul Hospital, 1935–50; Chief Medical Officer, National Health Service, Santiago, 1950–53; Director, Postgraduate courses for Latin American Health Educators, since 1957; Lecturer in Health Education, School of Medicine, University of Chile and Catholic University, 1960–66; Consultant in Public Health and Health Education, Department of Preventive Medicine, 1962–66. Member: WHO Expert Committee in Health Education of the Public, 1957–61; and Department of Public Health, Medical College, Santiago, 1960–66. WHO Fellow in Health Education, 1960, 1962 and 1965. Vice-President for Latin America of the International Union for Health Education; and President, Chilean Public Health Association, 1962–64.
Publications include: *Clinical Reports*, 1935–50; *Health Education in Hospitals and Outpatient Departments*, 1965; and various contributions to medical and other journals on public health administration and health education.

P. E. A. JOHNSON-MARSHALL
Professor of Urban Design and Regional Planning, Department of Architecture, University of Edinburgh, since 1964.
English—Educated Liverpool University School of Architecture. Senior Architect in charge of reconstruction of Coventry city centre; appointed to take charge of the London County Council Reconstruction Areas Group, 1948, including the preparation of Comprehensive Plans for the East End, Barbican, etc., for which he was awarded the Royal Institute of British Architect's Distinction in Town Planning. Later became Group Planning Officer for North-East London. Senior Lecturer, Department of Architecture, University of Edinburgh, 1959, Reader, 1963, and Professor of Urban Design and Regional Planning, 1964. Work in Edinburgh includes direction of the Planning Research Unit; the Lothian Regional Survey, jointly with the University of Glasgow, relating to the development of the new town of Livingstone, the Falkirk-Grangemouth Regional Survey and the West Borders Study. Member: R.I.B.A. Council; past member Town Planning Institute Council, and Board of Architectural Education; also member of WHO Expert Panel on Environmental Health and Planning.
Publications include: *The Rebuilding of Cities*, 1965/66.

L. A. KAPRIO
Regional Director of the Regional Office for Europe, World Health Organization, Copenhagen, since February 1967.
Finnish—Graduated in Medicine, University of Helsinki; Doctor of Public Health, Harvard School of Public Health, USA; Chief of the Public Health Section of the State Medical Board of Finland, 1952–56; with WHO since 1956, Eastern Mediterranean and

281

European regions, 1956–63, Division of Public Health Services, 1963–67. Member: Finnish National Medical and Scientific Associations; American Public Health Association; International Epidemiology Association; International Hospital Federation. Publications include: many articles on social medicine, public health and epidemiology.

H. KATSUNUMA

Professor and Head, Department of Public Health, Faculty of Medicine, University of Tokyo, since 1959.

Japanese—Graduated at the Faculty of Medicine, University of Tokyo, 1941; Research Assistant, Department of Public Health, University of Tokyo, 1949; Graduate School of Public Health, University of Pittsburgh, 1952–53. Participant: FAO/WHO Joint Seminar on Health and Nutrition Education, 1955, and WHO Seminar on "Role of Preventive Medicine in Medical Education", 1957, in Manila, Philippines; Chairman, WHO/ILO Seminar on Occupational Health, Tokyo, 1959. Professor and Head, Department of Radiological Health, School of Atomic Power Engineering, Faculty of Technology, University of Tokyo, 1961. Invited speaker and Councillor, General Congress of the Confederation of Medical Associations in Asia and Oceania, Manila, 1961. Chairman of symposium, International Conference on Health and Health Education, Philadelphia, 1962; Executive member of Board of Trustees: Japan Industrial Health Association; and Japan Medical Association, 1962; Japan Public Health Association, 1964. Invited speaker, 2nd General Congress of Australian Medical Societies, Perth, Australia; inspection visits to WHO, ILO and European countries as member of technical staff of Governmental Council for Industrial Safety; Delegate of Japan, General Congress of World Medical Association, London, 1965. Member: Permanent Commission, International Association of Occupational Health; and WHO Expert Advisory Panel on Professional and Technical Education of Medical and Auxiliary Personnel, 1966.

T. A. LAMBO

Professor of Psychiatry and Head of Department of Psychiatry and Neurology, University of Ibadan, since 1963; and Dean of the Faculty of Medicine, University of Ibadan, since 1966.

Nigerian—Graduated at Birmingham University, 1948; General Hospital and Midland Nerve Hospital, Birmingham, 1948–50; Medical Officer, Nigerian Medical Services, 1950–54; Specialist, Western Region Ministry of Health, Neuro-Psychiatric Centre, Aro, 1957, Senior Specialist, 1960, Consultant Psychiatrist, University College Hospital, Ibadan; Member of Expert Advisory Panel on Mental Health, WHO Geneva; Member, Scientific Council for Africa, 1960, Vice-Chairman, 1964, Chairman, 1965. Chairman, United Nations Permanent Advisory Committee on Prevention of Crime and Treatment of Offenders 1965. Awarded the Order of the British Empire, 1962.

Publications include: Neuro-psychiatric Observations in the Western Region of Nigeria (Br. med. J., 1956); The Concept and Practice of Mental Health in African Cultures (E. Afr. med. J., 1960); Further Neuro-psychiatric Problems in Nigeria (Br. med. J., 1960).

W. H. LE RICHE

Professor and Head of Department of Epidemiology and Biometrics, School of Hygiene, University of Toronto, since 1962.

Canadian—Epidemiologist, Union Health Department, South Africa, 1950–52; Consultant in Epidemiology, Department of National Health and Welfare, Canada, 1952–54;

Research Medical Officer, Physicians' Services Incorporated, 1954–57; Research Associate, Department of Public Health, University of Toronto, 1957–59; Professor of Public Health, University of Toronto, 1959–62; Member: Delta Omega Beta Chapter, Public Health Honour Society; American Epidemiological Society. Fellow: American Public Health Association; International Academy of Law and Science. Member: Research Committee, Canadian Public Health Association; Research Committee, College of General Practice; Committee for the Survey of Hospital Needs in Metropolitan Toronto; Panel on Antibiotics and Panel on Infection and Immunity, Defence Research Board; Advisory Committee on Epidemiology, Advisory Committee on Revision of the International Classification of Diseases and Subcommittee on Environmental Health and Epidemiology, Department of National Health and Welfare. Consultant, Medical Statistics, Hospital for Sick Children, Toronto.

Publications include: *Physique and Nutrition*; *The Control of Infection in Hospitals*; and 85 papers in medical journals.

PATRICIA J. LINDOP

Reader in Radiobiology, St. Bartholomew's Hospital Medical College, London, since 1955, engaged in research into the long-term effects of radiation, with special reference to ageing and carcinogenesis.

English—Ciba Foundation Award for Research in Ageing, 1957; William Gibson Scholarship, Royal Society of Medicine, 1957–60. Committee member: British Institute of Radiology; Association for Radiation Research; Section of Comparative Medicine, Royal Society of Medicine. Particular interest in the sociological implications of the advances of science and medicine. Assistant Secretary-General, Pugwash Conference on Science and World Affairs.

Publications include: papers on the biological effects of radiation in mouse and man and the radiobiological basis of radiotherapy.

A. M.-M. PAYNE

Assistant Director-General, World Health Organization, Geneva; and Anna M. R. Lauder Professor of Epidemiology and Public Health, Yale University and Chairman of the Department, 1960–66.

English—Educated at Trinity College, Cambridge and St. Bartholomew's Hospital, London. Formerly Senior Epidemiologist, Public Health Laboratory Service, Oxford; Chief Medical Officer, Endemo-epidemic and Virus Diseases, WHO, Geneva. Secretary WHO Expert Committees on Hepatitis, Influenza, Poliomyelitis, Respiratory Virus Diseases. Vice-Chairman Advisory Committee on Medical Research, Pan-American Health Organization. Member Technical Board, Milbank Memorial Fund. Has served on several committees of the US Public Health Service and the National Academy of Sciences, mainly in connexion with international health. Member Sigma Xi; Honorary Member Delta Omega Societies; Member American Epidemiological Society; International Epidemiological Association; Association of Schools of Public Health; Association of Teachers of Preventive Medicine; American Thoracic Society; New York Academy of Sciences; American Academy of Social and Political Sciences; Royal Society of Health. Fellow: American Public Health Association; Royal College of Physicians, London; Brandford College, Yale University. Has travelled widely in all continents on behalf of WHO, PAHO and the Milbank Fund.

Publications include: over 60 papers on biological and social aspects of epidemiology.

H. Pequignot
    Professor of Medical Pathology, Faculty of Medicine, University of Paris.
    French—Technical Adviser to several Ministers of Public Health in French Health
    Administration, 1945–55; Technical Director of the Medical Section of CREDOC, a
    centre for research into economic problems. Taught in Beyrouth, Saigon and Pnom-
    Penh.
    Publications include: *Une Introduction aux Etudes Médicales*; *Manuel de Médecine*; *Précis de
    Pathologie Médicale* (8 volumes); *Médecine et Monde Moderne*; *Eléments de Politique et d'Admini-
    stration Sanitaire*; *Notre Vieillesse*; and *Traité de Droit Médical* (with co-workers).

G. Pincus
    Research Director, Worcester Foundation for Experimental Biology, Shrewsbury,
    Massachusetts, since 1956; Research Professor of Biology, Boston University Graduate
    School, since 1950.
    American—Professor of Experimental Zoology, Clark University, 1938–44; Director of
    Laboratories, Worcester Foundation, 1944–56; Research Professor of Physiology, Tufts
    Medical School, 1946–50. Recipient: Oliver Bird Prize, 1957; Albert D. Lasker Award
    in Planned Parenthood, 1960; Honorary Professorship, San Marcos University, Lima,
    Peru; Modern Medicine Award for Distinguished Achievement, 1964; Barren Founda-
    tion Medal, 1966; Cameron Prize in Practical Therapeutics, 1966. Fellow: American
    Academy of Arts and Sciences; National Academy of Sciences. Special interests:
    physiology of reproduction in mammals, adrenocortical physiology, steroid metabolism.
    Publications include: *Recent Progress in Hormone Research* (editor); *The Hormones* (edited
    with Dr. Thimann and Dr. Astwood); *The Control of Fertility*.

A. Querido
    Professor of Medicine, University of Leiden; Chief, Department of Clinical Endocrino-
    logy and Diseases of Metabolism, since 1948; and Dean of the New Faculty of Medicine,
    Rotterdam, since 1966.
    Dutch—Trained in University of Amsterdam Medical School, 1929–37; Research in
    experimental nutrition, 1932–46; Research Fellow in experimental nutrition, Johns
    Hopkins University School of Hygiene and Public Health, 1936; Research Fellow, Pasteur
    Institute, Paris, in microbial physiology, 1938–39; trained in clinical medicine, Leiden
    University Hospital, 1939–42 and 1945–48. Rockefeller Fellow, Massachusetts General
    Hospital, Boston, 1949–50; Rockefeller Foundation Visiting Professor, All India Insti-
    tute of Medical Sciences, New Delhi, 1963–64. Member of the Royal Netherlands
    Academy of Sciences; Honorary member Association of American Physicians. Special
    interests: The relation of nutrition to diseases of metabolism; and medical education.
    Research on endemic goitre and cretinism in the Mulia Valley of the Central highlands of
    West Irian, New Guinea, 1962. Temporary consultant, Pan American Health Organiza-
    tion for goitre and cretinism in the Andean area.
    Publications include: papers on experimental nutrition and microbiological assay of
    vitamins in man; experimental and clinical endocrinology; genetic defects of the thyroid
    gland; and medical education.

A. Wolman
    Professor Emeritus, Sanitary Engineering and the Environment, The Johns Hopkins
    University, Baltimore, Maryland.

American—Formerly: Chief Engineer, Maryland State Department of Health; Chairman: National Water Resources Committee; Maryland Water Resources Commission; Maryland State Planning Commission. Consulting Engineer: Baltimore City, Baltimore County, Detroit, New York, Seattle, Portland, etc.; US Public Health Service, Army, Navy, Air Force, National Research Council, etc.; Calcutta, Formosa, Ceylon, Brazil, etc. Member: National Academy of Sciences; National Academy of Engineering.

G. E. W. WOLSTENHOLME
Director, Ciba Foundation, London, since its opening in 1949.
English—Educated University of Cambridge and Middlesex Hospital, London; Adviser in Transfusion and Resuscitation, Central Mediterranean, 1943–45; Organizer 1963, Haile Selassie I Prize Trust, Addis Ababa. Honorary Secretary, Royal Society of Medicine; Member of Council, Westfield College, University of London; Fellow, Royal College of Physicians; Fellow, Institute of Biology; Order of the British Empire (mil.); Chevalier, Légion d'Honneur; Gold medal, Italian Ministry of Education; Star of Ethiopia, 1966. Chief editor, Ciba Foundation symposia, colloquia and study groups since 1950; Editor, *Royal College of Physicians of London: Portraits*, 1964.

SIR NORMAN WRIGHT
Secretary, British Association for the Advancement of Science, London, since 1963.
English—Commonwealth Fund Fellow, USA, 1926–28 at Cornell University, New York and US Department of Agriculture, Washington; First Director, Hannah Dairy Research Institute, Ayr, 1928–47; Honorary Lecturer, University of Glasgow, 1932–47; Chief Scientific Adviser (Food) to the Ministry of Agriculture, Fisheries and Food, 1947–59; Special Adviser to Imperial Council of Agricultural Research, India, 1936–37; Member Scientific Advisory Mission, Middle East Supply Centre, 1944–45; Special Adviser to Government of Ceylon, 1945; British Member of FAO Mission to Greece, 1946; Chairman, Food Standards Committee, 1947–59; FAO Programme Committee (Rome), 1953–59; successively Chairman, Vice-Chairman and member of Committee for Colonial Agricultural Animal Health and Forestry Research, 1946–59. Deputy Director-General, Food and Agriculture Organization of the United Nations, 1959–63. Fellow, Royal Institute of Chemistry; Fellow, Royal Society of Edinburgh; Companion of the Bath, 1955; Created Knight, 1963.
Publications include: *The Development of the Cattle and Dairy Industries of India*; *The Development of Cattle Breeding and Milk Production in Ceylon*; *Report of FAO Mission to Greece* (co-author); Economics, Supply and Distribution of Foods in the United Kingdom, in *Food Science*; All Flesh is Grass, in *Research for Plenty*; The Ecology of Domesticated Animals, in *Progress in the Physiology of Farm Animals*.

INDEX OF CONTRIBUTORS*

*Numbers in bold type indicate a contribution in the form of a paper;
numbers in plain type refer to contributions to the discussions.*

Adrian, Lord   74, 107

Banks, A. L.   60, 61, 77, 100, 126, 158,
174, 216, **239**, 251, 253, 274
Beer, H.   157, 234, 266, 272
Beveridge, W. I. B.   **63**, 73, 74, 75, 76, 77
Burkitt, D.   97, 251

Candau, M. G.   43, 45, 59, 75, 100, 109,
124, 145, 146, 157, 162, 172,
233, 250, 251, 265, 267, 273
Cohen of Birkenhead, Lord   161

De Haas, J. H.   61, **79**, 98, 99, 100, 101,
109, 159, 262
Dogramaci, I.   **51**, 59, 99, 212, 231, 250, 263
Doxiadis, C. A.   155, 156, 173, **178**, 194, 216

Evang, K.   44, 73, 74, 76, 96, 97, 110,
125, 145, 156, 158, 160, 176,
196, 213, 214, 215, 249, 264, 272

Fanconi, G.   58, 75, 96, 144, 233
Florey, Lord   143, 146, 155, 160, 172,
173, 174, 175, 212, 215, 216

Garcia, Victoria   44, 96, 110, 125, 175, 248

Johnson-Marshall, P. E. A.   45, 99, 126,
172, 193

Kaprio, L. A.   43, 60, 75, 100, 101, 111,
157, 175, 212, 214, **218**, 237, 252
Katsunuma, H.   **113**, 124, 125, 126, 160,
161, 215

Lambo, T. A.   60, 98, **103**, 107, 108,
109, 110, 111, 159, 212, 235,
251, 263, 271
Le Riche, W. H.   1, 44, 45, 59, 107,
156, 177, 212, 249, 263
Lindop, Patricia J.   59, 74, 75, 124, 160
176, 177, 215, 264, 270

Payne, A. M.-M.   269
Pequignot, H.   43, 99, 108, 125, 214,
239, 248, 249, 251, 261
Pincus, G.   59, 96, 97, 98, 100, 108,
127, 144, 160, 236, 251, 269

Querido, A.   60, 98, 156, 161, 213, 214,
252, 265, 272

Wolman, A.   44, 45, 75, 101, 123, 124,
144, 158, **164**, 172, 173, 174
175, 176, 177, 248, 270
Wolstenholme, G. E. W.   74, **254**, 262,
263, 265, 266, 273
Wright, Sir Norman   143, **149**, 155, 157,
158, 194, 232, 272

* Author and Subject Indexes compiled by Mr. William Hill.

INDEX OF AUTHORS CITED

Numbers in italics indicate bibliographical references

INDEX OF SUBJECTS

Printed by Spottiswoode Ballantyne & Co.Ltd., London and Colchester